BRAIN BRILLIANCE

60 Nourishing **Recipes** and a **Nutritional Toolkit** for **Dyslexia, Dyspraxia ADHD, Autism** and all **Neurodivergent Kids**

LUCINDA MILLER

Foreword by Dr Richard Fry

Photography by Ali Allen

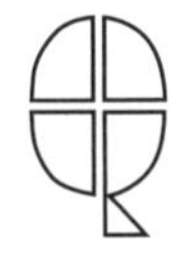

quadrille

Dedicated to my darling husband, Christopher, and his totally brilliant ADHD brain!

CONTENTS

SAVOURY SNACKS

SWEET SNACKS

BRILLIANT DRINKS

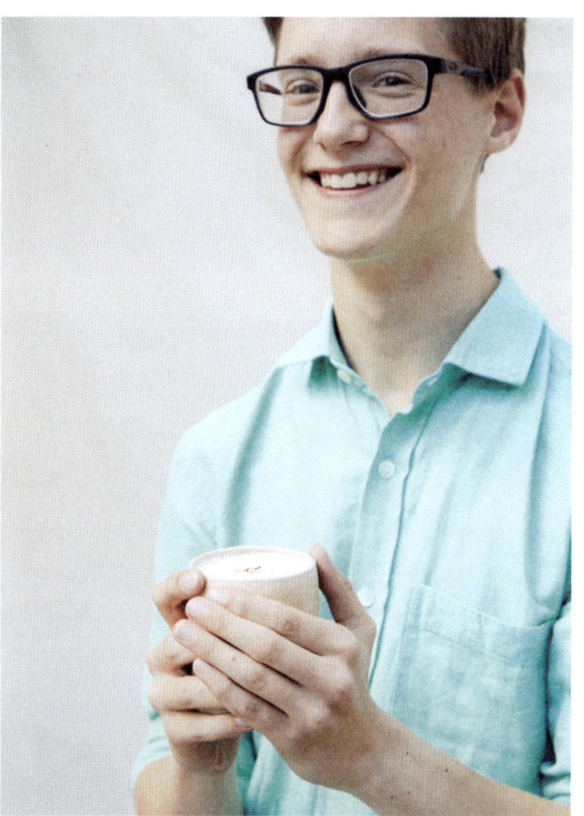

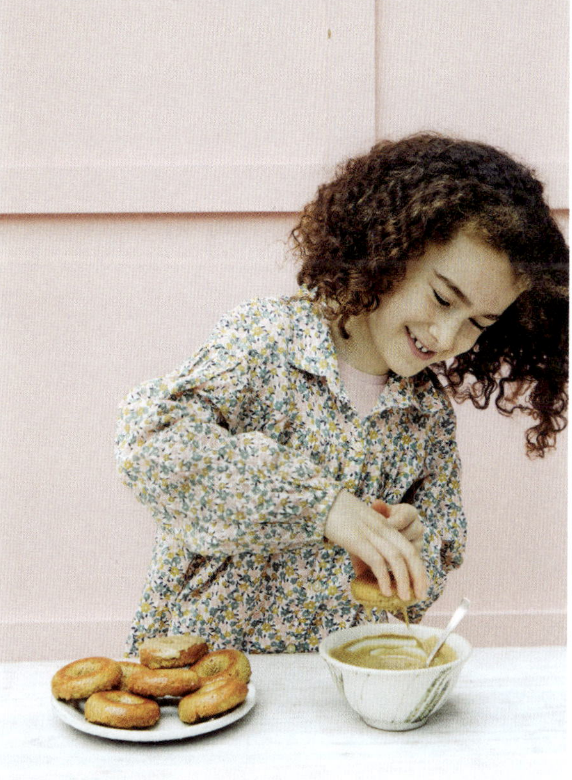

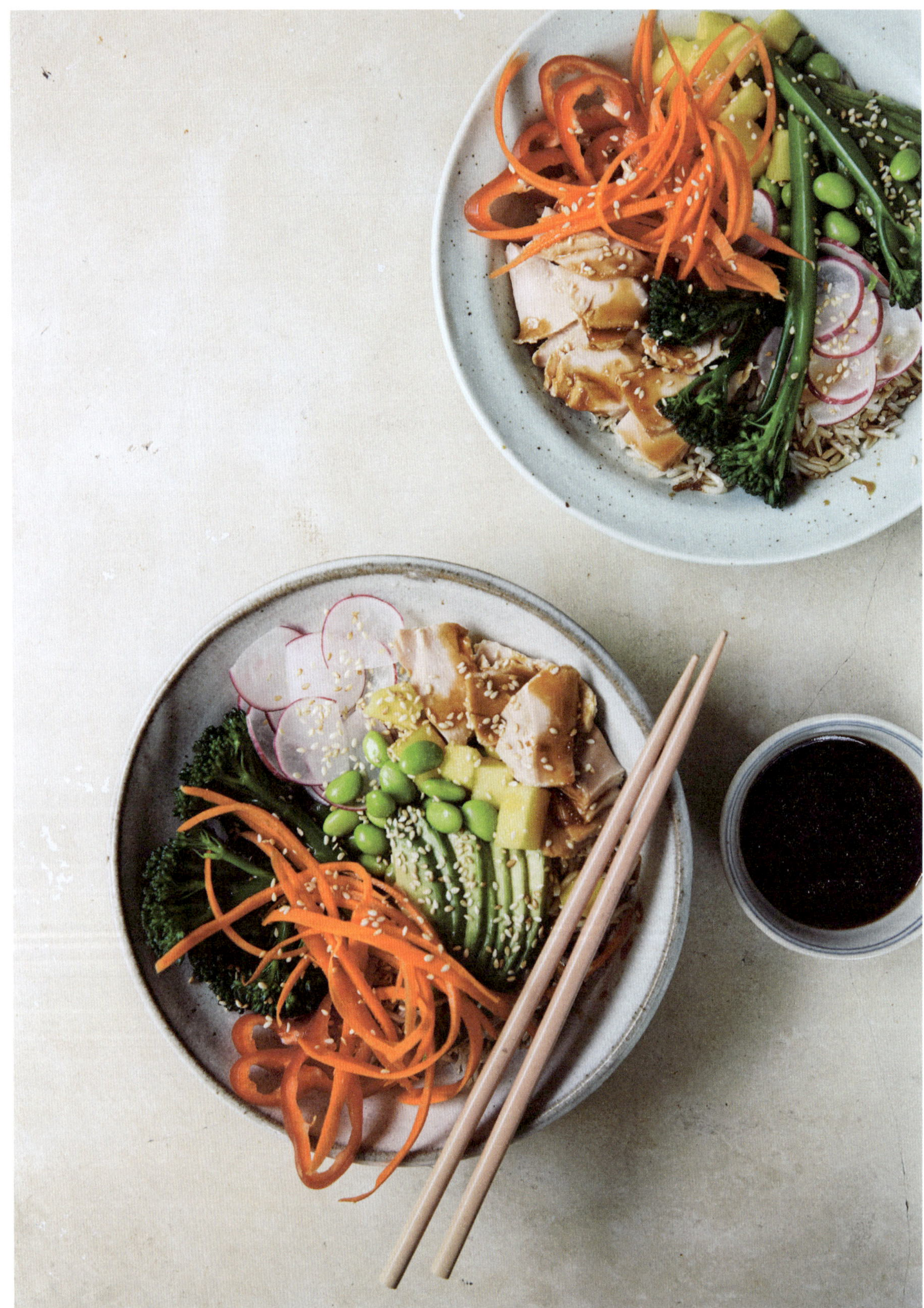

FOREWORD BY DR RICHARD FRY

The world is a very confusing place these days, and especially so for parents. With so much information out there and so little time to digest it, thank heaven that someone can write a fully referenced book that is easy to read, understand and put into action on the sometimes vexed subject of diet and neurodiversity. Lucinda Miller has, in *Brain Brilliance*, created a highly digestible guide to optimizing the neurodivergent brain through diet. Actually, neurotypicals can listen up too because it is also full of wisdom on how diet and nutrition affects the brain more generally!

When I was training as a doctor forty-odd years ago, there was nothing at all in the curriculum about food or diet apart from some things about sugar and diabetes, and a warning against fat. We then heard from some man called John Yudkin, who went on and on about how it was not fat that was the enemy but sugar. He was a prophet unhonoured in his own country, who turned out to be correct and is now fêted. Sugar is indeed our problem and inflammation our issue.

But so is the lack of micronutrients, the widespread consumption of ultra-processed foods and our increasingly challenging environment interacting with our genes. Here, Lucinda presents her easy-to-implement plans that will help you solve these issues and drop your kids' intake of ultra-processed food to 20 per cent or less.

In this book, she clearly and concisely spells out how to flex your child's diet to clear their brain fog, and support their neurotransmitter production and balance. She sets out what signs indicate they might need specific nutrients, and signposts what steps to take if they do. If you want a quick but thorough overview, you will have it by the end of chapter 2. If you want a deeper dive, look at the chapters later in the book. And if you want to know how to put all the theory into practice, keep reading all the way through to the end and enjoy her recipes.

Learn how an electric toothbrush can help encourage a broader and more varied diet; see how the right balance of foods can reduce after-school meltdowns; find out how cherries can help your child sleep better. All this and many more practical approaches are discussed. There are chapters on helping to read and write and how to reduce noise sensitivity and procrastination – these are day-to-day things that will be all too familiar to parents of neurodivergent children.

So many texts will give you facts; if you are lucky, they debate some of the research, but they leave you bewildered about what to do. In this book, Lucinda gives us the means of how to apply this knowledge – with real, practical and tasty recipes. See this book as an easy-to-action manual of how to move things forward for your child.

At last, here is an integrated and integrative look at the field of neurodivergence. I will be recommending it to parents and all my medical colleagues.

Dr Richard Fry, Consultant Integrative Child Psychiatrist MD

INTRODUCTION

We all have brilliant brains, whether we recognize it or not, and our minds are just as individual as our iris patterns and fingerprints. What a joy it is that we are all unique; and having a neurodivergent brain can add to this uniqueness. Neurodiversity is a relatively new collective term that embraces a multitude of cognitive characteristics. The best-known ones are Dyslexia, Dyspraxia, Attention deficit hyperactivity disorder (ADHD) and Autism, but there are many other learning or sensory differences. It's not nearly as lonely as it used to be, as neurodiversity is being recognized and accepted so much more. Welcome to our brilliant neurodiverse universe!

When our kids and teens are struggling with their learning, behaviour, development or mental health, it can be hard to see the upside. When the going gets tough for a child, they can find it hard to fit in and their frustrations spill out to affect the lives of other people around them. Sometimes, it can seem challenging and frustrating, and it can feel as if their neurodivergence is holding them back. But it does not need to be this way and I will show you how simple nutrition tweaks can provide some short- and long-term answers.

If you are reading this as an adult living with neurodivergence yourself, and you have grappled with cognitive or mental-health challenges over your lifetime, then you might also learn a thing or two from *Brain Brilliance*!

If you're wondering if your child needs a specific diagnosis to benefit from this book, the answer is no! Of course, many children will already have a diagnosis; others will be on an (often long) journey to it. This book is also for any parent, carer or teacher who even has an inkling that their child (or a child they are responsible for) is developing, learning or behaving on a different trajectory from the average 'neurotypical' child. Read this if you want to help them stay happy, healthy and gain the resilience to navigate life's inevitable ups and downs.

The best news is that no one needs to wait for a diagnosis to benefit from better diet nutrition. You can begin nourishing your child's brain cells right away, setting the foundations for a healthier and happier future. I have seen how a child's life, and their family dynamics, can so easily be derailed when you have neurodiversity in the picture, and equally how easily they can be perked up and rebalanced when you gain proper nutrition know-how.

For more than 25 years as a naturopath and functional medicine practitioner, I have put my heart and soul into supporting thousands of neurodivergent people through the gentle route of nutrition and natural remedies. It has meant many long evenings trawling through countless academic research papers and, more importantly, listening to every single individual, hearing their unique story and using this knowledge to help them become the best version of themselves. Now, in this book, I will share stories of hope from many of the families who have been under our care at my NatureDoc clinic.

My clinical work is dedicated to helping neurodivergent children and young people thrive using evidence-based nutrition. *Brain Brilliance* brings together my top nutrition and wellbeing tips to help kids of all ages shine with their very exceptional brains. See this book as a big warm hug to the neurodivergent community and a glow of positivity with lots of delicious recipes to nourish the brain and the soul. My mission is to make *Brain Brilliance* accessible to all and to highlight the everyday challenges that many neurodivergent children experience and struggle with, rather than focusing on the specific label or diagnosis. A love of food, and understanding its role in nourishing the brain, can help all brains to flourish, no matter what the diagnosis is.

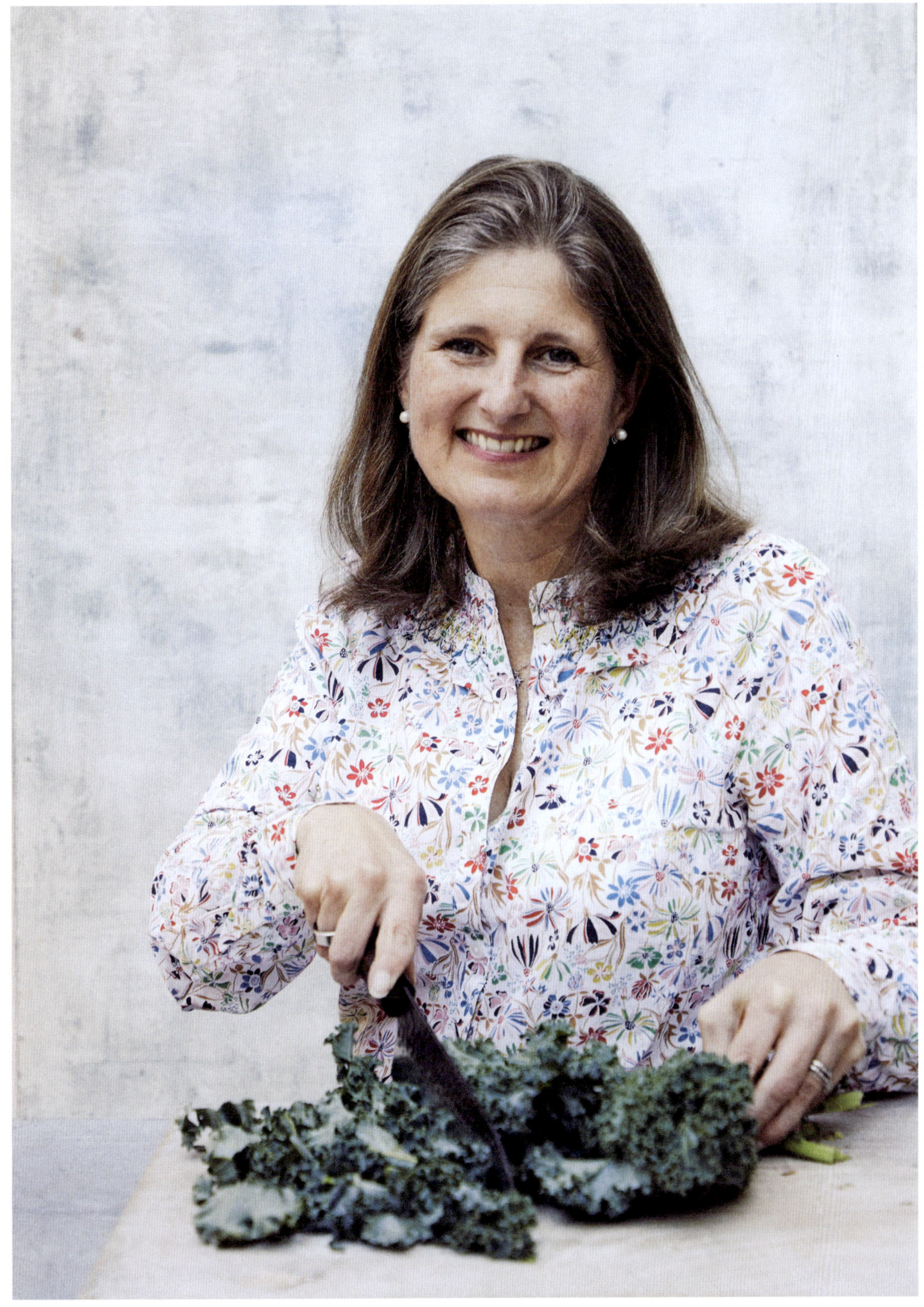

THE HIGHS AND LOWS OF HAVING A BRILLIANT BRAIN

The diversity of human minds and brilliant brains make our lives a little more exciting and complete. Our world would be boring and muted without the rich tapestry of exceptional people with distinctly different brains.

Difference can be positive and uplifting, whether someone has contributed to progress in science, technology, sport, the arts or music; or simply their uniqueness has touched their family or community. When your child is struggling, remember that some of the most successful individuals in the world, from entrepreneurs and Olympic athletes to talented artists and musicians, identify as neurodivergent, and plenty more are privately neurodivergent, or don't know it yet.

However, it is important to recognize that, equally, there are large numbers of neurodivergent children with significant special needs and disabilities who will need life-long care without ever being able to live independently. There are also, of course, a great many in between these two distinct ends of the neurodiversity spectrum. Once you have met one neurodivergent person, you have only met one presentation of neurodivergence, so understanding and respecting individuality is super important.

There are some incredible kids who endure long-term developmental, mental and physical health challenges with a smile on their face, despite huge adversity. You might think they are brilliant at masking their difficulties, but many are simply at ease with who they are, and they beam with positivity, often thanks to a great support network. However, plenty of neurodivergent kids find long periods of their life hard, and this can affect their family and other societal dynamics as well as future educational and work opportunities.

Big emotions can easily come alongside neurodivergence. Masking differences to fit into a world of 'neurotypical' people can be hard work and emotionally draining. Often it can seem that other people don't understand your child or the often hidden complexities of their needs. There are many challenges that neurodivergent kids face, which can influence their perspective of the world from childhood through to adulthood. Whether it is starting school with no voice or delayed speech, experiencing barriers to learning, being overwhelmed by the noise of school, not making friends or being bullied for being different – all these experiences can be traumatizing and give a nasty kick to self-esteem.

This is where emotional dysregulation, anxiety, meltdowns, behavioural outbursts, as well as physical and mental health problems, can develop and start to cause distress for neurodivergent kids and, in turn, affect the lives of those close to them. These early life experiences can shape how they navigate and thrive through their adult life, so getting it right early on can make a positive difference in the long term.

Feeling physically and mentally unwell or having chronic (long-term) learning or physical differences can be exhausting and debilitating for children. Finding yourself always the square peg trying to fit into a round hole can result in burnout. And, unfortunately, being in this state of inertia, isolation, or 'shut-down' for long periods of time can close doors to life opportunities – whatever those are to your child.

But it doesn't always need to be this way, and help is at hand via what you choose to eat. *Brain Brilliance* shares how nutrition and lifestyle changes can help your child navigate the highs and lows. After all, food is fuel for our bodies and what is in that food directly affects our brains and our mood, as well as our physical wellbeing. This book is going to show you that you really are what you eat.

WHY AM I INTERESTED IN HOW YOUR BRAIN TICKS?

I was diagnosed with ADHD in my early thirties, having had ups and downs at school and university. I just thought I was disorganized and scatty – any kind of paperwork was the bane of my life! My mental stamina was rock bottom, and I spent much of my teens and twenties feeling burnt out and exhausted from my busy brain.

Since then, it turns out that several of our wider family tick the boxes to some degree for being neurodivergent. These include ADHD, Autism, Dyspraxia, Dyslexia, sensory processing as well as chronic fatigue and depression. We are a family filled with very lovable, sensitive and interesting individuals. Although we know that our traits are strongly genetic, many of us have personally witnessed how important diet, nutrition and lifestyle can affect how we think and feel.

The positive changes in my own and my children's mental clarity, educational journeys and self-confidence after simple nutritional and lifestyle changes have been profound. This first-hand experience spurred me on to share this vital information and specialize in it professionally.

THE NEURODIVERGENT UNIVERSE

Thankfully, the ever-growing 'neurodiversity club' welcomes anyone who chooses to join, and individualism is celebrated and accepted. There is a dizzying list of conditions and neurodivergent traits that your child may be diagnosed with by a psychiatrist, educational psychologist, neurologist or medical doctor. And if you are at all worried about your child's development or symptoms, it is important to seek medical advice and diagnosis. Neurodiversity covers a whole host of neurological, neurodevelopmental and mental health labels, all of which can affect the mind. Here are very brief explanations of some of them if you have not come across the terms before:

Angelman syndrome – this genetic syndrome means the child is usually non-speaking but still good at communicating and able to get their needs met. Often, they are very delayed in their learning skills and overall development, and typically experience seizure activity. Known affectionately as 'angels', they tend to be very happy, smiley and calm souls.

Attention deficit hyperactivity disorder (ADHD/ADD) – this is when a child finds it hard to concentrate, gets easily distracted, and may also be very active, restless or impulsive. Some kids are not at all hyperactive and can be seen as daydreamers with active imaginations. ADD (without the hyperactivity) is now seen as a subdivision of ADHD. They might struggle to keep organized and can make decisions without thinking them through. But it's not all negative: children with ADHD can be highly energized, creative and full of fun ideas, making them great company, and as adults they are often successful in setting up their own businesses with an entrepreneurial flair.

Auditory processing disorder (APD) – with this condition the brain struggles to interpret sounds properly. As such, it's not a hearing problem but an issue with how the brain processes sound. People with APD might find it hard to understand speech, especially in busy, noisy places, because their brains confuse different sounds.

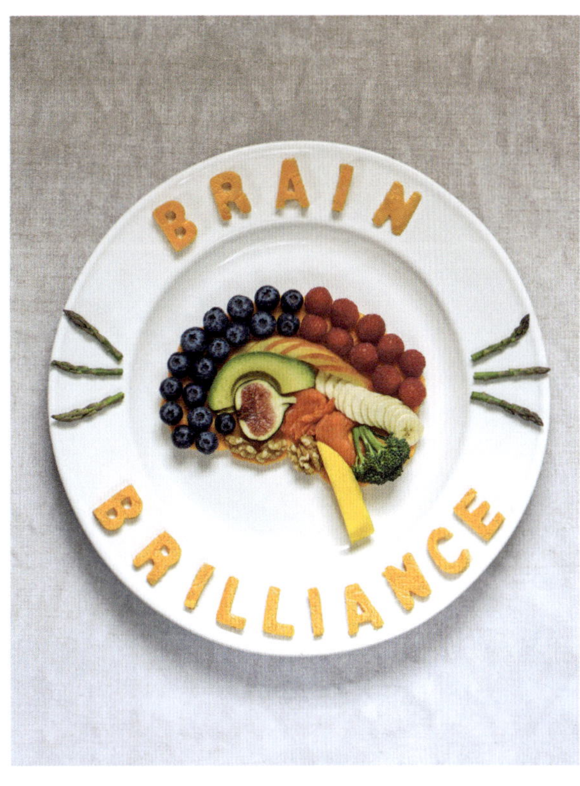

Autism – sometimes known as Autism spectrum disorder (ASD), it is a set of neurological differences that can affect how people communicate and interact with others. Autistic children might find social situations difficult, struggle to understand what others are thinking or feeling, and have a narrow set of special interests. They often prefer to stick to routines, or certain patterns of behaviour. These behaviours might seem rigid or repetitive, but they are ways for the child to make sense of the world around them. Some autistic people are academically able, social and can live independently and raise their own family, whereas others can be non-speaking with significant developmental delay and will never lead an independent life. And of course, the vast majority lie somewhere in between.

Brain injuries – many different scenarios can lead to a traumatic brain injury. It can often happen during pregnancy and/or around the time of birth if there is an interruption in supply of oxygen or other essential nutrients as well as birth trauma. Later, sports concussions, car crashes, falls, fights or accidents at home can cause brain injuries. They can also result from serious health problems like brain tumours, strokes, brain bleeds, or infections leading to brain inflammation. Such injuries can alter how the brain works and hugely affect memory, concentration, locomotor skills (movement and coordination) and even personality.

Cerebral palsy – this condition specifically affects a child's movement and coordination. It is usually caused by changes in the brain that happen before, during, or just after a baby is born. Such changes can make it harder for them to move their muscles as they wish. The condition is lifelong, but it can be managed by physical, speech and occupational therapies.

Chronic fatigue – also known as Myalgic encephalomyelitis or ME, this is a condition where a child feels constantly exhausted, and this doesn't improve with rest. It's not just about feeling sleepy; it's a deep, lasting fatigue that can make it very hard to do everyday tasks. The condition often lasts for several months or even years. Other symptoms can present alongside the fatigue, such as headaches, muscle pain or difficulty concentrating. A child with chronic fatigue may struggle with mood, sociability, brain fog and learning while they are unwell, and this is why it is sometimes included within neurodiversity.

Developmental coordination disorder (DCD)/ Dyspraxia – this affects both gross and fine motor skills – like riding a bike, tying shoelaces or using cutlery – and other physical movement and coordination. People with DCD might seem clumsy with their physical movements, but it also affects their planning and organization skills and ability to carry out daily tasks such as getting dressed or completing their homework.

Dyscalculia – kids with this condition find it hard to understand numbers, and simple maths concepts such as adding, subtracting, multiplying or dividing can be challenging. This makes everyday tasks like handling money or measuring ingredients for cooking difficult. It's not about being 'bad at maths', rather it's a specific learning difficulty that affects the way the brain processes numbers.

Dysgraphia – this condition makes writing difficult. Dysgraphia can affect handwriting, making it messy or tricky to read, and it also makes it harder for the child to put their thoughts down on paper. Like Dyspraxia, kids with Dysgraphia can struggle with fine motor skills.

Dyslexia – this learning difficulty can make it hard to write things down correctly and to understand written information. People with Dyslexia often mix up letters in their spelling or read words in the wrong order. But it's not about intelligence or effort: Dyslexia is a specific condition that affects working memory and how the brain processes language. It may co-exist with Meares-Irlen Syndrome, which affects vision or visual tasks and can include light-sensitivity, depth perception and visual distortions.

Executive function difficulties – a child might have trouble organizing tasks, managing their time, making decisions, and controlling impulses, often leading to difficulties in school and daily activities.

Fragile X syndrome – genetically acquired, this can lead to challenges similar to Autism, making social interaction and communication hard for those affected by it. The name derives from the fact that part of the X chromosome looks fragile under the microscope. Fragile X can present in either sex, but males are usually more affected. Apart from learning challenges, there may be associated physical characteristics, such as a long face or large ears.

Global developmental delay – this refers to when a child doesn't reach key milestones, such as crawling, walking, talking and social interaction, at the same rate as their age group. Essentially, they develop at a slower pace overall. This delay affects multiple areas of their development, and they may seem young and immature for their age, even when they grow up.

Highly sensitive person – this term is used for those who are particularly tuned in to social cues like voices or facial expressions. They can also be sensitive to sounds, light and smells, which can easily cross over with Sensory processing disorder. They often feel other people's emotions deeply, a sign they are very empathetic. Such heightened awareness also means they can become easily overwhelmed or overstimulated in busy or intense situations.

Mental health problems – mental health challenges that are chronic (long-term) can affect a child's day-to-day life. Conditions such as chronic depression, bipolar disorder and anxiety that also affects daily tasks and mental capacity are sometimes included under neurodivergence.

Misophonia – this refers to a strong negative reaction to specific sounds. It isn't just about disliking a sound, but Misophonia can make a person feel upset, stressed or angry. The condition can be standalone but is often found in people with other neurodivergence.

Obsessive compulsive disorder (OCD) – this is when someone cannot stop thinking about certain worries or fears, known as obsessions. It's a bit like having a song stuck in your head, but with worries instead of a tune. These repetitive thoughts can be very distracting and make the child feel the need to do certain actions over and over again; and these are called compulsions. OCD often presents alongside anxiety and tic disorders.

Oppositional defiant disorder (ODD) – this label is used when someone, typically a child or teenager, constantly misbehaves, argues and will not follow instructions from adults or those in authority such as teachers. It is as if they are in a permanently grumpy mood and often seem to be resisting anyone trying to assist or guide them; they can seem uncooperative, defiant and hostile. This can make it challenging for them to get on well with others.

Paediatric autoimmune neuropsychiatric disorders associated with or without Streptococcal Infections (PANS/PANDAS) – this is a misdirected autoimmune reaction to a streptococcus infection or other bacterial or viral infection in children, leading to rapid onset symptoms that include OCD, anxiety, tics, restricted food intake, emotional changes, irritability, a regression in behaviour or language skills, a decline in school performance, frequent urination, body dysmorphia, sleep disturbances and other symptoms. There are medical treatments, and symptoms can wax and wane.

Pathological demand avoidance (PDA) – an often overlooked yet profoundly challenging condition, it is characterized by intense unease, avoidance tactics or anxiety when confronted with the routine demands and expectations of daily life. Difficult scenarios may include going to school, shopping or interacting with other children. It's as if the brain's wiring interprets ordinary demands as significant threats. PDA should not be mistaken for unwillingness to comply; it stems from deep anxiety and a heightened fight-or-flight state so overwhelming that it becomes debilitating. This often comes hand in hand with Autism.

Post-viral illness and Long Covid – symptoms of these conditions can affect children and adults alike. Both are closely related to Chronic Fatigue and can cause problems with energy levels, resulting in persistent tiredness. Long Covid can be a more complex condition as it can trigger various additional health complications. Kids experiencing post-viral illness may fall under the neurodivergence umbrella while their mood, sociability, learning or focus are being affected.

Rett syndrome – this is a specific type of Autism that predominantly affects females and it is usually progressive. It is characterized by developmental delays, particularly in areas such as speech and motor skills. A child may experience a regression in their abilities and seizures after an initial period of typical development.

Selective mutism – with this severe anxiety disorder, a child may experience difficulties speaking in specific social situations, such as at school or at parties, despite being chatty and sociable at home or in other familiar settings or with close relatives. This often comes hand in hand with Autism.

Sensory processing disorder (SPD) – this condition affects the way the brain processes sensory information or stimuli. Those with SPD may experience heightened sensitivity to sensory inputs including what they see, hear, smell, taste or touch. These can include bright lights, loud sirens and fireworks, strong smells, food textures and labels on clothing. Sensations that may seem ordinary to others can feel overwhelming or intense to children experiencing SPD, which can affect their ability to navigate and engage with their environment.

Speech and language delay – this refers to when a child exhibits a slower pace in learning to use words or developing other forms of verbal communication compared to what is typically expected at their age. It involves delays in both expressive language (using words or gestures to communicate) and receptive language (understanding what is heard or read). Children with speech and language delays may stutter, struggle to form sentences, pronounce words incorrectly or find it hard to comprehend instructions or conversations.

Tourette syndrome (TS) and tic disorders – this involves sudden motor and vocal tics, repetitive movements or sounds that are out of a child's control. Motor tics can include eye blinking, facial grimacing or making jerking movements, while vocal tics may involve throat-clearing, grunting or repetitive sounds and even swearing. Tourette syndrome is generally diagnosed once the tics have been present for over a year.

Trisomy 21 (Down syndrome) – this is a genetic condition in which people have an extra copy of chromosome 21. They typically experience learning difficulties and may face challenges related to heart defects, thyroid problems, vision impairments and hearing difficulties. Down Syndrome is characterized by distinct facial features including almond-shaped eyes, a smaller nasal bridge, flattened cheekbones and often a protruding tongue.

Twice-exceptional (2e) – this term refers to kids endowed with great natural ability, intelligence or talent, often in one or a few specific areas, such as music, maths or art, but who, conversely, also face certain learning or developmental challenges. Such individuals are truly unique and talented or smart, and may also have Dyslexia, ADHD or Autism alongside. Their remarkable abilities can often mask their challenges, making it important for them to receive the right support.

Working memory difficulties – our working memory is like a mental notepad that temporarily stores and works with information to help us think and solve problems. A child with poor working memory may struggle to follow instructions, have difficulty with tasks that require remembering multiple steps like solving maths questions, and often forget what they were just doing or thinking about.

When assessing and supporting developmental differences, each condition has its own distinct diagnostic and management approaches. Dyslexia, for example, is assessed within educational psychology with a focus on literacy skills; Dyspraxia leans towards treatments like physiotherapy and occupational therapy to improve physical coordination; ADHD is primarily managed under psychiatry and can involve the use of prescription stimulant medications; while Autism blends medical diagnosis with a combination of educational, behavioural, speech and language as well as social skills therapies.

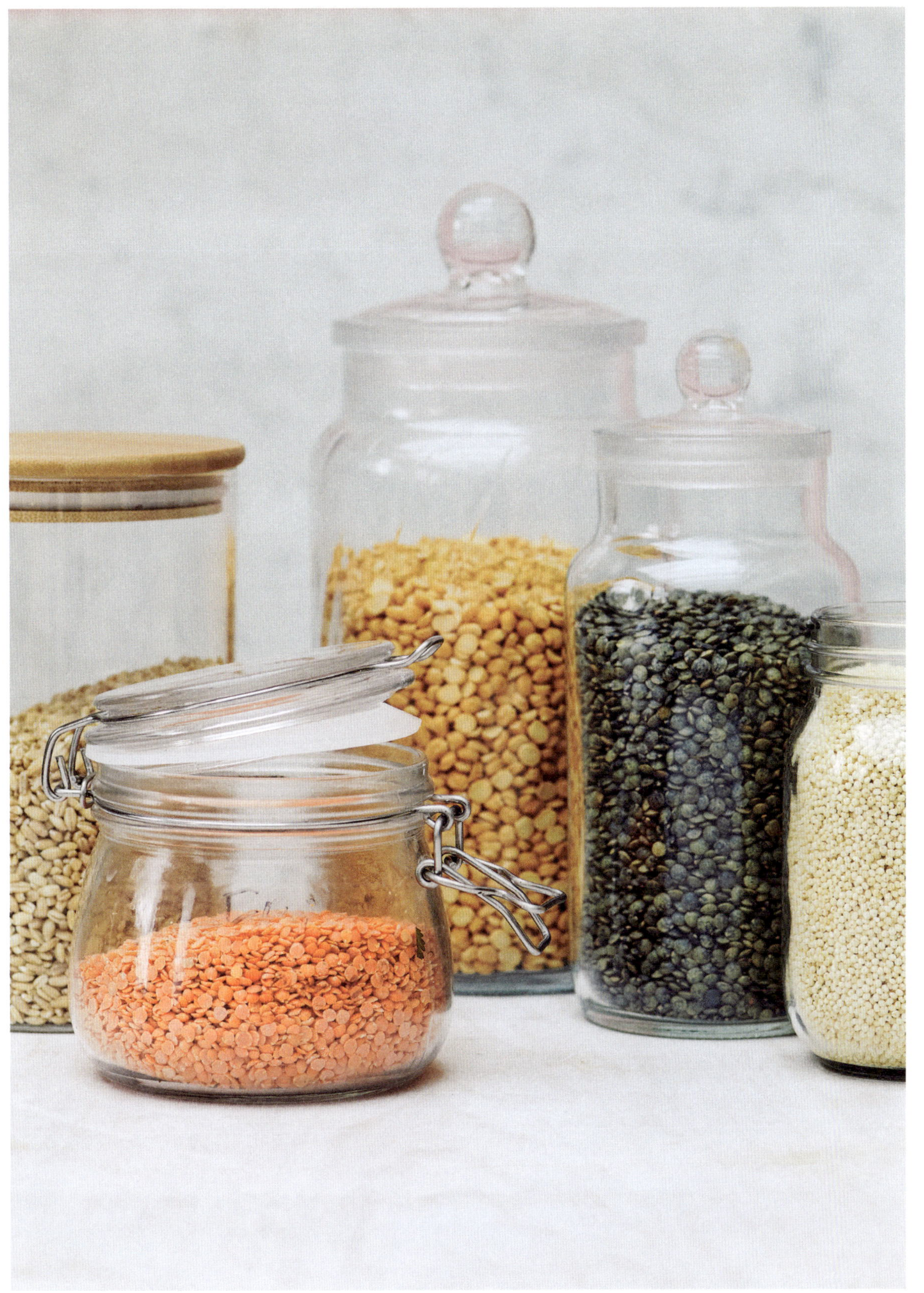

The reality is that many children who are diagnosed with one of the above also share traits with some of the others, and it is common for an educational psychologist's or psychiatric assessment to establish more than one diagnosis. For instance, you may embark on an educational psychologist's assessment assuming a child has Dyslexia and discover they also have Dyscalculia. Equally you may assume the condition is ADHD when seeing a psychiatrist and come out with add-on diagnoses of Autism and a tic disorder. Many kids are diagnosed with both autism and ADHD together and this is known as AuADHD.

There is no blood test to diagnose any of these neurological differences; it is up to the skills of the professionals involved to evaluate how your child presents at the time of the assessment, which usually cross references with a report from school or another expert who knows them well.

WHY READ BRAIN BRILLIANCE?

The wrong food choices can really affect a developing brain, and this is all the more important when someone is struggling to reach their potential. But by eating the right foods and optimizing nutrition you can create the scaffolding to help the brain flourish, meaning that learning, communication and social interaction are not so challenging or overwhelming. And if a child gets optimal nutrition while they are developing, it can be a lasting benefit that helps them achieve their true potential in the long term.

A diverse diet packed with healthy nutrition is the cornerstone for feeding a developing neurodivergent brain. The ideas in this book are affordable and easy switches. Given that children eat at least three times a day, these are three opportunities a day to nourish them so they flourish. Nutrition is not the only therapy to support neurodivergent kids and teens – far from it – but many people find that when they get the nutrition right it becomes easier to access some of the other therapies and educational support.

All the tips and hacks here are safe and simple dietary and lifestyle changes that can make a difference to your loved ones, even if specific research has not been carried out on their unique combination of neurodivergence. The majority of the scientific literature surrounding diet, lifestyle and environment influencing neurodivergence focuses on Autism or ADHD, which are often more complex to unravel and come under the umbrella of psychiatry. However, if your child does not have either of these, it should not pose any barriers to benefiting from this book, as the right nutrition can help everyone.

And don't worry, eating more nutritious foods will not mute their super skills, talents and unique characteristics – you will find that their individual, exciting and interestingly wired brains will still be there, fully intact and able to shine through even more brightly. The right nutrition can simply help to dial down the background noise, so that life becomes less overwhelming, exhausting and distracting.

The individual chapters set out the key nutrients and lifestyle changes that have been found to help many children, teens and young adults, according to scientific studies and our clinical experience and extensive lab testing. Importantly, because nutrition can be complex, I explain how to spot if your child is deficient in specific nutrients, so you can focus in on the individual support they need.

The book is divided into three main parts. The first introduces the essentials of nutrition and the key nutrients we all need to thrive. It looks at how ultra-processed foods affect the brain and the importance of a healthy gut microbiome and balancing blood sugar levels. Even our immune system affects the brain – once you understand how, you'll appreciate the significance of what you eat even more.

The second part takes a deep dive into the common challenges experienced by neurodivergent children, from highly selective eating, emotional dysregulation, anxiety and tics to speech delay, difficulties with reading and writing, apathy and lack of concentration. I share my top nutrition tips to help you and your child navigate these challenges.

Finally, you will find 60 nutritious and delicious recipes that will help your child to become their best selves, one tasty mouthful at a time.

LEARN TO PUT YOUR OXYGEN MASK ON FIRST

The first step is looking after yourself so that you can keep calm, strong and resilient for your child both in the short and long term.

As parents supporting complex kids, we can become hypervigilant and easily overwhelmed. This is especially so at the outset when we are first getting our head around the fact that our child is taking a different developmental pathway from their peers and siblings or struggling with their physical and mental health.

If you are anything like I was when I realized my kids needed more input to help with their learning, focus and coordination, I went on a mission to help them as best I could, and in the meantime overlooked my own health and wellbeing. This meant I got burned out and exhausted, and this in turn exacerbated my own ADHD, so I became less 'on it' for my kids. When I stood back and I started to look after myself, I was able to make much more progress with them, as I had much more calm energy and mental clarity.

So, my advice to you, just as you are advised on an airplane, is to 'put your own oxygen mask on first' when you are on a journey to support your neurodivergent child. It can seem like a marathon to get them on track, and you need the mental and physical stamina to fight for the therapies and the education that they need to blossom and thrive. This can mean prioritizing time for yourself every single day. For me it began with a warm bath before bed, as it was the only time in the day that I could squeeze in for myself. It became my sacred sanity time and meant that my busy brain was able to wind down and then sleep came more easily.

Here are some other things to put in place to help build your resilience:

▸ Prioritizing sleep is super important, even if your child is not sleeping that well or needs you by their side when they are in bed. Do your best to get the rest and sleep you need to function. This may seem near impossible at times and my tips in chapter 11 should help everyone to get a better night's sleep.

▸ If you set out to feed your kids a healthier diet, then do the same for yourself, and I recommend that you eat as a family whenever possible, so you are all getting nourished by the good stuff. The recipes I have developed for this book are for everyone to enjoy together so you only need to cook once for you and your gang.

▸ Light exercise, whether this is walking in nature, going for a bicycle ride with your kids or practising yoga, can really help ease you through the ups and downs of parenthood. Everyone feels better after some exercise as it lifts the endorphins.

▸ Laugh and keep things light – even when you are going through dark days, try to weave in something light hearted and uplifting. Do something small that sparks joy every day.

▸ Making changes for your child can seem quite alienating at first and you can feel quite alone. It is therefore important to find your parent tribe and share the highs and lows of having a neurodivergent child with like-minded souls going through the same journey as you. I have set up an online community, NatureDoc Live! Q&A but many people also hook into local or global social media or messaging groups. Raising kids is so much easier when you have someone to turn to when your child is having a rubbish day.

If you have got this far, congratulations! You have taken the first step to making positive changes. Let's now get started, digging deeper into the foundations of nutrition!

1 HOW TO READ & USE THIS BOOK

This book is your friendly guide to unravelling the emerging science that explains the important interplay between nutrition, gut health and immunity and their influence on how the brain ticks. There are now dedicated global research teams digging deeply in fields such as nutritional psychiatry, psychobiotics, immunopsychiatry and neuroinflammation. This new research helps us to understand how nutrition, the balance of gut microbes, infections and allergies, as well as inflammatory processes in the body, interact with the brain. These in turn may provide clues on how to help neurodiverse children unlock their full potential and thrive in their own special way.

It can seem complex at the outset, and hard to work out where to start. My advice to you is to read through this book once from cover to cover. Then go back and highlight the parts that you feel are most relevant to your child and write these down in a list. Then start to make one new change at a time, which could be supercharging their breakfast with one new ingredient such as ground flax seeds in their porridge, or adding in one new food supplement into their orange juice, such as a few zinc drops. Or get your kids to look through all the recipes and choose which ones appeal to them most.

All my recipes in *Brain Brilliance* are nutritionally packed, simple to make and have got the thumbs up from our brilliant children's taste team.

MY CHILD IS A HIGHLY SELECTIVE EATER. I WON'T BE ABLE TO MAKE CHANGES!

You might be wondering how new food ideas can help your child if they are a highly selective eater, they are grappling with a complex relationship surrounding food or have disordered eating habits. It's no secret that many neurodivergent children have a rather limited diet, and any changes can become an uphill battle. If this describes your child, and they only live off a handful of foods, learning about nutrition and gut health is even more important. This is because certain food supplements and home remedies can prevent nutrient deficiencies and support intestinal health if the diet remains restricted or haphazard.

The beauty of this gentle approach using food supplements is that these additional nutrients and live bacteria can help to enhance your child's appetite, stimulate gastric juice production, optimize digestion and even modulate the brain's perception of the food they are consuming. Over time, many parents discover that this approach can alter their child's taste buds, sense of smell and even the sensation of different food textures in the mouth – and ultimately, they start to eat a much broader range of foods.

Certain exercises can also help with oral tone to help with chewing and swallowing over the longer term. Over time, better oral tone can take away the fear of trying new foods and so widen food choices. These include simple things like drinking through a curly wurly straw, having fun with party blowers, musical pipes and blowing bubbles. They all strengthen the muscles in the mouth, which in turn help with chewing, swallowing and texture perception. (See chapter 8 for more information.)

A neurodivergent brain needs a diverse and wholesome diet to thrive! So, you will be relieved to know that my food and nutrition mantras are not about strict diets or banning certain foods forever – quite the opposite. My tried-and-trusted method is all about learning exactly what a young brain requires to flourish, and finding easy ways over time to incorporate a child's nutritional needs into lifestyle and eating habits that are enjoyable, sustainable and truly nourishing. Above all, it's about feeding them food that they will actually eat!

'BUT MY CHILD EATS A BRILLIANT DIET ALREADY!'

Bravo, if this is your child! A varied, wholesome diet is a great start and probably means that they have the foundations of good nutrition already. That said, I usually find there is room for improvement and just small tweaks can still make useful differences.

What is important to get your head round is that eating what most people would consider a 'healthy' diet doesn't necessarily guarantee that your child is avoiding nutritional pitfalls. Several factors come into play – their body's ability to absorb and digest nutrients, the freshness and quality of the food they are consuming, and any competition in the gut from parasites or other unwanted microbes. Certain medical conditions, such as Crohn's or Ulcerative Colitis (inflammatory bowel disease) or Coeliac disease (an autoimmune reaction in the gut to consuming wheat and gluten), can also adversely affect a young person's absorption of nutrients, and so too can external factors, such as stress. Stress and trauma also affect how well we assimilate and digest nutrients from food, and when children are in a flight-or-fight state, their digestion can slow up quite a bit.

The very acts of smelling food as it is cooking, as well as salivating and chewing food well, send important signals to make enough enzymes further down the intestines. These enzymes break down the food efficiently, meaning you get the most nutrition from your food. This is why it is important to avoid eating on the run, bolting down meals too quickly or eating food directly from a packet – all of which can surprise your digestion so that the gastric juices are not ready to do their best job.

Once food is digested in the gut, the nutrients are absorbed into the bloodstream – the body's natural transport system – and then specific vitamins and minerals help to make special chemicals that transport fats, carbohydrates and proteins as well as micronutrients into our cells. The cells are where all the magic happens, and our energy and vitality are created. Cells that are well nourished play a vital role in maintaining a child's mental stamina and abilities.

The efficiency of all these vital bodily processes – the gut, the bloodstream and the cells – can be altered or even blocked by genetic factors, nutrient deficiencies, chronic inflammation, oxidative stress and even the presence of environmental pollutants. All of which will be discussed in this book.

Thankfully, the difficulties of getting nutrients from mouth to cell can often be temporarily overcome by taking food supplements, such as vitamins, minerals, amino acids, essential fatty acids, enzymes and herbal support. Over time these helping hands are either no longer needed or only on an ad-hoc basis during times of significant challenges or change.

IT'S ALL GENETIC, ISN'T IT?

Genetic testing has revolutionized our understanding of why some children are either born with or develop certain neurological conditions or neurodivergence. This is an emerging science and there are still only a handful of conditions where one specific inherited gene mutation or chromosome difference has been identified, such as Rett Syndrome, Fragile X and Down Syndrome.

Research into genetic testing for predicting Dyslexia, Autism and ADHD has found several common shared genes, but none that directly dictates that your child will have these conditions. While genetic testing is still in its infancy, many people will not have the opportunity to be tested and thus be unaware whether they carry this potential in their DNA.

However, many people can spot signs of neuro-divergence in several generations and in the wider family, even if those family members don't have a diagnosis. Parents of neurodivergent children often say that, on reflection, their child was born with it, and there were soft signs from an early age. I believe genetics plays a critical role and our knowledge will increase as testing is more widely used.

We all carry a mixed bag of genes and many of us will have genetic tendencies towards acquiring certain diseases and metabolic problems. But just as family members who share the same DNA can experience a viral infection such as Covid 19 differently, the expression of neurodivergence can also differ. Some neurotypical parents may have neurodivergent children, and some neurodivergent parents may have neurotypical children.

The number of kids diagnosed with the many presentations of neurodivergence is now huge – and growing rapidly.[1] Despite better awareness and improved diagnosis, the total figure is increasing faster than a genetic blueprint alone could ever explain. And our medical and education systems are now struggling to accommodate the enormous influx of children with severe challenges in language, socialization, learning and behaviour, which will impact on their opportunities in adult life.[2,3]

EPIGENETICS IS KEY

Epigenetics refers to the interplay between a child's genetic blueprint and their diet and environment. It refers to the potential for a much wider variation in neurodevelopmental outcomes than stems from a child's fixed inherited genes. Many studies have found that epigenetics may explain why neurodivergence is now more common and more strikingly apparent.[4,5,6]

It is now well established that how our genetic blueprint is expressed can change with our diet, lifestyle and environment. A child carries a gene pool similar to that of their parents and grandparents, but things can be magnified if their diet is poor, there are elevated levels of stress, they experience trauma, catch a significant infection, or are exposed to high amounts of environmental toxins. All or any of these factors can negatively influence the child's development and learning and can exacerbate neurological challenges.[7,8] These changes, unlike mutations, don't alter the actual DNA sequence, but instead alter how the body interprets this all-important genetic information.

It must be emphasized that none of this is the parents' or anyone's fault. The reality is that most humans on Earth today face a life peppered with stress, illness and environmental pollutants and are increasingly consuming a diet of ultra-processed foods. Even some baby foods have been found to contain high levels of arsenic, lead and cadmium as our soil is increasingly polluted.[9]

A healthy diet and lifestyle can have a very positive influence on epigenetics. Certain nutrients and daily healthy habits can potentially turn gene-expression off – or at least suppress it or slow it down. This is called DNA methylation, and the right food, clean water and air, enough sleep, supporting the immune system and helping stress response are all incredibly important. So a child's genetic blueprint does not necessarily dictate everything about them, and their inherited pool of genes do not always determine their future health. The right diet, lifestyle and environment can help them thrive. Positivity is incredibly important here. According to research, just knowing your genetic risks can be self-limiting, and positive belief in your genes releases improvements.[10]

The main nutrients that are known to help DNA methylation are essential fatty acids, choline, B vitamins, vitamin D, and the brightly coloured pigments called polyphenols within fruits and veg. In chapter 2, I will go into much greater depth on these.

NEURODIVERSITY CAN BE ACQUIRED

Some neurodivergence is less obvious from birth and can reveal itself as a child develops. Typically, parents may notice signs of Autism when their child is around 18 months old and teachers may flag Dyslexia, Dyspraxia or ADHD within the first few years of a child starting at school. Many kids mask their neurodivergence until a time when they are highly stressed; commonly, the time for ADHD and Dyslexia to be formally diagnosed is the mid-teens, when public exams are looming.

Regressive Autism occurs when a child appears to develop typically but then starts to lose social and communication skills as well as developmental milestones, often between the ages of 1 and 3 years. This can seem to happen 'almost overnight', or more slowly, over several months. The loss of skills or abilities is not unique to Autism and can sometimes occur much later in childhood. At my NatureDoc clinic, I have seen kids who have regressed out of the blue at the ages of 7, 9 and even 12 years.

Signs of a child regressing in their skills can vary but generally include:

SOCIAL SKILLS

a child might become less responsive to their name, make less eye contact, or have reduced interest in people, including parents and siblings. They may stop waving goodbye or engaging in social games they previously enjoyed.

COMMUNICATION

previously acquired language skills may be lost. A child may stop using words or phrases they were previously able to say, might start babbling again, or stop making sounds entirely. Non-verbal communication (gestures, such as pointing and clapping), may also decrease.

REPETITIVE BEHAVIOURS

repetitive behaviours may start to emerge out of the blue, such as spinning, lining up toys, or hand flapping.

PLAY SKILLS

a child might show reduced interest in different play activities, preferring repetitive activities, and may stop playing with toys. For example, rather than pushing a toy car, they might just spin its wheels.

EMOTIONAL CHANGES

an increase in tantrums or seemingly unprovoked crying may be apparent, or the child might become more passive, withdrawn and shy.

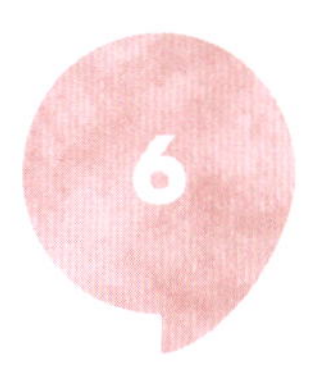

MOTOR SKILLS

occasionally, children may lose motor skills they had previously developed, such as the ability to feed themselves or to be able to hop or skip. Some may even lose the ability to walk.

Sometimes these regressions can wax and wane and children with PANS/PANDAS (see page 11), for instance, can start talking in a baby voice when they are experiencing a flare-up alongside their other symptoms. Kids with Long Covid can find that they develop brain fog and poor word retrieval which can affect their socialization and use of language. There can be noticeable changes in a child's development shortly after a severe infection, which can lead to neuroinflammation, and if seizures develop as a result, this can also play a role in a regression of skills, particularly speech and language skills as well as sociability, and this is why it is important to seek medical advice.

Children can display a subtle loss of skills over longer periods of time or a stalling in development. For example, reading skills may not progress or writing and drawing skills might seem to be less advanced than previously, or the child may just seem less mature than their peers. These examples are often flags for nutrient depletions, gut-microbiome disruptions and chronic inflammation from diet or environmental stressors.

Every individual has a unique story, and it is important to look at the whole picture rather than assume their neurodivergence is purely genetic – it can, of course, be genetic in origin, but there may be other factors that you can work on and support. And these are the things that are explained in greater depth in chapters 2 to 7.

2 THE KEY BASICS OF NUTRITION & NEUROTRANSMITTERS

'My child is neurodivergent, but that's got nothing to do with what they eat,' is a sentiment I hear frequently in the neurodivergent community. Well, it turns out there are quite a lot of connections between food, mood and mind! Scientists are now finding that the food our children eat can play a significant role in how they think, feel and function. Food can also help to make neurotransmitters, which are brain chemicals that support mood, learning and development. So, in turn, quality fuel from the right foods and targeted nutrients can enhance focus, improve memory and even ease some of the big emotions that often accompany neurodiversity.

Before going deeper into the specific metabolic and nutritional needs of a neurodivergent brain, it is important to understand the key basics of nutrition for physical, mental and cognitive health. This is a whistle-stop tour of the elements of food that crop up repeatedly throughout this book. Later in this chapter I introduce you to the naturally occurring vitamins, minerals, fats, specialist foods, herbs and spices which have been found to have a positive or balancing effect on the brain. I also explain about neurotransmitters and some metabolic differences shared by quite a few neurodivergent children.

MACRONUTRIENTS AND MICRONUTRIENTS

When talking about nutrition, two terms that frequently come up are 'macros' and 'micros', which are short for macronutrients and micronutrients. These are the main families of nutrients that our bodies need to function optimally. Understanding their roles can help us make the right dietary choices for us and our kids to help them flourish.

MACRONUTRIENTS

Macronutrients are the nutrients that our bodies require in large quantities. They are the foundation of our diet, providing the bulk of the energy we need to go about our daily lives. The three primary macros are carbohydrates, proteins and fats.

Carbohydrates act as the powerhouse for the body, providing the energy we need to function. When we consume any carbohydrates, our bodies break them down into glucose, a type of sugar that their cells can use as a direct energy source. Not only do carbohydrates fuel our bodies, they also play a critical role in brain function. In fact, the brain favours carbohydrates, in the form of glucose as its main energy source. Sources of this include sugar, fruit and starches, such as bread, pasta, rice and potatoes. Fibre-filled carbohydrates such as vegetables, wholegrains and pulses release carbohydrate more slowly, which helps to create a better balance of energy over the day and would be the better choice.

Proteins, on the other hand, are essential for muscle growth, repair and maintaining good health. They supply amino acids, the building blocks for cells. Importantly, these amino acids are necessary for the creation of neurotransmitters, those vital chemicals that allow brain cells to communicate with each other. Proteins are nutrient-dense foods such as meat and offal, fish and seafood, eggs, dairy products (milk, cheese and yoghurt), legumes and pulses, nuts and seeds.

Fats and oils often get a bad rap, but the brain is 60% fat and they are essential for the body. They provide a concentrated source of energy, help with the absorption of certain vitamins, and contribute to the structure of our cells. Among the vast family of fats and oils, the omega-3 fatty acids and phospholipids, such as choline, are crucial for the neurodivergent brain, as they form an integral part of the brain cells' structure, supporting cognitive function. Healthy fats are in extra virgin olive oil, coconut oil, avocados and cocoa butter, and there are good-quality fats and oils in eggs, dairy, grass-fed meats, fish and seafood, nuts and seeds.

Most foods contain a little of each of these key macros, but in different proportions. For instance, pulses contain both carbohydrate and protein while eggs and seeds contain both protein and fat.

MICRONUTRIENTS

While macronutrients are the basis of our diet, equally important are the micronutrients. These include 13 essential vitamins and 24 key minerals. Although they are needed in far smaller amounts, a deficiency in one or more micronutrients can lead to serious health issues. For instance, B vitamins are essential for energy production and maintaining healthy brain function, and there is a Vitamin D receptor on every single cell in the body. Minerals like magnesium help nerve function and muscle contraction, while zinc supports the immune system, growth and neurotransmitter synthesis.

Micronutrients are individually and collectively catalysts for thousands of functions in the body and the brain. They are involved in myriad chemical reactions, facilitating the conversion of food into energy, the repair and growth of tissues, and the strengthening of the immune system – so getting enough of these is crucial for how our kids feel day to day as well as for their long-term health. Macros and micros have distinct roles, but they also work synergistically to ensure cells function efficiently. A balanced, varied diet is the best way to ensure our children get a good mix of both. Understanding how these nutrients influence physical, mental, emotional and cognitive health is a crucial step towards motivating us to make better dietary choices for our kids to keep them strong and resilient.

What does all this mean for the neurodivergent mind? Nutrients are the brain's best friends, of course! Every mouthful of food our kids eat can either support their brain, making them feel switched on and positive, or neglect it, leaving them feeling low and slow. The right nutrition can help balance mood, sharpen focus, boost energy and much more.

WATER, YOUR BRAIN'S LIFEFORCE

Water is not just a thirst-quencher; it is the very essence of life and especially vital for brain function. Imagine your child's brain as a sponge, soaking up water to help make all the neural connections. Water is the main medium for all the biochemical reactions that occur within the brain. It facilitates the smooth transit of nutrients, hormones and oxygen to cells, while also carrying away waste products. Thus, keeping our cells functioning efficiently, supporting overall brain health and cognition.

Even mild dehydration can have a significant effect on both body and brain. We can experience symptoms such as fatigue, headaches and poor concentration. These symptoms are alarm bells, alerting us that our cells aren't getting the hydration they need to function optimally.

So, how much water should our children be drinking? Well, it can vary depending on a few factors like age, activity level, and the temperature, but a good rule of thumb for teens is to drink about 2 litres or 8 glasses a day. Most younger kids thrive on 6 glasses a day.[11] But you can 'read what they need' from the colour of their urine. Aim for straw yellow: too dark, and they need to hydrate; too light, and they may be drinking too much.

Ideally, drinking water should be filtered to reduce exposure to environmental pollutants such as microplastics and heavy metals. Emerging research has found a potential link between exposure to microplastics and heavy metals in the womb and the trajectory of neurodevelopmental differences. Exposure to these pollutants can be reduced simply by filtering the water you drink at home.

THE KEY BRAIN NUTRIENTS EVERYONE NEEDS TO KNOW ABOUT

Which key nutrients do you need to focus on if your child has a neurodivergent mind? Here are the stars of the show, which are important to learn about and to try and include in your child's diet or supplement regime. I have gone into quite a bit of depth, as I refer to these throughout this book, so these should become well-thumbed pages for you!

I have included key body signs your child might be displaying if they are low in these key nutrients – see these as barometers for an understanding of whether they need more or less. Ideally, nutrient levels would be checked via blood test or comprehensive nutrient testing by a nutrition professional. I appreciate, however, that this may not always be possible; sometimes you need to use common sense but also remember never to go overboard either.

See the appendix at the back of this book for age-appropriate dosages if you are using food supplements (see page 232).

OMEGA-3

Omega-3 is now a very well-known nutrient. It's a fatty acid that is crucial for brain health and can make a huge difference to learning, mood and behaviour.[12, 13, 14, 15] This amazing fat feeds the prefrontal and frontal lobes of the brain and is key for social, emotional and behavioural development[16] as well as executive and complex cognitive activities including sustained attention, planning and problem solving.[17]

It is described as an 'essential' fatty acid because we can only obtain omega-3 from food. There is a special type of omega-3 that is most important during preconception, pregnancy and breastfeeding as well as the child's early years called docosahexaenoic acid (DHA). DHA is the predominant omega-3 oil found in the brain and is critical for both eye and brain development.[18,19]

The other two key members of the omega-3 family are eicosapentaenoic acid (EPA) and alpha-linolenic acid (ALA). They occur only in small amounts in the brain and are more helpful for reducing chronic inflammation (see chapter 5). Most foods rich in omega-3 contain a combination of omegas; supplements will contain a different balance depending on their purpose.

The main dietary sources of DHA and EPA are oily fish, such as salmon, mackerel, sardines, anchovies, trout and shellfish. Other sources include some eggs laid by chickens fed on flaxseeds,[20] as well as organic whole milk and meat from grass-fed animals.[21] Omega-3 fish oil supplements are popular and convenient if your child does not eat these foods on a regular basis.

What if you are plant-based, vegan or vegetarian? In theory, the body can convert plant-based ALA omega-3 from foods such as walnuts, flax, hemp and chia seeds into the DHA form, but to do so the body needs to be well nourished and unstressed.[22] At best, conversion is only around 10 per cent; males and babies convert as little as 1 per cent of dietary plant-based ALA into DHA. If your child consumes too many processed foods or if they are deficient in nutrients such as zinc, calcium, magnesium and some B vitamins, conversion will be extremely low.[23]

In such scenarios it would be almost impossible to get enough omega-3 from diet alone. Marine algae omega-3 food supplements can come to the rescue for plant-based diets or non-fish eaters. This naturally DHA-rich oil is extracted from vegan marine algae – the nourishing food that oily fish eat, which gives this type of fish its concentrated abundance of omega-3.[24]

It is easy to tell if your child is low in omega-3 because the body can be helpful at showing even minor shortfalls.[25,26] The following signs are all indicators that your child may need to consume more omega-3:

- Dry skin
- 'Chicken skin' (see box opposite)
- Eczema
- Excess thirst
- Dry hair
- Dandruff
- Brittle nails
- Frequent urination and bed-wetting
- Asthma
- Blood sugar highs and lows 'hyper then hangry'
- Chronic pain

CHOLINE

Acetylcholine is a critical neurotransmitter for neurodevelopment,[30] including learning, memory, executive function, motivation and emotional regulation. Choline-rich foods fuel the making of acetylcholine and it is one of a group of important phospholipids that help to keep brain cell walls flexible. This in turn can lead to more flexible thinking.

Choline is also thought to be a healing nutrient when the unborn child has had any kind of developmental issue or trauma within the womb.[31,32] Choline via food is key for neurodevelopment during the first 1,000 days of life – from conception until a child's second birthday[33] – and low levels of this nutrient are linked to a higher likelihood of Autism, ADHD and Dyslexia.[34] Children who consume choline-rich food tend to have better written and spoken language,[35] and choline can help with visuospatial learning such as thinking in images and pictures,[36] which can in turn help with their spelling and handwriting skills.

Choline plays an important role in stress response and in sensory processing. Neurodivergent children with the highest difficulties surrounding their sensory needs often have low levels of phospholipids.[37]

Choline can be sourced from a wide range of foods – liver, beef, egg yolks, dairy products, soya beans, sunflower seeds, quinoa and peanut butter – and these ingredients need to be eaten in abundance when the focus is on nourishing the brain, which is the one of the purposes of the recipes in this book.

Our gut bacteria also contribute to producing acetylcholine. One of the reasons for eating live yoghurt and kefir is because the *Lactobacillus* strains they contain are the building blocks for making acetylcholine. This gut–brain link is explored in more detail in chapter 4.

'CHICKEN SKIN'

If you rub the skin on the tops of your child's arms, does it feel a little rough like sandpaper or is it smooth? Raised red bumps on the upper arms are thought to signify inflammation and can indicate depletions in nutrients such as Vitamin A and omegas, which are important skin nutrients.[27] Some kids with gut malabsorption issues, including coeliac disease,[28] can also develop this 'chicken skin' and similar skin conditions. Your child's skin is a good barometer for whether they are getting enough nutrients from the food they eat.[29] I have found in our NatureDoc clinic that chicken skin is very common among the neurodivergent kids that we support, and often it is obvious on the face, upper legs and torso as well as the arms. In many cases, increasing the intake of foods naturally rich in omega-3 and Vitamin A as well as taking a cod liver oil or fish oil supplement over several months can lead to smoother, less bumpy skin... as well as a sharper brain!

IRON

Iron is a critical trace mineral that transports oxygen around the body and brain via the bloodstream, and we all know that oxygen is essential for life and vitality. Iron is also important for many different processes in the body, supporting energy levels and the immune system. It is the most abundant mineral in the central nervous system and a shortfall in iron can lead to emotional and psychological difficulties such as anxiety, depression and OCD.[38,39,40]

Low iron levels can also affect focus and attention. I have observed iron-deficiency in a number of children who find it hard to maintain good levels of dopamine and have an ADHD diagnosis or associated symptoms.[41,42] This may be because iron specifically helps to convert the amino acid tyrosine (found in protein-rich foods) into dopamine. So, it is key to build up their iron stores if a child struggles with focus and attention as well as impulsivity.

Key reasons for low iron levels

It comes as a surprise to many parents to learn how much iron kids need to maintain a healthy store. As a guide, they should consume at least two servings of food that contain good levels of iron every day. Iron-rich foods include offal, red meat, pulses, eggs, green vegetables, dates, prunes and apricots. Ideally pair these foods with ones that are high in Vitamin C, like oranges, strawberries, (bell) peppers or parsley, as the vitamin enhances iron absorption, ensuring your kid gets the most out of every meal.

Why do our kids become low in iron? Here are some reasons why your child might be deficient:

► Modern dietary choices and the movement towards eating white meat and plant-based options rather than red meat or offal.

► Many kids choose 'beige' crunchy processed foods that are devoid of iron. When this becomes a habit, it is very easy for iron levels to drop.

► Adolescent girls often become low in iron or anaemic due to menstruation, especially if the flow is heavy, long or frequent. Paradoxically, low iron can lead to heavier periods, which is why the daily recommendation for iron intake is much higher for tween and teen girls whose periods are regular.

► Children who eat lots of milk and dairy products are prone to iron-deficiency, as these foods can block the absorption of iron from their food. If trying to top up iron levels, aim for a maximum of 2 glasses of milk each day and take iron supplements at a different time from eating dairy products.

► The tannins in tea and coffee can also block iron absorption, so look out for this with your teenagers.

Possible signs and symptoms of low iron

► Paler-than-usual skin on areas like the face, lower inner eyelids, or nails.

► Unexplained fatigue, lack of energy, and a general feeling of weakness.

► Shortness of breath, chest pain, or headaches, particularly after exertion or exercise.

► Rapid heartbeat and sensations of pounding or whooshing in the ears.

► Hair loss or brittle nails; excessive hair in your child's hairbrush or shower plug hole could indicate a need for more iron.

► 'Pica' where a child might start to crave or put non-food items in their mouth (see box on page 26).

► A sore or smooth tongue.

► In children low iron can lead to frequent tummy aches and a lack of appetite.

Although mild iron deficiencies can be corrected by eating plenty of iron-rich foods, the reality is that this can take a long time. This is where prescription iron and iron supplements can help.

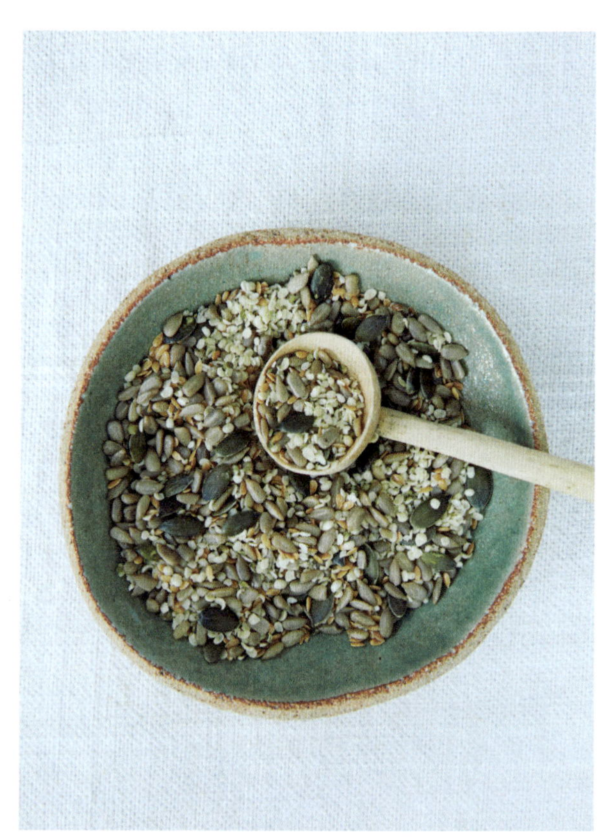

ZINC

Zinc is the second most dominant trace mineral within the central nervous system.[43] It has widespread functions and is critical for overall child development including fine and gross motor skills as well as cognitive development.[44] It has been well established that kids with Dyslexia are often very deficient in zinc[45] and that children and young people with ADHD[46] or Autism[47] are also prone to low zinc levels and benefit from supplements.[48] Low zinc levels have been found in the hair[49,50] of very young babies as well as the baby teeth[51,52] of little ones who later are diagnosed as autistic.

Zinc is key to keep neurotransmitters, such as acetylcholine, in balance, which is important for maintaining cognitive abilities such as executive function and working memory as well as mental health.[53] It can help with mood swings, self-regulation and emotional regulation.

It supports a robust immune system, protects from significant infection and helps with skin conditions such as acne and eczema. One of the key reasons why tweenagers and teenagers are prone to low zinc levels is because their zinc stores are being sucked up more rapidly while they are undergoing the rapid hormonal and physical changes from childhood to adulthood.

Furthermore, zinc is needed to help kids grow and it can stimulate appetite and aid digestion. A zinc deficiency is also suspected if there is dysregulated eating or an eating disorder such as Anorexia nervosa[54,55] – the symptoms of zinc deficiency and an eating disorder are very similar.[56] Zinc is a key nutrient to consider supporting if there are problems with lack of morning appetite, especially during puberty and also when taking ADHD stimulant medications if the child is not growing or is losing weight.

This mighty mineral also supports the neurological system and can cultivate and support a healthy sense of smell and taste and I have also found it helps the perception of texture. Kids with a neurodivergent brain are often very sensitive to even small shortfalls in zinc, which is why it's one of the first checks I make when a child is a highly selective eater or is struggling to expand their food repertoire.

Alongside poor growth and selective eating, key signs and symptoms that your child might be low in zinc are white flecks on the nails which tend to be more obvious when a child is going through a growth spurt or puberty. This is known as leukonychia[57] and is a generalized mineral deficiency sign, so if these are obvious and, on several nails, then do also consider other mineral support such as selenium, calcium and magnesium.

Quite marked low zinc levels can also lead to pica (see overleaf) and this can occur alongside an iron-deficiency or by itself. This is why it is important to carry out lab tests for both iron and zinc levels at the same time.

Possible signs and symptoms of low zinc

- Poor working memory
- Executive function difficulties
- Mood swings or emotional dysregulation
- Poor sense of smell or taste
- Low morning appetite
- Picky eating
- Slow growth
- Loose bowel or frequent tummy bugs
- Constantly catching colds, coughs
- Acne
- Eczema
- White flecks on the nails

The main dietary source of zinc is oysters – not usually a child's first choice of food! However other zinc-rich foods include nutrient-dense seafood such as shellfish and fish, as well as red meat and offal, eggs and dairy products, nuts, seeds, wholegrains and pulses. Soaking and sprouting your own seeds, nuts and beans, or buying sprouted wholegrains can help to optimize zinc absorption.

MAGNESIUM

Magnesium is another key mineral that assists hundreds of actions in the body, including supporting the nervous system, regulating sleep and energy, and regulating hyperactivity.[62] It is also important for balancing blood glucose.[63]

Research reveals that many people with ADHD have a shortfall in their magnesium levels[64] and that supplementing magnesium alongside vitamin D can help reduce behavioural and social problems, anxiety and shyness.[65] Magnesium can be taken with ADHD medications to reduce overall symptoms of ADHD, such as hyperactivity and irritability.[66]

PICA: DOES YOUR CHILD CHEW ON THEIR CLOTHES?

Does your child incessantly put non-food items in their mouth such as toys, stones, sand, ice cubes, tissues or paper? Do they love sucking or chewing on the collars and cuffs of their clothing? This may be a sign of the condition called pica, which is more common in neurodivergent children.[58]

While it's natural for babies to put everything in their mouth, if this behaviour persists in children older than two years, it could be indicative of cravings for important nutrients. Pica is the body's way of flagging up a significant deficiency in certain nutrients, usually iron and/or zinc.[59]

There are of course potential risks associated with pica. Eating non-food items such as soil or stones can increase the risk of parasitic infection. Some children might swallow items they put in their mouths, which could potentially block the intestine or puncture the gut lining. Lead toxicity from ingesting non-food items is also a risk, and high levels of lead can hamper intellectual development and growth. Lead is still found in some old toys, household paint and soil. Interestingly, lead exposure can lead to anaemia,[60,61] which in turn can trigger pica behaviours.

Correcting these deficiencies is crucial for the child's development. This can be done by a combination of dietary changes and supplements and can be guided by a qualified nutritional therapist, naturopath or functional medicine practitioner.

Possible signs and symptoms of low magnesium

- Regular tics
- Eye twitches
- Restless legs
- Growing pains
- Difficulty sleeping
- Muscle aches
- Hyperactivity
- Inability to wait for food
- Anxiety
- Constipation

Nuts, seeds, green veggies and dark chocolate are all great sources of magnesium.

VITAMIN D

Vitamin D and magnesium are co-dependent, so it is important to consider both at once.[68]

Every cell in our body has a Vitamin D receptor, which you can visualize as a socket, helping this fat-soluble vitamin to connect to the cell and work its magic. Many people carry a genetic blueprint, making it much harder for Vitamin D to attach to the cell, which is why, irrespective of sunshine exposure, some people need ongoing monitoring and support for their vitamin D levels.

Vitamin D is necessary for calcium metabolism to help with growth. Insufficient Vitamin D means bones will not form properly and the condition known as rickets, with its hallmark bowed legs, is exhibiting

EPSOM SALT BATHS

A lovely relaxing way for children (and adults!) to replenish their magnesium levels is to add a couple of cups of calming Epsom salt or magnesium flakes to a warm bath. Let them play or soak for at least 20 minutes so that the skin absorbs the magnesium from the water.[67] Magnesium-rich baths are also good for sporty kids who are prone to muscle cramps and injuries because the mineral helps to relax the muscles. My daughter when she was little used to say she always had happy dreams after having an Epsom salt bath.

a resurgence among children even in developed countries. Vitamin D supports the immune system to fight off infections and also helps to dial down brain inflammation and chronic pain.[69,70] Low vitamin D blood levels are common in depression and anxiety.[71] Interestingly, Vitamin D can support gut health and improve diversity within the gut microbiome which in turn can help with brain health in neurodivergence.[72]

Vitamin D deficiency is more prevalent in children with ADHD compared with neurotypical children[73] and supplements like Vitamin D sprays, drops or capsules have been found to lead to significant improvement in the ADHD symptoms of the children studied, especially during evenings when they tend to be quite wired and find it hard to get to sleep.[74] Autistic people are also often low in vitamin D blood levels,[75,76] and it seems that low vitamin D status runs in families where Autism features. Vitamin D supplements have also been found to help with a number of the core features of Autism in some people.[77] This may be because the majority of Autism-related genes are Vitamin D sensitive, therefore even small shortfalls of this vitamin could influence the expression of those genes.[78]

Picky eating may also lead to a Vitamin D deficiency.[79] Our primary source of Vitamin D is exposure to sunlight, but some can be obtained from foods such as oily fish, egg yolks, the meat from outdoor-reared pigs[80] and whole milk from grass-fed cows who have spent time in the sunshine.[81]

The amount of Vitamin D that the body can synthesize depends on the amount of UVB light that penetrates the skin. It can be blocked by wearing clothing and sun cream as well as excess body fat. As more kids choose to spend time indoors in front of screens rather than outside in the sun, Vitamin D deficiency is a growing problem worldwide.

Skin colour, determined by the skin pigment melanin, really makes a difference to Vitamin D uptake from the sun. The paler your child's skin, the greater the amount of Vitamin D is absorbed by exposure to the summer sun.[82]

The British NHS suggests that because of our long dark and cloudy winters, we should all top up with at least a 400iu Vitamin D supplement daily from October to March to prevent deficiency.

B VITAMINS

One family of vitamins that work in harmony with each other come under the umbrella term 'B vitamins'. Often all the key B vitamins are available in a multivitamin supplement. Individually they support a wide range of bodily functions – I will explain the role of each in turn.

Vitamin B1 (Thiamine)

Thiamine is important for a host of pathways in the body and can regulate the nervous system as well as support energy levels and mental health.[83] It is also important for allergies: stabilizing histamine and mast cells (see chapter 6)[84] which can help with car sickness, sea sickness and overreaction to insect bites. Thiamine is also very important for helping carbohydrate reach cells to make energy.[85]

Some kids are sensitive to even a mild shortfall in vitamin B1, and it can be associated with mental fuzziness and subtle difficulties in memory, along with loss of appetite and sleep disturbances. Gastrointestinal discomfort, slow digestion and constipation are also common symptoms. Food intolerances and vomiting may develop as deficiency increases.[86,87]

Thiamine is found in pork, fish, beans, lentils, brown rice, green peas, sunflower seeds and yoghurt. Vitamin B1 is added to baby cereals because these products tend to use very refined grains.[88] Because thiamine is a water-soluble vitamin, it is hard to take too much – any excess is passed away through urine.

Vitamin B2 (Riboflavin)

Vitamin B2 is key for supporting energy and helping fatty acids pass from the bloodstream into our cells. It also helps to fuel the mitochondria which are the powerhouses or 'batteries' within our cells that create energy and vitality.[89,90] Vitamin B2 also helps with blood glucose regulation and immunity.

Riboflavin is present in a number of foods, including eggs, offal, meats, yoghurt, milk as well as some fortified foods like bread and cereal. When anyone takes a vitamin B2 supplement their urine turns bright neon yellow, and while this can be alarming at first, it is totally normal and harmless.

Vitamin B3 (Niacin)

Niacin is another B vitamin that often needs supplementing when neurodiversity is present. Like riboflavin, it is key for creating enough mitochondrial energy to complete daily tasks[91,92] and many people with chronic fatigue or post-viral illness benefit from one of the various forms of vitamin B3.

The main dietary sources are meats, fish, brown rice and peanuts. Care is necessary if taking some of the niacin-based supplements, which, at higher amounts, can cause temporary hot flushing. This can be alarming, even if it is totally harmless. The niacinamide form, however, is non-flushing.

Vitamin B6 (Pyridoxine)

Vitamin B6 is a primary nutrient for making many neurotransmitters and helping to regulate the nervous system;[93] a deficiency of this vitamin can be one reason for dysregulation difficulties that neurodivergent children can experience.[94] Shortfalls in Vitamin B6 can be due to genetic predispositions such as Pyrrole disorder (see page 35) alongside a need for zinc.

Vitamin B6 also plays a role in breaking down histamine in the gut (which in excess can make us sneeze and itch, and kids can get very hot and sweaty at night). Many people with allergies together with hyperactivity can find it hard to regulate histamine.

Vitamin B6 in food and supplements has been found to help both verbal and non-verbal communication, repetitive behaviours and social skills in autistic people and it seems to be better tolerated when calming magnesium is given at the same time.[95,96] Taken together, these two nutrients can also help with noise sensitivity (see chapter 13).

Other possible indicators of a low Vitamin B6 status can be anger outbursts and sleep issues. A sign you might need more vitamin B6 is if you have no dream recall[97] and, when you step up the vitamin B6, you remember your dreams more easily. However, if you take too much, dreams can become very vivid.

Often, low Vitamin B6 might show as cracked lips at the corners of the mouth, which can also be an overall sign to support B vitamins.[98] Tingly fingers or toes are signs of too much B6: if you or your child experience this, you need to stop taking the supplements immediately. The Pyridoxal 5 Phosphate form of B6 supplements rarely gives these side effects and would be my choice over standard pyridoxine supplements.

Foods that are abundant in Vitamin B6 include salmon, tuna, chicken, turkey, beef, liver, chickpeas (garbanzo beans), potatoes and bananas.

Vitamin B9 (Folate)

Folate or Vitamin B9 is needed to support our neurological system. You find folate in green 'foliage' foods like salad leaves and green veg, which is why we are all told to eat our greens regularly. Many neurodiverse kids lack the ability to methylate B9 efficiently.[99] (Methylation is a complicated biological process that involves the conversion of dietary folate into methyl tetrahydrofolate, the type of folate that our bodies can use most efficiently.) Once the folate is methylated and goes through many more complex processes, it then helps to create a powerful antioxidant known as glutathione. This, among other antioxidants, is super important, helping to repair cells, and protects from inflammation, oxidative stress, neurological and cellular damage as well as autoimmunity (see chapter 6).

Synthetic folic acid is the most difficult form of folate to methylate and synthesize, especially for one of the many people carrying the Methylenetetrahydrofolate Reductase (MTHFR) genetic variation[100] and this form of folate is the one used in most standard multivitamin supplements and fortified foods, such as breakfast cereals and some flour.

One way to circumvent this is to consume foods naturally rich in folate – which I appreciate is not most kids' immediate favourite, but you can get smart and grate or blend these into the foods they do like. Folate-rich foods include mixed salad leaves, leafy green vegetables, broccoli, cabbage, green beans and other legumes, pulses and eggs. If a folate supplement is necessary, opt for one labelled as methyl tetrahydrofolate, folinic acid or calcium l-folinate, and avoid those containing the folic acid form.

Vitamin B12 (Cobalamin)

Vitamin B12 is a key nutrient for forming healthy red blood cells as well as the neurological system.

A deficiency in Vitamin B12 is well documented

in research on Autism and ADHD[101,102] and optimizing levels of this vitamin has been found to improve sleep and help with gastrointestinal symptoms, hyperactivity, tantrums, non-verbal IQ, vision, eye contact, echolalia (echoing heard speech) and bed-wetting.[103] The development of obsessive and compulsive behaviours may sometimes be an early hallmark of a Vitamin B12 deficiency.[104]

Many neurodivergent children feel better once their levels of Vitamin B12 are supported properly, and it has been found to help many aspects of neurodivergence, such as improved expressive communication, better personal and domestic daily living skills, as well as interpersonal skills, the ability to enjoy play and to cope with social situations.[105]

Vitamin B12 is sourced mainly from animal products such as meat, seafood and eggs. We ideally need to eat this together with folate-rich foods – the 'meat and two veg' meal! Together, folate and Vitamin B12 work with iron to create healthy blood and help to build the nervous system.

Many other vitamins and minerals in addition to those highlighted above are involved in supporting health and vitality. They act together, working in harmony with each other. Natural foods contain a whole host of different nutrients that the body can assimilate and metabolize. This is why a good diet is one that includes a wide variety of nutrient-dense foods to ensure all these nutrients are kept in balance.

MOTHER NATURE'S BRAIN FOODS

As well as omega-3, vitamins and minerals, several plant-based foods, herbs and spices can help to nourish and balance the brain. These are usually only needed to be taken in the short term and can, I find, make a significant positive difference to mood, focus and stress quite quickly. Many children start off with taking them daily for three months and others feel they only need to take them on an ad-hoc basis when they are going through stressful or challenging times. See them as a hug from Mother Nature when your child feels discombobulated! Here are my favourites and the ones that most frequently benefit NatureDoc clients. They can be taken solo or as blends; some will suit some kids better than others.

SAFFRON

Saffron is the deep orange spice that adds flavour and vivid colour to paella and some curries. The tiny strands are the dried stigmas of a flower, *Crocus sativus*. This spice is also used as a natural remedy for anxiety,[106] depression[107] and insomnia.[108] More and more people are discovering that it also helps to increase focus levels and provide support during stressful times or if prone to panic attacks. Studies show that saffron supplements also play a role in supporting children with ADHD and concentration problems as well as hyperactivity.[109,110] It can help with winding down for bed and promotes better sleep patterns, sleep quality and restorative sleep.[111,112]

Some NatureDoc clients have described the change in their child's outlook on life to be quite dramatic in terms of improving their mood and stress control[113] and have said they no longer need to be in fear of their mood swings.

Saffron supplements can be a neurodivergent female's best friend to help ease the menstrual cycle.[114,115] Not only does it help with period pain, but it can also help to ameliorate premenstrual irritability, anxiety, anger and depression.[116] Some who suffer with extreme mood swings and psychological distress called Premenstrual Dysphoric Disorder (PMDD) find relief from taking saffron.[117]

Look out for my Saffron & Cardamom Latte on page 216 and Chicken, Apricot & Saffron Tagine on page 155.

L-THEANINE

L-Theanine, often known as just theanine, is the amino acid found in black and green tea. If hot drinks are not their thing or your child is too young, theanine supplements are available. It is what eases the jitters after a shock, by providing that same zen-like feeling of having mediated or done a yoga class.

Theanine helps to promote the neurotransmitter called GABA (see page 33), that helps with sleep, anxiety, the stress of exams or deadlines etc, which is very calming on the nervous system.[118] It can help hyperactive kids to get to sleep and enjoy better-quality sleep.[119] It is now thought to lift the mood and ward off depression.[120] Drinking green tea has been found to reduce anxiety, and help with working memory and attention.[121]

Some teens and young adults with ADHD benefit from the combination of theanine and caffeine[122] and may therefore do well by drinking tea. Caffeine does not suit everyone, however, and can overstimulate some people. Educate your kids to drink tea in the morning, so the caffeine it contains does not disturb their sleep patterns. You may find that this approach improves their daily routine, and disordered sleep if they are activated earlier in the day by caffeine, and then they will be more subdued later, ready for bed.

LION'S MANE

Lion's mane (*Hericium erinaceus*) is an amazing edible mushroom with both neuroprotective[123] and anti-inflammatory[124] properties. It has been found to have a calming effect on the brain and can be helpful for spatial memory[125] – like remembering where your keys are. Most research on lion's mane has been conducted on the elderly who experience cognitive decline.[126] However, it is also used by younger people to support low mood and depression and sometimes to recover from traumatic brain injury.[127]

Some people describe lion's mane as toffee flavoured. It often comes in powder form to which you add hot water, or you can stir it into hot chocolate. It is also sold in capsules, and often combined with other neuroprotective nootropics such as bacopa (brahmi) and turmeric.

BRAHMI

Bacopa, also known as brahmi or *Bacopa monnieri*, is water hyssop, a wildflower from the tropics. It comes from the Indian Ayurvedic tradition and has been described as a calming cognitive enhancer. It is helpful with anxiety and insomnia, word recall and memory.[128] It has been shown to improve students' memory skills[129] – even to help with multi-tasking.[130] It has been found to help improve vocabulary and verbal comprehension as well as reduce hyperactivity and inattention.[131]

PASSIONFLOWER

Also known as *Passiflora incarnata*, you may be familiar with this beautiful trailing vine in gardens. Passionflower is very rich in GABA (see page 33), which helps to regulate the nervous system and help kids feel more connected and centred.[132] It can help with focus and calm, making day-to-day tasks more manageable and can reduce anxiety and nervousness.[133] A small study found that it helped children with ADHD just as much as the medication Methylphenidate but without the side effects of appetite loss, anxiety or nervousness.[134] It is well known as an aid for a better night's sleep[135] and to rebalance the circadian rhythm.[136]

A cup of steeped passionflower tea can be very soothing for the mind. If your child is not a herbal tea drinker, then steep some passionflower tea in hot water, let it cool and then blend with fruit to make a smoothie or freeze as an ice lolly (popsicle).

LEMON BALM AND VALERIAN

These two herbs are both rich in calming GABA (see page 33), which can help anxious souls and people who struggle to sleep.[137,138] They can be taken separately but are often taken together.

Even little children can benefit from these herbs when they worry too much or need a little dose of calm. A combination of lemon balm (also known as Melissa) and valerian has been found to help reduce restlessness and impulsiveness as well as improve concentration difficulties in primary school children[139] and kids with ADHD.[140] It can also help them get to sleep and stay asleep.[141]

WHAT ARE NEUROTRANSMITTERS AND WHY ARE THEY SO IMPORTANT?

Our brains are controlled by a family of brain chemicals called neurotransmitters that do their best to keep our minds happy, healthy and well. When these neurotransmitters are out-of-sync a person can develop 'brain fog', and feel flat, anxious and distracted. The nutrients in food feed these neurotransmitters, and when we are fully tuned in to our kids, we can observe that they can feel low and slow after eating some foods, and then become wired and agitated after others.

Neurotransmitters are essential chemicals that aid cell communication within the brain and help with regulating mood, appetite and sleep, as well as controlling movements and sensory perception. They also enable memory, learning and recall. They are primarily produced in the neurons of the brain as well as in the intestines by our gut bacteria. There is a two-way communication system between the gastrointestinal tract and the brain known as the gut–brain axis. It is not entirely clear how these neurotransmitters reach the brain from the gut, but it is thought that the vagus nerve, which connects the brain and the gut, plays an important role.

Eating enough of the right micronutrients, such as vitamins, minerals and certain fats, plays a crucial role in maintaining the correct levels of neurotransmitters in the brain, enabling them to function optimally. Certain foods contain the building blocks of neurotransmitters, which is why a varied diet is so important.[142] Imbalances or disruptions in neurotransmitters can contribute to various mental health or neurological disorders, including some of the more pronounced challenges faced by neurodivergent kiddos who tend to be very sensitive to even small disruptions of neurotransmitters and can find it hard to keep the right balance.

Learning how neurotransmitters assist the brain can help to optimize the way your child interacts with the world. Here are the key ones, together with foods that naturally contain these vital chemicals.

ACETYLCHOLINE

What does it do?	• Working memory, processing information, self-regulation and emotional regulation. • Muscle movement to regulate the heartbeat and gut peristalsis.
Symptoms of too much	• Excessive salivation, tear production, bowel movements and a slow heartbeat.
Symptoms of too little	• Difficulties with memory, processing and thinking, executive function. • Muscle weakness, a sluggish gut, fatigue and problems with coordination and movement.
Foods that provide it	• Peas, spinach, radishes, mung beans, aubergines and squash. • Choline-rich foods include eggs, meats, fish and whole grains.

DOPAMINE

What does it do?

- Dopamine is involved in motivation, memory, and movement coordination.
- A 'reward chemical' because it is released in the anticipation or excitement of something good happening and helps you to feel pleasure.
- Many people with ADHD find it hard to regulate dopamine.

Symptoms of too much

- Feelings of euphoria, aggression, or intense sexual feelings.

Symptoms of too little

- Tiredness, lack of motivation and focus, difficulty experiencing pleasure.

Foods that provide it

- Avocados, bananas, plantain, apples, oranges, peas, aubergine, tomatoes and spinach.
- Tyrosine, an amino acid, is the building block of dopamine that you get from meat, fish and eggs.

GLUTAMATE

What does it do?

- The most abundant amino acid found in the human diet, it helps with learning and memory, and stimulates the brain; it is also the most concentrated amino acid in the brain. Most people nowadays have far too much glutamate and need to reduce the amount they are consuming.

Symptoms of too much

- Abnormally high concentrations can act as an 'excitotoxin' within the body and brain,[143] leading to migraines, irritability, anxiety, aggression and depression.
- Seizure activity[144] as well as tic disorders.[145,146]
- OCD symptoms, along with a love of fixed routines.[147]
- Being more introverted and anxious.[148]
- High risk-taking in kids who have no sense of danger or get involved with addictive substances.

Symptoms of too little

- This is very rare and can lead to some cognitive impairments.

Foods that provide it

- Monosodium glutamate (E621), yeast extract, citric acid and hydrolysed protein ingredients in ultra-processed foods.
- 'Umami' foods: Parmesan cheese, seaweed, soy sauce, fish sauce, concentrated tomato purée (paste) and ketchup.

GABA

What does it do?	• The calming opposite to glutamate is GABA, and most neurodivergent brains need much more of this neurotransmitter! It helps to slow down brain activity. It is vital for relaxation, reducing stress and promoting sleep. Think of GABA as a child's inner 'yogi' keeping them chilled and calm.
Symptoms of too much	• This is rare and can look like excessive sedation, fatigue and muscle weakness, as well as difficulties with concentration and memory.
Symptoms of too little	• Increased anxiety, restlessness, and a heightened stress response, as well as insomnia or disturbed sleep patterns.
Foods that provide it	• GABA is abundant in oats, barley, buckwheat, brown rice, spinach, potatoes, sweet potatoes, yams, kale and chestnuts.[149] Also try broccoli, cabbage, cauliflower, rocket, Brussels sprouts and beans. • Certain gut microbes can directly make GABA, via live strains of bacteria in yoghurt and kefir which contain *Lactobacillus* and *Bifidobacterium*.[150,151] • Also try theanine (the main component of green tea), chamomile, passionflower (*Passiflora*), *Ginkgo biloba*, rosemary, sage, thyme and lemon balm[152] as well as the mineral magnesium, which is known to be calming. • Find some natural GABA calm by walking in nature, meditating or practising yoga.

NOREPINEPHRINE

What does it do?	• Also known as noradrenaline, this is often referred to as a 'stress hormone' as well as a neurotransmitter. It is involved in the body's 'fight or flight' response, where it increases heart rate, releases glucose for energy, and increases blood flow to muscles. It also plays a role in attention and focus.
Symptoms of too much	• Feelings of anxiety, hyperactivity or being on edge. • Physically, symptoms are a rapid heart rate, high blood pressure or sweating.
Symptoms of too little	• Tiredness, have difficulty in concentrating and focus, or experience low mood. • Physically, it can lead to low blood pressure and a low heart rate.
Foods that provide it	• Foods that can help keep norepinephrine in balance include apples, avocados, bananas, pineapple, green veggies, nuts, cheese, fish, meat, liver, poultry, tofu and wholegrains.

SEROTONIN

What does it do?	• Serotonin is often called a 'feel-good' hormone or neurotransmitter because it helps with mood regulation, making us feel happier and more stable. It's also involved in other functions, like sleep, digestion and bone health, as well as learning, cognition and memory via the gut–brain axis.[153]
Symptoms of too much	• Agitation, restlessness, confusion, rapid heart rate, high blood pressure, dilated pupils, loss of muscle coordination.[154]
Symptoms of too little	• Feeling flat, down or depressed. • Anxiety, difficulty sleeping or having a low appetite. • Physical symptoms can include constipation, fatigue or a lack of interest in daily activities.
Foods that provide it	• Serotonin is synthesized from the amino acid 5-hydroxytryptophan (5-HTP), and tryptophan. • High levels of tryptophan are present in a variety of foods, such as chicken, turkey, bananas, avocado, cashew nuts, strawberries, passion fruit, pineapples, papayas, pomegranates, kiwi fruit, plums, spinach, tomatoes, onions, chicory, lettuce, potatoes, wild rice, coffee and paprika.

METABOLIC FACTORS

As well as eating more nutritious foods, there are metabolic reasons why we need more of certain nutrients to help us to thrive. There are two common metabolic challenges that can affect a broad number of kids and can be supported through nutrition.

PYRROLE DISORDER

A very frequent reason why parents seek support from my NatureDoc team is because their child displays persistent uncontrollable and 'predictably unpredictable' mood swings. They can seem jolly and happy one moment, and the next they flip to a state of rage. This can have a ripple effect on the whole family, and they soon learn to approach them 'as if walking on eggshells' to try and keep the peace. We see parents who are genuinely petrified living under the same roof with a child who has a violent temper and destructive behaviours.

Frequent meltdowns and a significant inability to manage stress could be due to a metabolic issue known as Pyrrole Disorder or Kryptopyrrole (KPU). This is a genetic condition that causes deficiencies in major nutrients such as zinc and Vitamin B6. Raised pyrroles may be more likely if someone is in a high histamine allergy state (see chapter 6) and, as well as zinc and Vitamin B6 deficiency, it might also indicate a need for manganese, Vitamin B3 and Vitamin C.[155]

Interestingly, kids who carry this genetic predisposition often have beautiful porcelain-like skin and bright eyes and look well-nourished and healthy. So, from their appearance they are not obvious candidates for additional nutrition.

Mood swings are the most highly reported symptom of KPU, followed closely by social withdrawal, compulsive behaviour and emotional eating.[156] Poor stress control, nervousness, anxiety, inner tension, episodic anger, picking arguments, poor short-term memory and depression are other common signs of KPU. Violent and destructive behaviours can be reduced dramatically by addressing nutrient imbalances which may partly stem from KPU.[157]

In clinic, we have found that both carbohydrate craving and sugar sensitivity are also common when a child is KPU-positive, along with a number of food and environmental allergies and sensitivities. They may be highly selective eaters or very particular about what they will or won't eat. There are often difficulties with aspects of learning, and they find it hard to focus. They may be slow to grow, and puberty may be delayed.

Another consideration is a slow but steady decline in mood, cognition or demeanour, as these nutrient depletions happen gradually over time. This might look like temper tantrums as a toddler and then magnify into school exclusion during the primary years and culminate in more significant behavioural or mental health challenges as a teenager.

As an aside, adults with KPU can become increasingly eccentric, cantankerous and unconventional as they age. This can give them unique artistic, musical and academic brilliance, but usually goes hand in hand with some pretty tough mental health challenges. There also may be a strong family history of alcoholism or other addictions.

Testing for KPU can be done via a simple and affordable urine test, and kids with a positive test result can be easily supported with high-dose supplements of vitamin B6 and zinc, under the supervision of a naturopath or nutritional therapist. Being a genetic condition, it is often wise to test other family members too.

The great news is that the disorder is relatively quick to rebalance and the difference in mood can be quite dramatic within a few weeks or months. This is achieved by making positive diet changes to include plenty of zinc, B6 and omega-6 rich foods (eggs and meat) as well as supplementing with zinc and vitamin B6. Subsequently, all that is usually needed is maintaining this nutrient-rich diet, as well as keeping oxidative stress under control by eating plenty of brightly coloured foods. However, during growth spurts, such as puberty, or times of illness or high stress, it is important to go back to supplementing. Some people find they need to keep up their supplementation to sustain mood and demeanour over the longer term. It is all very individual.

BRILLIANT STORY OF HOPE – KPU

Flora, aged 13, was diagnosed with Sensory Processing Disorder and found school and making friends very hard. She would often retreat from her family into her own room and would find any small demands put on her very overwhelming. She was highly anxious and sensitive. She tested positive for KPU and started to take zinc and B6, as well as saffron because she was having some hormonal challenges while going through puberty. Her mother emailed me a month later to say that there had been a 'humongous change' in her daughter – she seemed to control her moods better, was chatting more, having a laugh and being helpful around the house. They were no longer treading on eggshells around her!

INSUFFICIENT CHOLESTEROL

While many adults are working to prevent their cholesterol levels from becoming too high due to the cardiovascular risk, persistently low cholesterol in children can greatly affect mood and brain function.[158,159] It can lead to hyperactivity, irritability, difficulty sleeping and poor social interactions.[160]

You are aiming for higher levels of HDL (high-density lipoprotein) cholesterol, which is known as 'good' cholesterol as it helps to remove the less healthy LDL (low-density lipoprotein) cholesterol from the bloodstream. HDL also has significant antioxidant and anti-inflammatory effects. Natural and minimally processed foods help to boost 'good' HDL and it is the highly processed foods that increases the 'bad' LDL.

What is less well known is that cholesterol is a key brain food, and it is used to produce vital hormones, especially testosterone and oestrogen as well as cortisol. It also helps to synthesize Vitamin D.

Low levels of cholesterol are sometimes associated with increased impulsivity, aggression and violence[161] as well as depression.[162] Behavioural problems, such as repeated self-injury, biting and head-banging are sometimes improved by normalizing cholesterol levels.[163,164]

Low cholesterol levels can be driven by a host of nutritional and metabolic factors, such as manganese deficiency, coeliac disease, hyperthyroidism, liver disease and malabsorption, as well as poor nutrition or choosing a low-fat diet. Highly selective eating can also play a role.

If your child does not regularly eat eggs or offal, and has ongoing anxiety or is prone to self-injury, consider checking cholesterol levels through a blood test. The good news is that in most cases, cholesterol levels can be raised quite quickly through eating plenty of egg yolks[165] as well as offal, which might need to be hidden in other foods such as bolognaise. Getting it right can lead to a calmer and better-regulated disposition quite fast.

THE ROLE OF ULTRA-PROCESSED FOODS

3

Our overall eating habits have changed rapidly in my lifetime, much more than in any previous generation. Today we cook less from scratch than ever before, and we've lost a lot of connection with food origins, when so much arrives conveniently in packets.

Ready-made meals and snacks are available everywhere – from supermarkets, fast-food restaurants and takeaways, canteens, petrol stations, gyms and small corner shops. With just a tap on a mobile app, we can get food conveniently delivered to our door. It's hard to ignore the mountains of crisps (potato chips), biscuits (cookies), chocolate, sports drinks, cereals and sweets (candy) that are tempting us to buy and eat them there and then. And because they are so moreish, all we need to do is rip open a packet and they are down our throat before we can blink.

It is common knowledge that people who mainly consume a diet of junk foods and packaged foods are generally not in the best of health. Populations of the most developed countries are now buying and consuming way more convenience, shop-bought foods than they should. These shifts in eating patterns are thought to be a key contributor to developed world obesity rates as well as metabolic illnesses such as type 2 diabetes and cardiovascular disease. However, what is less well known is the effect of ultra-processed foods on the brain and how we think and feel when we eat too much of it.

WHAT ARE ULTRA-PROCESSED FOODS?

Most of us instinctively know that the classic junk foods, such as pizza, burgers, chips (fries), doughnuts and ice cream are not healthy options to choose all the time. In the past, healthy eating messages have all been about reducing consumption of fat, sugar and salt – and junk foods are obviously high in some or all of these. However, fat, sugar and salt may not actually be the bad guys after all.

Few people are aware of the high level of processing of ingredients in the food we buy. The latest thinking is that these processed foods, known as ultra-processed foods (UPFs),[166] contain artificial ingredients that may be far worse than natural fat, sugar or salt. After all, there are foods that contain lots of fat like avocados and nuts, there is natural sugar in fruit, honey and milk, and foods like olives, anchovies and capers are cured in salt, yet all of these foods are healthy for us and our brains.

Ultra-processed foods[167] are those items that have been manufactured by food corporations using ingredients and methods that we could never mimic in our own homes. These are often ready-to-eat foods, drinks and snacks with extensive lists of ingredients that might not be instantly recognizable as food. They include emulsifiers, artificial sweeteners, preservatives, flavourings, acidity regulators and food extracts, which are frequently found on the labels of most pre-packaged foods.

Even some of our basic foods can now contain a whole host of ingredients that are not found in a domestic kitchen, and many have undergone industrial processes to make them more palatable but not necessarily that healthy. These foods include staples such as bread and yoghurt. And I find that foods containing these ultra-processed ingredients seem to affect kids and teens who have highly sensitive brains, more than the general population.

The creation of these ready-made food products involves sophisticated machinery and technology to enable, for instance soybeans to be transformed into soy milk, vegetable oils into margarine, or grains to be puffed up into manufactured breakfast cereals.

Vegetable oils often undergo refinement, with bleaching, deodorizing and hydrogenation so they do not affect the taste of the food item they are added to and they can be used to firm up the texture. Maize and soya proteins are also often hydrolysed, making them more palatable and easier to blend in with other foods. The starches derived from these foods are often modified, which can increase their 'blissy' sweet and soft appeal, which can affect blood glucose when consumed in high amounts.

Compare these 'refining' processes with more traditional practices like blending, pickling, drying and smoking foods, which have been used for centuries, and are techniques that we still use in home kitchens and that continue to be good ways to prepare and store food.

UPFs create highly profitable products for the manufacturer – food that is cheap to produce with a long shelf life, ready to consume and highly palatable. This movement towards ultra-processing is also partly driven by consumer demands for the 'perfect' crunch, mouth feel or taste as well as needing to comply with the ongoing lobbying for a reduction in fat, refined sugar and salt.

UPFs are typically high in calories in the form of modified starches, unhealthy fats and artificial additives, and low in fibre, protein, omega-3, choline, vitamins and minerals – the important nutrients that fuel the brain and mood. Eating these refined ingredients can cause spikes in blood sugar levels, which can lead to type 2 diabetes in the long term and also pose a higher risk for cardiovascular disease.[168]

Overconsumption of UPFs can also lead to mood swings, even feelings of anxiety and depression.[169] Over time, the consistent consumption of such nutritionally poor foods can alter brain development[170] and cognitive performance.[171] These ingredients can also be highly addictive and this can lead to a vicious cycle of overeating and unhealthy dietary habits such as binge eating.[172]

Clearly, this relatively new way of eating is affecting us all in many ways; and because more of our food is packaged and less cooked from scratch, our daily nutrient intake has suffered and so have our children's brains.

Not every food that you buy in a supermarket or local store is ultra-processed, and obviously some foods have undergone a greater complexity of ultra-processing than others.

Ideally, less than 20 per cent of our children's calories would come from ultra-processed food, but the reality is that these days for many kids that figure can be much higher. For an average British toddler almost two-thirds of their diet is thought to be made up of UPFs; for primary-school-age kids this is more like 75 per cent and for secondary school children as much as 83 per cent.[173] The figures are equally high in the US[174] as well as in many other modern countries.

If you can aim to feed your tribe 80 per cent cooked from scratch and 20 per cent ultra-processed, you will probably be getting a good nutritional balance. But switching from UPFs to home-cooked meals can initially be very hard and overwhelming. To make it much easier for you to make this positive change I have included lots of delicious recipes for your family to enjoy in this book. I have kept the preparation simple and there is no need for special cooking equipment.

CATEGORIES OF PROCESSING

The first three categories are healthy and should comprise 80 per cent of the diet:

▸ **Unprocessed and minimally processed foods:** these foods are eaten whole or have had less processing such as chilling, slicing, grating (shredding) and packaging. Examples include fresh meat, poultry, fish, seafood, eggs, fruits, salads and vegetables, unsalted nuts and seeds, pulses, wholegrains and unpasteurized milk.

▸ **Processed culinary ingredients:** these foods undergo a bit more processing, which can include drying, freezing, pasteurizing, gas- and vacuum-packing, bottling, fat-reduction and fermentation. Examples of these are frozen fruits and vegetables, dried beans and fruits, unsweetened fruit juices, pasteurized milk, coffee, plain yoghurt and kefir.

▸ **Processed foods:** these are ingredients that originally come from plants, animals or fungi, which are then milled, pressed, ground, stabilized or purified for use in cooking or baking. They include flour, cooking oils, butter, cream, sugar or nut butters. The category also includes preserving techniques, such as poaching, salting, pickling, smoking and curing. Examples include fruits preserved in syrups, canned fish in brine, ham, salami and cheese.

▸ **Ultra-processed foods:** these products are created with few wholefood ingredients and a high number of additives, including artificial flavours, colours and sweeteners, emulsifiers and preservatives, or industrial processes to alter the texture or shape of the product. Ultra-processed products can be fortified with vitamins and minerals and are designed to be ready-to-eat versions of wholefood items. Examples are breakfast cereals, grain snack bars, hot dogs, low-fat yoghurts, plant-based cheese and milks, biscuits (cookies) and crackers, crisps (potato chips), sweets (candy), fizzy drinks and ready-made condiments and sauces.

WHY UPFs CAUSE NUTRITIONAL PROBLEMS

There are numerous reasons why ultra-processed foods are not doing us any favours. Here are a few of the principal ones:

DISPLACEMENT OF KEY NUTRIENTS

Food-processing can strip out the fibre and nutrients from the original wholefood ingredients such as omega-3, vitamin B1, iron, selenium and zinc.[175] This displacement, from nutritious food to processed food, can result in a deficit of these essential brain-boosting nutrients in the diet, potentially affecting mental health and overall wellbeing. And, because ready-made foods are convenient and easy to consume, kids may end up eating smaller quantities of other foods that naturally contain more of these nutrients. The UK government has put in place laws so that refined grains are fortified with Vitamin B1, but to date there is nothing formally set in stone for the other essential fatty acids, vitamins and minerals that can disappear when processed.

A SUGAR ROLLER COASTER

Ultra-processed foods are usually loaded with sugars and starches. This high sugar and starch content can cause problems with a child's blood glucose levels and is associated with increased inflammation as well as a higher likelihood of gaining too much weight or type 2 diabetes.[176] Less reliance on processed foods and cooking from scratch more often will help to prevent the development of metabolic health problems in children.[177]

If you check the labels on most UPFs, you'll often find starches (maize, rice and potato starch, modified starches or flours) as well as several types of sugar among the main ingredients, which means the bulk of the product is made from them. Many times, the names of these sugars end in '-ose', like glucose, fructose or dextrose so you may not always realise they are sugars.

Because UPFs are so high in carbohydrates and often low in protein and healthy fats, they can cause a child's blood sugars to go on a bit of a roller-coaster ride. After eating these foods, their blood sugar levels can spike rapidly, giving them a quick burst of energy. But then they crash back down, leaving them feeling tired and sluggish and even 'hangry' for more.

EXCESSIVE GLUTAMATE

Ultra-processed foods can also over-produce a neurotransmitter called glutamate which can overstimulate our kids' brains (see chapter 2). When brain pathways stimulated by glutamate become too active, problems ensue, for instance difficulty sleeping, oppositional behaviours (defying rules or authority), lack of fear or increased risky behaviours, such as running across the street or climbing on the roof. And also getting stuck in a loop of repetitive thoughts and even OCD.

SNACK ADDICTION

Ultra-processed foods are often extremely tasty and addictive,[178] affecting the reward pathways in our brains. They are specifically designed to be delicious and hard to resist – one reason why we can become so hooked on them.

When we eat a cookie or a packet of crisps (potato chips), for example, the brain releases dopamine, the chemical that makes them feel good. This is the brain's reward system and it's why we want to repeat the behaviour that led to the reward.[179] ADHDers often have a tendency to consume and crave more snacks and ultra-processed foods because they are seeking this dopamine hit, which, sadly, is usually very short-lived, and so the behaviour is repeated over and over again. We've all been there and and wolfed a whole family pack of crisps (potato chips) at a sitting; but this is a problem when it's the norm.

HOW ULTRA-PROCESSED FOODS SPECIFICALLY AFFECT THE BRAIN

Are UPFs affecting how our kids develop, think and feel? It's only relatively recently that scientists have become aware that these foods are also affecting general intellectual and mental health just as much as physical health. There is also emerging evidence that UPFs are affecting children's neurodevelopment,[180] IQ and academic achievement[181,182] as well as their mental health.

SPEECH AND LANGUAGE

It seems that ultra-processed food may play a role in how a child develops speech, language and communication skills. The research is still in its infancy, and so far, it has mostly been carried out by observing the eating patterns of pregnant women; and then their offspring are tracked for several years to record their development. The purpose of these studies was not to make mums feel guilty about what they ate when they were pregnant, they are conducted because scientists are interested in any changes that could occur during pregnancy and the early years.

These studies have found that women who consume the most UPFs during pregnancy often find that their child struggles with their neurodevelopment[183] and verbal communication, such as slower speech and language development in early childhood.[184] They may not eat enough zinc and protein which has also been associated with developmental delay in children.[185] This could also be due to the pro-inflammatory nature of these foods (see chapter 5 to learn more).[186]

DEVELOPMENTAL DELAY

Research has gone so far as to suggest that the rise in UPF consumption and findings of heavy metals in baby food may in part explain why developmental delays and demands for specialist education provision are both rising. This takes into consideration factors over and above what can be accounted for through genetics and better diagnosis and awareness. Obviously, this is a complex and potentially emotive subject, and many reasons are being considered for why the number of autistic children who also have special educational needs in the UK has almost tripled, developmental

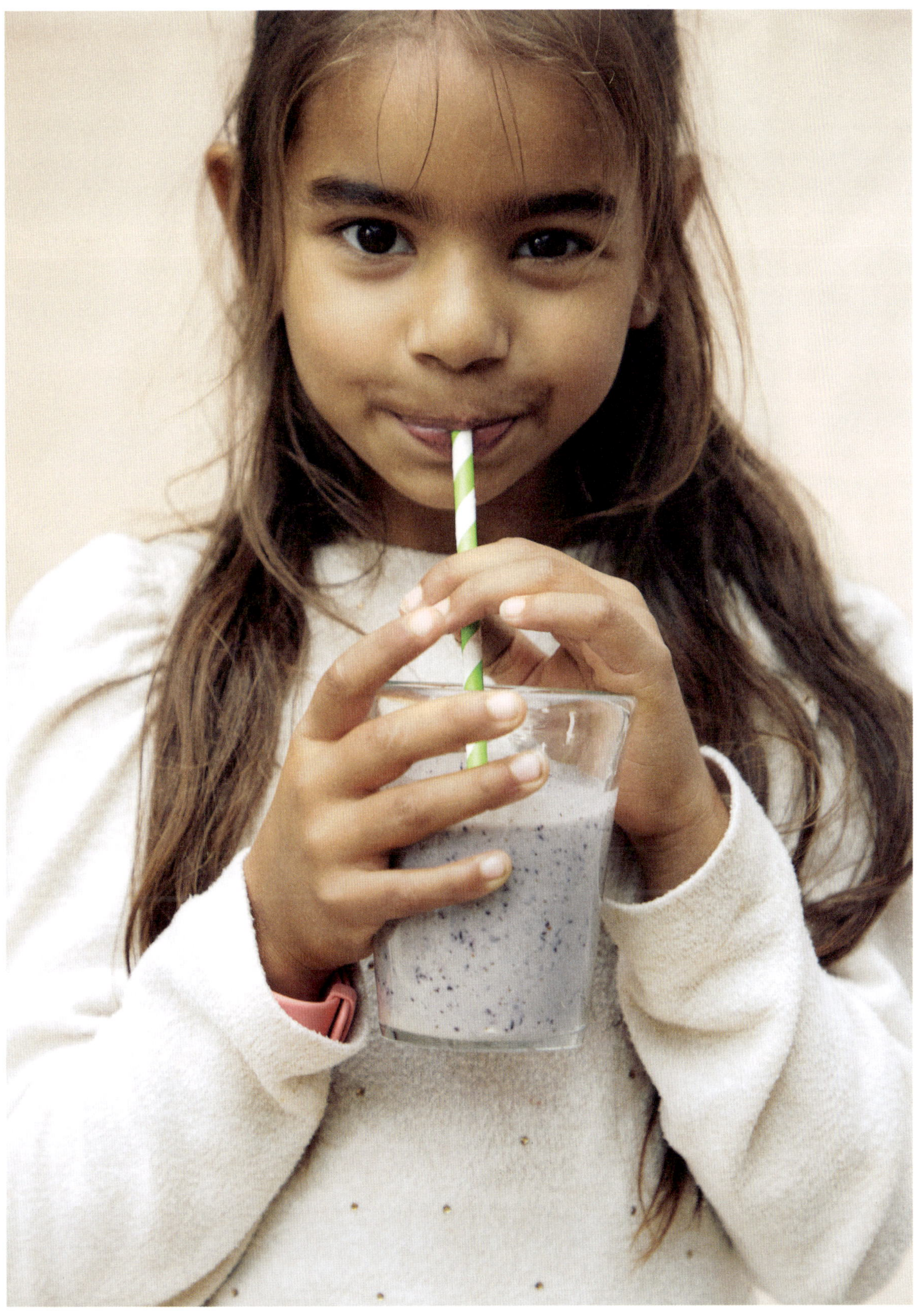

delay has quadrupled, and ADHD has risen from 10 to 16 per cent over the past 20 years.[187] The numbers are also climbing rapidly in the US, where about 1 in 6 (17 per cent) children aged 3–17 years are diagnosed with a developmental delay.[188]

Mercury, lead, arsenic and cadmium are now very prevalent in our food chain. It is hard to avoid them entirely as, sadly, they are found in much of our soil and thus contaminate some fruits and vegetables, even if they are organic. Simple changes to daily habits, such as washing and peeling fruits and vegetables, can help to reduce exposure.

LOCOMOTOR SKILLS

As well as affecting speech and communication, an over-consumption of UPFs during the early years may also affect the way a child develops important locomotor skills, such as learning to hop, skip and jump as well as throwing and catching a ball, which are key for coordination and learning.[189] They need to develop balance, hand-eye coordination and agility skills as well as physical fitness. Without these core locomotor skills, a child may well go on to receive a diagnosis of Dyspraxia or Developmental Coordination Disorder later in childhood. However, they can be helped by supporting the maturation of primitive reflexes (see right) as well as occupational therapy. Locomotor skills also help the brain to develop neural connections which, over time can help with further executive function and focus.

HYPERACTIVITY AND IMPULSIVITY

Eating a lot of processed foods and fizzy drinks or having a 'junk-food' diet is well known to cause children's blood sugar levels to rise and fall sharply. These swings can make them hyperactive at times, and lethargic at others, and can exacerbate impulsivity. One study found that children who ate more processed foods lacking in key brain nutrients by the age of 4 were more likely to be hyperactive aged 7.[190] If you have an ADHD child, you will know all too well that these foods can make them wired and struggle to focus.[191,192,193] The connection between early-years nutrition and child behaviour is now quite clear: kids whose diet lacks essential vitamins, minerals and omega-3, and instead is abundant in UPFs may be more likely to have conduct problems such as fighting, lying or stealing later on in childhood, and greater emotional difficulties as adolescents.[194,195,196]

INSOMNIA

Some research shows that if you eat a lot of UPFs, it could your sleep. Specifically, it could change how long you sleep as well as the quality, and this seems to be true for all age groups. Sleep challenges seem to be a real problem for many neurodivergent kids, and cutting back on the consumption of UPFs may

WHAT ARE RETAINED PRIMITIVE REFLEXES?

Retained primitive reflexes are baby movements that stick with the child longer than usual, affecting how they learn to move, balance, and react to the world around them.

An example is the Moro reflex, also known as the startle reflex. It is an involuntary response in babies where they suddenly extend their arms and legs, arch their back, and sometimes cry when they feel like they are falling or are startled by a loud noise or sudden movement. This reflex is a normal part of infant development and usually disappears around 4 to 6 months of age. A persistent or retained Moro reflex can interfere with a child's motor development, balance, coordination, and even sleep patterns, potentially leading to challenges in later life such as difficulty in focusing, heightened sensitivity to stimuli, and poor impulse control.

There are a number of clinics who now specialize in therapies to help mature these retained primitive reflexes.

make a difference – especially around the evening meal or snacks before bed.[197,198,199]

MENTAL HEALTH

An over-consumption of UPFs is now thought to be closely linked to psychological and social challenges in teenagers and young adults. Psychological issues might include mental health problems such as depression and anxiety,[200] or personality disorders, which can affect emotional stability and mental wellbeing. Eating too many UPFs might also make it difficult for someone to think clearly, manage their feelings, make decisions, or cope with stress.

Researchers from different countries have observed that regularly consuming lots of UPFs is associated with significant depression[201,202] and psychological distress up to fifteen years later.[203] So the effects of UPF on children and teenagers are not just short-term but can affect their mood and mental health many years on. This is why more education on the link between eating healthy food and mood is essential. Imagine the positive difference in overall mental health if all school children learned to cook from scratch? Prioritizing a healthier diet might mean a better trajectory for everyone.[204,205]

HOW TO CUT BACK ON EATING ULTRA-PROCESSED FOODS

Here are my top easy tips to reduce the amount of UPFs your child eats – take one step at a time and before you know it you will all be eating much more home-cooked nutritious food:

- Prioritize cooking from scratch – the more you cook food yourself the more likely you will be making more nutritious choices for your family. Aim for one new recipe a week.

- Read the label and buy foods containing fewer than one or two UPF ingredients – these will be names you don't recognize as food, and you wouldn't normally find in a domestic kitchen.

- Avoid emulsifiers, acidity regulators, artificial sugars, food dyes and preservatives where possible.

- Try to feed your child a protein-rich breakfast. This keeps them fuller for longer, so they are less likely to snack on UPFs between meals.

- Send them to school with a home-made packed lunch if possible.

- Pack them enough snacks and enough food for school if the lunch options are likely to be UPFs.

- Ideally make or assemble snacks yourself. This will save some money too.

- Switch from energy drinks to fizzy water or filtered water to reduce their intake of sugar, artificial sugars, preservatives and caffeine.

- Think ahead – plan to fill their tummies up before your kids go out to a party or event, so they don't end up bingeing on the sugary junk.

- Start to make a connection between the foods your child eats and their mood – identify those that buoy up their mood, brain and energy and others that make them low, foggy and tired. This will help you all make more positive choices over time.

4 THE SECOND BRAIN IN YOUR GUT

We all have billions of bacteria, yeasts and other micro-organisms living in our gut, which together form a delicate ecosystem known as our gut microbiome. This complex 'soup' of different microbes within our intestines is essential to life and is now recognized as of primary importance for overall physical, mental, emotional and neurological health and wellbeing. It has a huge influence on our mood, behaviour, how we think and interact with the world around us and not least our children.[206]

There is increasing research linking the health and diversity of the gut microbiome with how the brain operates[207] – termed the gut–brain axis.[208] From ADHD[209] to Autism[210] as well as depression and anxiety,[211,212,213] a growing body of evidence shows that the balance of microbes in the gut may amplify how these conditions affect individual people.[214]

Beneficial gut bacteria help to create the building blocks for the production of our brain neurotransmitters:[215] approximately 95 per cent of serotonin, for instance, is manufactured in the gut.[216] And these neurotransmitters help our brain cells to transmit signals between each other. As well as serotonin, the gut also makes GABA, acetylcholine, dopamine and norepinephrine, all of which help our kids access learning and development as well as regulate their mood, sleep and behaviour patterns. This goes some way to explain why our gut has been dubbed our 'second brain'.

There is a long wandering nerve linking our brain and our gut called the vagus nerve – see this as a super-highway sending signals up and down. This bi-directional communication may well be responsible for what is known as the gut–brain axis.[217,218] Around 10–20 per cent of these signals send messages from the brain to the gut to control the muscles responsible for creating gastric juices and moving food through the gut. However, most of these signals (80–90 per cent) pass sensory information from our stomach and gut microbiome to the brain via the vagus nerve.[219] Since our gut bacteria make neurotransmitters, which are so important for mood regulation, cognition and learning (see chapter 9),[220,221,222] it is thought that these can also reach the brain via the vagus nerve. So it seems that what goes on inside the belly is of huge influence on the brain and it needs to be nourished on a daily basis.

GOOD GUT BACTERIA VS THE BAD GUYS

Certain strains of gut bacteria can help reduce inflammation and promote a healthy gut–brain axis. For example, *Bifidobacterium* and *Lactobacillus* strains have been shown to have anti-inflammatory effects and can help regulate the immune response in the gut. These strains have also been associated with improved mood and reduced symptoms of anxiety and depression.[223]

Abundance of unwanted bacterial strains, such as *Clostridium*,[224] which has been linked to inflammation, have been found to be more prevalent in people

PREBIOTICS VS PROBIOTICS

Probiotics are beneficial live bacteria typically found in cultured and fermented foods such as live yoghurt, kefir, pickles, apple cider vinegar, miso, sauerkraut, and kimchi as well as in supplements. They are essential for maintaining healthy gut flora and aiding in digestion and immunity. They dial down inflammation, and some strains can help to make B vitamins, which are also the building blocks for neurotransmitters and positive mental health.

Prebiotics are dietary fibres that nourish and feed these good bacteria. Found in foods such as garlic, onions, chicory and bananas, they help probiotic bacteria to thrive and improve gut health.

Together, probiotics and prebiotics synergistically support a balanced microbiome in your gut.

with mood disorders and neurodiversity.[225,226] These bacteria can produce neurotoxins, which can affect the brain, and other harmful by-products, which contribute to inflammation of and damage to the gut lining. See these as the 'bad guys' that need crowding out by the 'good' bacteria. This is why building up beneficial bacterial diversity in the gut through eating a healthy diet really counts!

It's important to understand that your gut usually has a mix of many different types of good and bad bacteria. When bad strains become dominant, problems can occur; but also, you want diversity among the good strains for optimal gut health.

Specific strains of good gut bacteria that provide the building blocks for neurotransmitter production include:[227,228,229,230]

- *Lactobacillus* helps make acetylcholine and GABA.
- *Bifidobacterium* helps make GABA.
- *Escherichia* helps make norepinephrine, serotonin and dopamine.
- *Streptococcus* and *Enterococcus* help make serotonin.
- *Bacillus* helps make norepinephrine and dopamine.

THE EFFECT OF THE GUT ON CHILD DEVELOPMENT AND BEYOND

How a baby is born and fed in their early months can be critical for developing a healthy and diverse gut microbiome. Babies born vaginally and/or who are breastfed might get a head start in building a varied microbiome early in life over those who are born via caesarean section and bottle-fed. This is because the mother's own microbiome is transferred to her child via the birth canal and breast milk.[231]

Studies also suggest that a child's gut microbes might have a big influence on their personality, temperament and brain development.[232,233,234] It is thought that toddlers who find it hard to handle their mood may have imbalances of bacteria in their gut microbiome.[235] For instance, a baby with a more diverse gut microbiome including an abundance of *Bifidobacterium* tends to be calmer, cuddlier and will probably soothe more easily – and usually smiles and laughs more.[236]

One explanation could be that *Bifidobacterium* might help shape the nerve connections in a baby's brain as it produces and regulates GABA, the relaxing neurotransmitter. This vital gut microbe also protects from significant infection[237] and antibiotic-resistant bacteria[238] as well as inflammation,[239,240] which can pose a risk for child development. Overall levels of *Bifidobacterium* in the gut have reduced significantly and today's breast-fed babies have less in their gut than bottle-fed babies a century ago, which could have far-reaching implications.[241,242]

Interestingly the diversity of the bacteria in the gut microbiome can also affect sociability in teens and young adults; people with larger social networks tend to have a more diverse microbiome, whereas social anxiety and stress are linked to reduced diversity and less healthy microbiome composition.[243] It can be hard to get one's head around the idea that a thriving and diverse community of microbes within the gut can influence how a child develops friendships and social skills!

Many other factors can shape the microbiome in a child's early years. For instance, the use of antibiotics for bacterial infections[244] and proton pump inhibitors[245] for reflux can negatively affect a healthy gut microbiome.

Changes in a child's digestion and bowel habits, such as yellow 'ochre' coloured poo beyond the age of 6 months old or seeing undigested food in their poo, may indicate maldigestion or malabsorption, which can easily lead to nutrient deficiencies and may be due to a disrupted gut microbiome. Frequent gastric or viral infections could also mean that their microbiome needs extra care, as the gut is also an important part of our immune system.

HOW TO SUPPORT THE GUT MICROBIOME

▸ Serve up plenty of wholefoods: fruits, veggies, nuts, seeds, pulses and wholegrains.

▸ Avoid processed foods, such as white flour and refined sugars where possible.

▸ Make sure your home is well aired – open those windows and let the microbes in!

▸ Get your kids outside into the fresh air and encourage outdoor play.

▸ Excite them with a 'rainbow' of fruits and veggies every day. Be creative with things like smoothies and ice lollies, or get smart at hiding nutrition in treats like muffins and pancakes.

▸ Vitamin D and omega-3 can support a healthy microbiome, so try to include these in their diet as food via organic whole milk, oily fish or supplements – and through exposure to sunshine.

▸ Introduce a variety of foods as early as possible to develop their acceptance of different foods.

▸ Consider adding cultured and fermented foods to their diet like live yoghurt, kefir, apple cider vinegar and miso.

▸ If your child was born prematurely or by C-section, or received antibiotics in the first six months, you might want to consider a *Bifidobacterium*-based probiotic supplement.

▸ If you or your child is dairy-free or chooses not to eat many dairy products, consider topping up with a *Lactobacillus*-based probiotic, which can be grown on a dairy-free medium.

It's never too late to improve your child's eating habits. The gut microbiome can be nurtured and reset at any age, which can potentially influence mood, learning, behaviour and overall development. Your child's brain keeps developing into their mid-twenties and, thankfully, is still malleable and 'neuroplastic' throughout their lifetime. But that said, the sooner you start, the easier it will be and they may catch up sooner.

Importantly, our child's gut microbiome is an ever-changing and evolving ecosystem that we can influence and improve by making changes to diet, stress management, and by spending more time in nature. Over time, it is possible to build a healthier and more diverse microbiome. Small changes can make a big difference over the long term.

THE MYCOBIOME – THE YEAST BEAST!

As well as bacteria in the gut, yeast overgrowth can be one of the key challenges for neurodivergent children, and, once you understand the dynamics of the 'yeast beast' and how yeast in the gut can affect behaviour, cognition, learning, energy and mood, you will probably spot this in other kids. It is quite a bit to get your head around but do read to the end of this section to get a full understanding of the implications and how to keep the beast in check.

The mycobiome or mycobiota is a community of fungal and yeast microorganisms that normally live in harmony with the gut microbiome in the digestive tract – but it can get out of balance very easily. Like bacteria, the composition and number of yeast and fungal species can vary enormously. Research has identified at least 200 distinct fungal species that can be living in our bellies.

Candida albicans is the most prevalent and extensively studied type of yeast found in the gut, while other common yeasts include *Geotrichum*,

THE DAIRY-FREE–ANTIBIOTIC–NEURODIVERSITY CYCLE

Lactobacillus is a key building block for creating enough acetylcholine, which helps with working memory, executive function, self-regulation and emotional regulation. It is also important for making GABA, which helps us to stay calm, emotionally regulated and sleep well.

So it seems obvious that parents would want abundant levels of *Lactobacilli* in their child's gut if they are to develop without too many worries, behavioural challenges or learning difficulties. However, gut microbiome tests find it is quite scarce these days. Here is a typical scenario I see all the time, which goes a long way to explain why so many people are low in *Lactobacillus*:

▸ The baby was born by C-section, so did not benefit from their mother's natural flora from the birth canal.

▸ The baby was exposed to antibiotics within the womb or shortly after birth, which will have reduced any *Lactobacilli* that had been populated in the gut by that point.

▸ One of the key roles of *Lactobacillus* is to digest milk products. Kids depleted in *Lactobacillus* often show strong signs of cow's milk allergy or intolerance. Often, the advice is to go dairy-free, which in the short term can help them feel more comfortable and may make a difference to their immunity at that point in time.

▸ However, a dairy-free diet will most likely be devoid of *Lactobacillus*, and without finding an alternative source of this strain it is much harder to populate in the gut and, consequently, far harder to create the neurotransmitters acetylcholine and GABA.

▸ The infant then experiences persistent ear, nose and throat infections, such as tonsillitis or *otitis media* (middle ear infection), and may be given repeat courses of antibiotics, each time further lowering the levels of *Lactobacillus*.

▸ Fast-forward a few years and the child shows all the symptoms of low acetylcholine and GABA – anxious, overwhelmed, disorganized and struggling with working memory and cognitive processing.

Explaining this vicious cycle to parents helps them to understand why their child may be finding regulating their mood or learning a challenge. The great news is that, over time, those *Lactobacillus* levels can be rebuilt. There are now dairy-free probiotic yoghurts and water kefir, and most live bacteria probiotic supplements will contain *Lactobacillus* strains. And the upside is that the added *Lactobacillus* might even help to rebuild dairy tolerance over time.

Penicillium and *Cladosporium*, all of which can cause havoc if they get out of control.[246]

Normally, these yeast organisms are well controlled by the naturally occurring yeasts, prebiotics and probiotics in the gut, but sometimes these overgrow and can cause problems systemically.

Antibiotics can create the ideal conditions in the gut for yeast to replicate and can lead to thrush.[247] Children with a compromised immune system or an autoimmune tendency may create the perfect environment for *Candida* to thrive.[248,249] Some children have limited ability to digest carbohydrate in the gut, which can lead to fermentation of the partially digested sugars and yeast. What's more, some autistic people,[250,251,252] those with ADHD,[253,254] as well as others who struggle with their mental health can be particularly sensitive to the effects of yeast overgrowth.

Yeast overgrowth can be detected both in stool tests and urinary organic acid tests. A medical doctor can do basic swabs for fungal infections on the skin, ears and mouth as well as genital areas. So, it is good to test your child if you are unsure. But here are some common physical symptoms that may well mean yeast overgrowth is part of the picture:

► White tongue: a thick, white coating on the tongue, often accompanied by bad breath.

► Skin rashes and vaginal infections: yeast overgrowth can cause athlete's foot and ringworm as well as vaginal thrush and nappy rash.

► Bloating and gas: excess yeast can disrupt the balance of gut bacteria, leading to digestive discomfort, gas and bloating. Sometimes there is associated gut pain.

► Itchy skin: a common symptom of yeast overgrowth is persistent itchiness and irritation of the skin, usually without a rash.

YEAST OVERGROWTH AND AUTO-BREWERY SYNDROME

An overgrowth of *Candida albicans* and other yeast infections in the mouth and the gut can cause a condition called Auto-Brewery Syndrome (ABS),[255,256] which can affect both adults and children. Yeast overgrowth ferments carbohydrates in the digestive system, producing ethanol (alcohol) as a by-product, which enters the bloodstream causing symptoms similar to alcohol intoxication:[257] a low-grade feeling like a hangover – mildly nauseous, brain fog and yo-yo energy levels.

THE EFFECT OF YEAST OVERGROWTH ON NEURODIVERGENT CHILDREN

Yeast overgrowth presents with disparate symptoms in children and sometimes it is hard to join up the dots and associate them with the same cause.[258,259] This is because *Candida albicans* and other yeast infections and the ethanol they produce can affect the central nervous system.[260] These infections can also cross the blood-brain barrier (see page 51)[261] and disrupt the brain's 'housekeeper cells', the microglia[262] that help to mop up inflammation as well as infections. When the blood-brain barrier is compromised and the microglia are put under pressure, brain function can be affected and may be associated with a wide range of behavioural and neurological symptoms.

High levels of ethanol produced by the yeast overgrowth can often exacerbate some of the existing symptoms of kids with neurological differences. Parents report that symptoms are usually more pronounced shortly after a child has been on a course of antibiotics or when they eat lots of sugar and white carbs, because both antibiotics and sugar can exacerbate an existing low-grade yeast infection. These symptoms include:

► Laughing or giggling out of context: this can seem quite cute! However, ethanol emitted by yeast overgrowth can induce sudden, uncontrollable laughter at random times, perhaps in the middle of the night or out of the blue during the day.

► Brain fog: the effects of ethanol on cognitive function can lead to difficulty concentrating, memory issues and confusion.

► Poor sugar balancing: yeast overgrowth can disrupt the body's ability to regulate blood sugar levels, leading to fluctuations and related symptoms, including sugar cravings.

▶ Mood swings: the effect of ethanol on neurotransmitter levels can cause rapid shifts in mood and emotional instability.

▶ Sleep disturbance and bed-wetting: ethanol is well known for disrupting sleep and increasing the need for urination in the middle of the night.

▶ Hyperactivity and climbing/jumping off things: ethanol can bring on hyperactive behaviour and give a short-term dopamine surge.

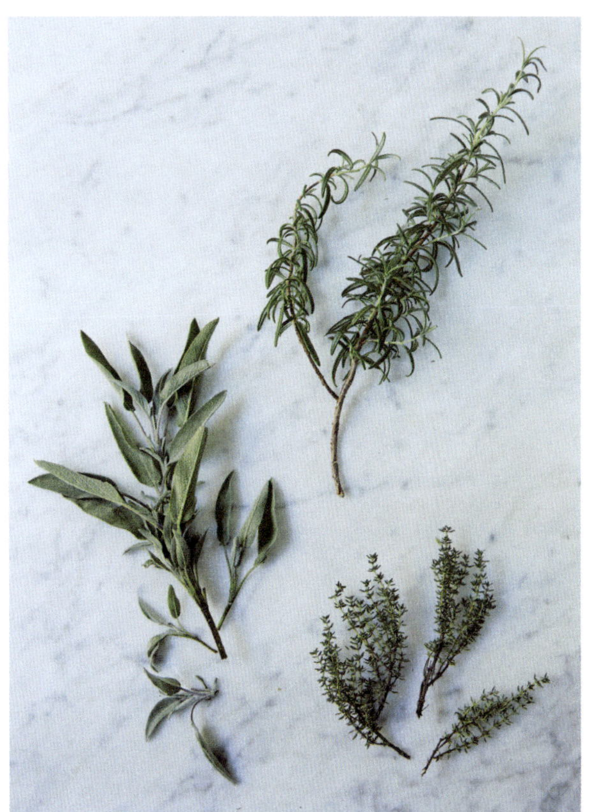

MANAGING YEAST OVERGROWTH

To combat yeast overgrowth and minimize its effects on sensitive kids, here are my top tips:

1 Adopt a low-sugar diet. Reducing the intake of white sugar and refined carbohydrates can help starve the yeast and prevent overgrowth. Your child does not need to stop eating fruit, as the natural fructose may help to inhibit *Candida* growth.[263]

2 Introduce beneficial bacteria through diet or supplements. This could be simply a few spoons of live yoghurt or kefir daily. Probiotics can help restore the balance of gut flora and inhibit yeast growth. Include strains of good yeasts and live bacteria such as *Saccharomyces Boulardii*, *Lactobacillus* and *Bifidobacterium*.[264]

3 Identify if your child has a zinc,[265,266] biotin,[267] or selenium[268,269] deficiency. These three nutrients are important in the control of yeast levels.

4 Incorporate herbal antimicrobial agents. Natural antimicrobials are found in food ingredients, such as garlic, cinnamon, thyme and coconut, and many others can be bought as concentrated herbal extracts, teas and capsules to help control yeast overgrowth.[270,271,272] Diet-wise, introduce garlicky pesto, salsa verde made from fresh herbs, and add ground cinnamon to porridge, pancakes and muffins.

5 Introduce milk protein supplements for those who can tolerate dairy products. The supplements colostrum[273] and lactoferrin[274,275] can help with *Candida* infections.

5 CHRONIC INFLAMMATION & ITS EFFECTS ON THE BRAIN

Have you ever noticed how a sudden physical pain, such as a nasty burn or a twisted ankle, can drag your mood down, leaving you feeling exhausted and withdrawn? And, when the pain lifts, so do your energy levels and your spirits? This connection isn't just anecdotal: there is a scientific explanation which links our physical and mental states and it's called inflammation.[276] This can affect your children too.

When anyone injures themselves the body's response is to inflame the injured area. This is called acute inflammation, and it's a normal part of the healing process. We recognize acute inflammation by its redness, heat and swelling, symptoms that subside once the injury starts to heal.

However, when we experience continuous mini injuries or damage to our cells, the body keeps responding by releasing small proteins called cytokines to try and control inflammation. Repeatedly releasing cytokines can cause chronic inflammation, autoimmunity and lead to numerous different physical, mental and neurological changes in the body.[277] These health knocks can be the result of poor dietary, lifestyle and environmental choices, for example inadequate nutrition, dehydration, stress, lack of sleep, infections, pollution, exposure to allergens or a high histamine state.

Infections are a major driver of inflammation and while the body is recuperating from an infection, there will be some degree of active inflammation and cell damage, known as oxidative stress. It can take weeks to fully recover from some infections and, as we have learned from the Covid 19 virus, a cytokine storm can lead to oxidative stress manifesting as prolonged symptoms collectively termed 'Long Covid'.

Usually, we associate inflammation with pain or conditions like arthritis or fibromyalgia, but it's also believed that medical conditions, such as type 1 and type 2 diabetes,[278] obesity, heart disease,[279,280,281] asthma[282] and eczema[283] are also connected to chronic inflammation.

These conditions affect lots of children these days, but signs of inflammation can be more subtle. Before the more significant health challenges kick in, look out for long-term persistent but relatively low-grade inflammatory symptoms such as: fatigue, brain fog, difficulty concentrating, aches and pains, increased belly fat, acne and skin rashes, wheezing and digestive problems such as a persistent tummy ache. These are little niggles that many children experience, including neurodivergent kids.

HOW CAN CHRONIC INFLAMMATION AFFECT THE BRAIN?

Traditionally, the medical world viewed the brain and body as entirely separate entities, divided by the supposedly impenetrable 'Berlin Wall' of the blood-brain barrier. Therefore, physical and mental illnesses have always been treated independently – medical doctors for physical health, psychiatrists for mental health and neurodivergence. However, disciplines such as neurology and immunology have important crossovers between the two. Research now suggests that inflammation can affect both the body and the brain, and that the permeability of the blood-brain barrier can be compromised by chronic inflammation, leading to mood and neurological changes.

The interplay between inflammation, the brain, the immune system and the neurological system could explain why people with long-term disabilities are more prone to mood disorders and why so many with mental illness also suffer with chronic pain or an inflammatory-related illness. If chronic inflammation isn't kept in check and rebalanced with a healthy lifestyle, it can become a ticking time bomb, resulting in a plethora of issues including chronic fatigue, depression, OCD and anxiety.[284,285]

A growing number of psychiatrists from around the world believe there is a significant bi-directional connection between chronic inflammation and depression.[286,287] Research suggests that for some people, depression may be caused by underlying chronic inflammation and immune dysregulation,[288] rather than a problem with serotonin regulation. This could be a game-changer for those kids and teens who don't respond to traditional antidepressants that work on the serotonin pathways.[289]

One large-scale study carried out in the UK found that the inflammatory markers serum interleukin 6 and C-reactive protein can be found raised in children as young as 9 years old. Even if they seem perfectly happy, healthy kids at this stage and show no signs of mental illness, these raised markers predict a higher risk of mental health issues, including depression and psychosis in their teenage years.[290] The study highlights the importance of helping to educate our children to lead an inflammation-free life by instilling positive dietary and lifestyle habits from the start.

Inflammation can affect the brain, leading to brain fog, which is reduced cognition with the inability to concentrate and multitask, as well as some loss of short- and long-term memory.[291] Long Covid is now known to be linked with chronic inflammation, and one of the hallmarks is brain fog.[292]

It is common for people with mental health issues to report inflammation-related sleep disturbance[293] and fatigue[294] during the period leading up to the appearance of their symptoms. If inflammation can be nipped in the bud, it stands to reason that mental-health challenges may not occur at all or may only be fleeting. So, this is a big reason to take nutrition and an anti-inflammatory approach seriously.

CHRONIC INFLAMMATION AND NEURODIVERGENCE

Autism and ADHD often go hand in hand with inflammation,[295,296] which may be related to a misdirected immune system.[297] Many neurodivergent kids suffer from chronic pain,[298,299] another indicator of chronic inflammation. They can also experience pain very differently from neurotypical people,[300] a phenomenon that may well be due to changes in the neurological system that can increase their pain signal, along with a less effective pain-inhibition mechanism, which alters their perception of pain. Simple routine self-care tasks such as brushing teeth, clipping nails or having a haircut can bring an overbearing feeling of pain or discomfort. Often when neurodivergent children are in any kind of pain, all other demands in their life can seem totally overwhelming and they can show signs of pathological demand avoidance.[301]

Conversely, other neurodivergent kids hardly feel pain at all, and a significant injury can go totally unnoticed. Low perception of pain can be risky, especially if a child or teen has unknowingly broken a bone, suffered a deep cut or serious burn, and potentially serious if they do not realize that they need urgent medical care.

A high proportion of the neurodivergent population are born hyperflexible, with hypermobile joints, which make them more prone to dislocations and joint pain.[302] Hypermobility can bring problems with swallowing and bowel motility, allergies, dizziness and blood pressure changes and fatigue, as well as joint pain and inflammation. Chapter 12 takes a deep dive into hypermobility and how nutrition can help to support children experiencing difficulties associated with an overly bendy body.

Neurodivergent kids often suffer from other chronic inflammatory disease states known as co-morbidities. These can include inflammatory bowel disease (IBD), such as Crohn's or ulcerative colitis,[303] and well as painful migraines and headaches.[304,305]

BRILLIANT STORY OF HOPE – INFLAMMATION

From my clinical experience I would say that inflammation is one of the key drivers of many of the challenges associated with neurodivergence. A toddler, Axel, is one of my little heroes, for whom inflammation has played a significant role. Axel's symptoms included highly selective eating and his nursery had identified difficulties with emotional regulation and social skills. He was highly sensitive to food textures and touching certain textures. It was assumed this was all behavioural. We found that not only did Axel have significant gut inflammation, he also had various inflammatory markers which suggested low-grade brain inflammation. Because his diet was so limited, I introduced omega-3 fatty acids, turmeric and a generalized anti-inflammatory approach (see right). Within a few weeks he was eating much better and tolerating more textures. He started to find his time at nursery much easier and he became more interactive with everyone.

HOW TO REDUCE INFLAMMATION

Here are the key things you can do to help reduce inflammation. Over time if you can adopt these daily dietary and lifestyle habits, they will be more likely to keep inflammation at bay. It can take time to weave these things in, and every single step counts.

- Adopt the anti-inflammatory principles of the Mediterranean diet at home as much as you can and refer to the recipes in this book, which will help tick these boxes.[306]

- Avoid ultra-processed foods (UPFs) as much as you can, as these can exacerbate inflammation.[307]

- Support the diversity of the gut microbiome by including cultured or fermented foods like kefir, yoghurt, pickled cucumbers, kimchi and sauerkraut.[308]

- Focus on omega-3 rich foods, such as oily fish, organic milk, omega-enriched eggs and walnuts, and take a supplement if it is hard to be consistent.

- Add in anti-inflammatory ingredients to your family's meals and drinks, such as turmeric, ginger, fenugreek, garlic and rosemary.[309]

- Encourage drinking plenty of filtered water: dehydration is very pro-inflammatory.

- Work on sleep quality and duration, which will help to reduce inflammation overnight.

- Spend time in nature, as plenty of fresh air can help to bolster the gut microbiome and reduce inflammatory stress.

- Take steps to help manage stress levels – try breathing techniques, yoga,[310] meditation or mindfulness.[311]

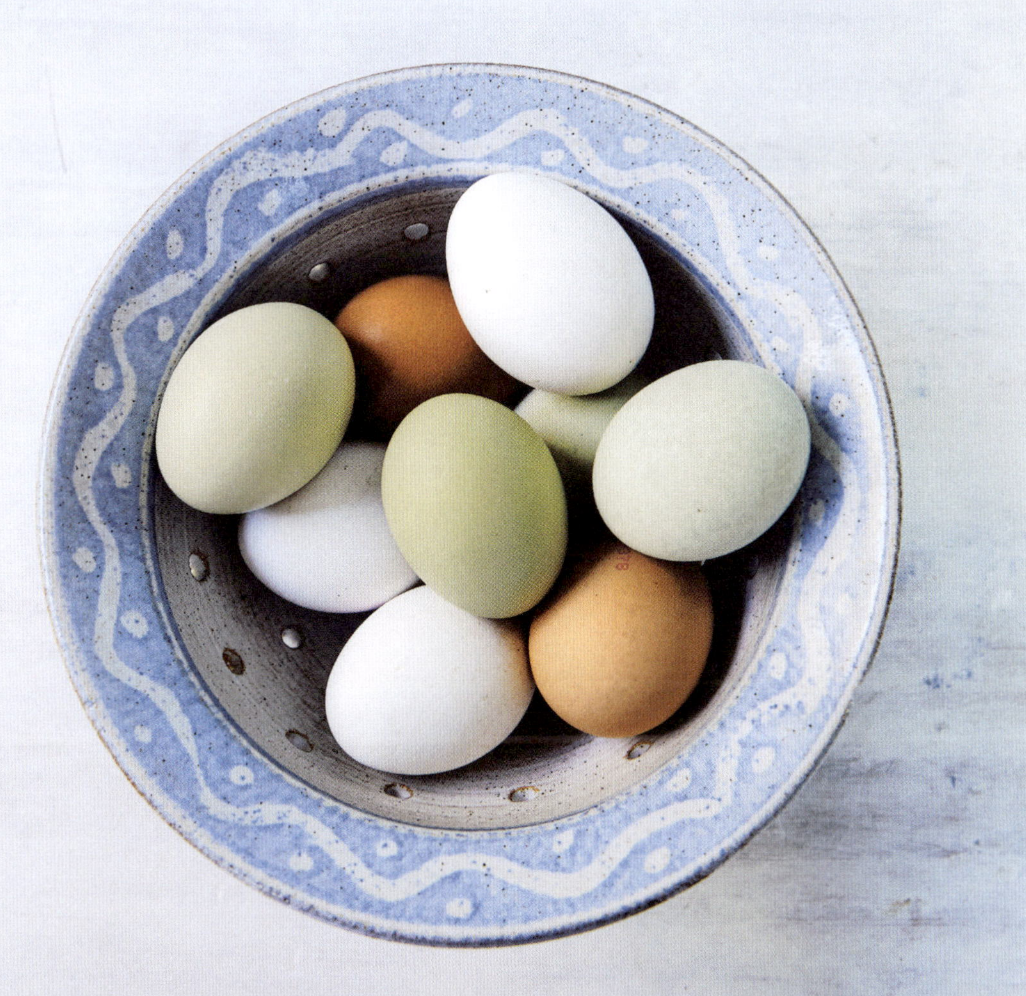

6 A HAYWIRE IMMUNE SYSTEM

The human immune system is fascinatingly complex and can influence both neurodivergence and mental health. An out-of-sync immune system not only affects physical health but also how we think and feel, and this is where the growing science of immunopsychiatry[312] is making strides into understanding why.

Our children's mental health[313] can be affected when we experience autoimmunity,[314] are in a high histamine state[315,316,317] or even suffer badly from viruses[318] or bacterial infection.[319] These autoimmune and inflammatory knocks often go hand in hand with neurodiversity and may also influence how the brain develops.[320,321,322,323]

You may recall from the last chapter those friendly cells in our brain called microglia, which act as housekeepers for the brain and central nervous system.[324] These are constantly on the lookout, scavenging for damaged cells and infections, keeping our nervous system and brain in balance, and protecting us against chronic brain inflammation. Microglia can be very sensitive to the state of the immune system and can sometimes become dysfunctional or overactive[325] in neurodivergence, resulting in less protection from neuroinflammation.[326,327]

UNRESOLVED INFECTIONS

Growing up, we were taught that once we contract an infection, our immune system generates a memory of it, preventing us from catching the same disease again. However, scientific understanding of immunity has evolved; we now realize that the immune system may not always function as efficiently as we would wish, and that infections morph and adapt over time, either continuously or repeatedly challenging our body's defences. For instance, my clinical team sees children who have contracted chickenpox not once but multiple times. Shingles, which 'should' normally only appear later in life when you are run down, is affecting more children and can wax and wane in adults, never quite going away entirely.

We also see many kids who are constantly battling low-grade viral or bacterial infections, never entirely free from symptoms such as a runny nose, bunged-up nose, sore throat or swollen glands. Of course, these symptoms are inevitable from time to time and can be more common during nursery and early school years. However, some kids seem to be hit harder than others and being dragged down by infection can easily affect their mood and performance.

If these infections are not effectively addressed, they can accumulate, layer upon layer. This build-up can reduce their vitality and siphon off essential energy that could otherwise support brain function.

When we run a full battery of tests at my NatureDoc clinic, we often find there are active viral, bacterial, yeast and parasitic infections. By working to reduce the overall load of these infections and help support the immune system to fight them effectively, we find very often the energy lifts, the brain becomes less foggy and the mind less dysregulated.

Certain specific infections have been more closely associated with some of the more marked traits and challenges that neurodivergent children can experience. For instance, pro-inflammatory bacteria such as *Streptococcus* and *Mycoplasma* have both had long-term associations with the onset of anxiety, OCD and tics.[328,329] The Epstein-Barr virus (glandular fever) and Cytomegalovirus are thought to kick-start autoimmunity[330,331] and are associated with the onset of chronic fatigue;[332] and raised antibodies, suggesting previous viral infection, are common in autistic people.[333] Overgrowth of bacteria in the small intestine has been associated with anxiety, stress and neuroticism.[334]

AUTOIMMUNITY

Autoimmune disorders occur when the immune system mistakenly attacks the body's own cells. Recent studies suggest that autoimmune disorders may be intertwined with neurodivergence. These conditions are often seen alongside Autism, for instance, not as a cause but as a co-morbidity, which means they come hand in hand.

Interestingly, parents and close family members of autistic children often have at least one diagnosed autoimmune disease or some symptoms of autoimmune activity. These can include type 1 diabetes, Hashimoto's thyroiditis, rheumatoid arthritis, ulcerative colitis, multiple sclerosis and coeliac disease.[335,336,337] We often see these theories borne out in our neurodivergent clients when we start to ask questions about their family medical history.

Paradoxically, many kids with autoimmunity don't display illness symptoms such as a fever or a sore throat. Instead of getting physically unwell, the autoimmune reaction to the infection may make their brain seem foggier or magnify any social problems – they may feel a bit low and find social situations harder. Many parents will say that their neurodivergent child has never had a day sick, even when the rest of the household picks up regular infections, but they notice that their mood and behaviour can decline for several weeks or months afterwards.

One condition, called PANDAS (Paediatric Autoimmune Neuropsychiatric Disorders Associated with Streptococcal Infections),[338,339] characterizes a misdirected neuroinflammatory autoimmune reaction to a streptococcus infection. PANS (Paediatric Acute-onset Neuropsychiatric Syndrome) can manifest with similar symptoms to PANDAS, but the trigger can be other infections, such as mycoplasma or Covid 19.

With these conditions, rather than fighting the infection, the immune system starts attacking the brain, leading to rapid onset symptoms such as OCD, anxiety, urinary incontinence and food restrictions or disordered eating – mimicking *Anorexia nervosa*[340] or Avoidant Restrictive Food Intake Disorder (ARFID).[341,342] Affected children can suddenly seem more immature, adopting a baby-like voice, or skills such as handwriting and drawing can go downhill. This sudden change in behaviour can be alarming and the symptoms can wax and wane depending on future infection exposures, often intensifying in response to new infections. This intensity of symptoms or an abrupt onset is known as a PANDAS flare.[343,344] The average age at which the condition develops is thought to be around the age of nine, though it can present in much younger children.

It is important to remember that PANS/PANDAS might well mimic or exacerbate mental-health issues and neurodivergent presentations, so if you feel your child has abruptly changed in their demeanour or regressed in their development, this is something to investigate.

THE INFLUENCE OF ALLERGIES ON BRAIN FUNCTION

The spring and summer are generally fun and enjoyable seasons most of us look forward to, but for many, this time of year signals high pollen levels and associated allergies. Common allergy symptoms include sneezing, a runny or itchy nose, and irritated eyes. However, these allergies can also cause headaches, nausea, coughing and a sore throat.

Seasonal allergies occur when the immune system overreacts to environmental pollens, usually from trees and grasses (hence the term hay fever). However, some people are more affected by allergy symptoms in autumn and winter, typically due to sensitivity to mould, which thrives in cold and damp conditions and also when leaves fall from trees and decompose.[345,346,347]

BRILLIANT STORY OF HOPE – PANS/PANDAS

Elena, aged 16, is one of the sweetest young ladies with a calm disposition. She has Global Developmental Delay (see page 11) but normally shines through each day with positivity and joy. Whenever she is exposed to a viral or bacterial infection, she rarely gets a sore throat or a temperature. Instead, her overall disposition rapidly goes downhill – she stops sleeping and starts getting repetitive thoughts. These thoughts get so stuck in her head that she is unable to access her schoolwork, or her hobbies, and she also cries all day.

Elena has been under the care of an immunologist and has been diagnosed with PANS/PANDAS. By taking a holistic, anti-inflammatory approach to her diet and cooling down the autoimmune response with supplements such as omega-3, turmeric and palmitoylethanolamide (PEA). Elena can usually get back to baseline. Her parents have learned how to keep things in check, and to act before a flare gets out of hand.

Obvious environmental allergies are not the only cause of these symptoms. There are some immune cells, called mast cells, that also play a key role in allergic reactions and inflammation, releasing histamine. Mast Cell Activation Syndrome (MCAS) is where the body releases allergy-like substances in response to a wide range of foods as well as environmental chemicals, such as ingredients in soaps, shampoo and household cleaning products, tobacco smoke and artificial fragrances. This overactivity of mast cells often coincides with hypermobility[348] as well as chronic pain and fatigue.[349]

Histamine intolerance is a condition where the body can't break down histamine (naturally occurring in foods) in the gut. This can then build up in the system over the day and lead to a whole host of allergy-type symptoms such as skin rashes, sneezing, itchy eyes, insomnia and feeling very hot and sweaty at night, as well as a foggy brain[350]. Foods with high levels of histamine include tomatoes, spinach, avocados, bananas, oranges and strawberries.

Histamine, mast cells and allergies seem to be very significant factors for many of our young NatureDoc clients with Long Covid;[351,352] we are seeing more histamine-related issues in our neurodivergent clients too since the pandemic. It is too early to say exactly why this should be the case, but I do know that when I take an overall antihistamine approach to kids with high histamine levels who are also neurodivergent, they often find that they sleep better, feel calmer and can focus better. It's been described to me several times that the brain has stopped jumping around or skipping ahead so that thoughts can be processed and organized better.

Luckily, many natural remedies can help to dial down inflammation triggered by histamine and mast cell activity. Here are my natural approaches to keeping histamine at bay:

1

First, ensure your child is consuming enough vitamin C and magnesium through diet and food supplements. These nutrients help to stabilize the histamine pathways in the body.

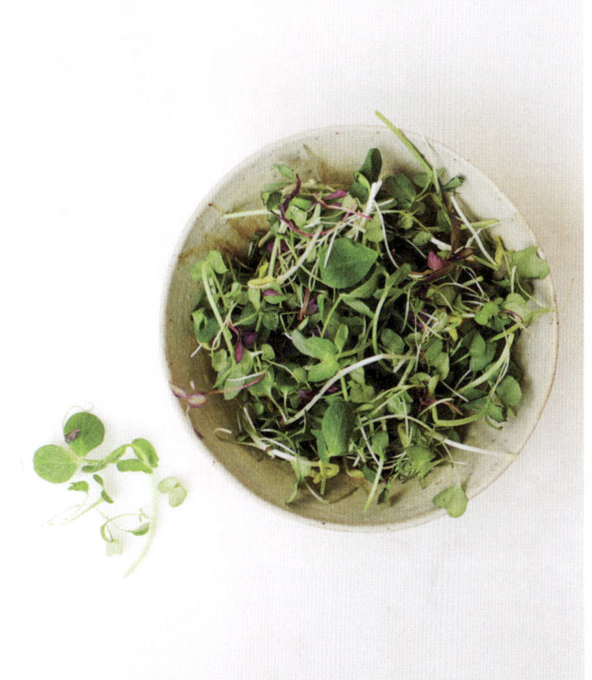

2

There is substantial evidence to show that quercetin, a pigment naturally found in foods such as pea shoots, red onions, red (bell) peppers and apples, and extracted from the flower of *Sophora japonica*, commonly known as the Japanese pagoda tree, has natural antihistamine and anti-inflammatory properties.

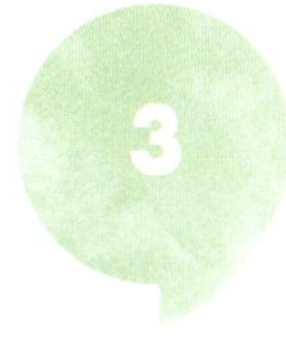

3

Ocimum tenuiflorum, better known as holy basil or tulsi, is native to India and a popular Ayurvedic herb that also helps with inflammation related to a high histamine state. This can be taken as a supplement or drunk as a tea.

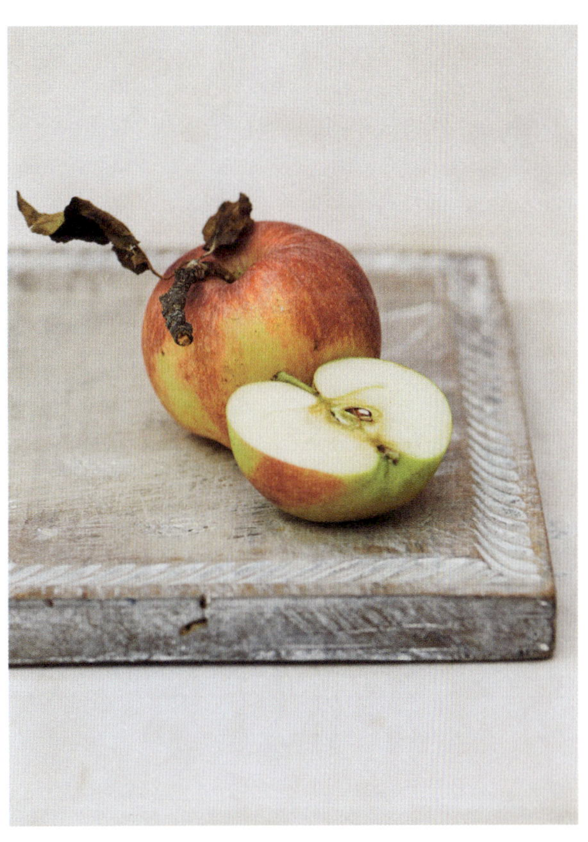

4

Palmitoylethanolamide (PEA), found in foods such as egg yolks and peanuts, is one of the key supplements that is used for neural inflammation related to high histamine or mast cell response. It may be helpful for people with chronic pain. Supplements are available.

7 BLOOD GLUCOSE DYSREGULATION

Do you ever feel 'hangry'? It describes that weak, wobbly feeling coupled with irritability or zoning out if a meal is running late or you have forgotten a snack. Then, do you feel so much better once you have eaten? If this happens a lot, it is a sign that you might have blood glucose dysregulation, and it is also extremely common among neurodivergent kids.

Blood glucose dysregulation, meaning poor blood sugar balance, can affect us all to some degree – it influences mood, focus, energy and sleep patterns and there is usually an immediate positive difference when a child starts to eat foods that help them to optimize their blood sugar. Some parents describe the contrast like night and day, and once they see their child have a good blood sugar day, they never look back. I would say that putting in place a diet that balances blood glucose can be the most important and positive dietary step that anyone can make for their kids if they are struggling with their physical, mental and emotional health or need to build general resilience.

It is well known that kids with ADHD[353,354] can be drawn to consuming excessive amounts of refined sugar and are also quite sensitive to it. This sugar sensitivity has been associated with hyperactivity, impulsivity and inattention. Dyslexic kids may also have dysregulated glucose metabolism in the brain, which can affect their ability to process sounds and access words automatically, meaning they can struggle to have a good mental dictionary and might find it hard to spell words easily.[355] It is also thought that many dyslexics carry genes that are shared with people who develop type 2 diabetes, a condition related to poor glucose tolerance.[356]

Neurodivergent kids can find they struggle with impulsivity and self-control, which can lead to aggression. Self-control can be a limited resource, and when people engage in one act of self-control, they may have less self-control for subsequent tasks. This could be because self-control takes up a lot of energy and blood glucose, as well as brain glycogen which provides brain energy for sustained effort.[357] A child who puts a lot of effort into self-control, such as sitting still in class, may easily become aggressive when they have not eaten or become angry when their blood sugar dips too low. Episodes of early-life hypoglycaemia (extremely low blood sugar) is one of the many risk indicators for a child developing Autism.[358]

Almost every other disease state associated with chronic inflammation can creep up if blood glucose dysregulation continues to be out of whack. Addressing blood glucose dysregulation is especially important because, as I mentioned above, neurodivergent kids are often more sensitive to refined sugars and starches but, paradoxically, they crave these same foods because they provide a short-term dopamine hit.

INSULIN RESISTANCE

Insulin resistance occurs when the body's cells struggle to respond properly to insulin, the hormone responsible for regulating blood sugar levels. When this happens, blood sugar levels can become imbalanced, which can exacerbate symptoms of dysregulation. Here are some key indicators of insulin resistance or poor blood glucose regulation.

- Tiredness: you feel as if your child is constantly running on empty and is exhausted.

- Hunger: if your child has just eaten a meal but almost immediately, they are raiding the refrigerator for a snack, or they are planning what to eat at the next meal. If they get peckish or sluggish within 2 hours of eating a meal, this is likely to be insulin resistance and indicates that they ate too much carbohydrate (sugar or starch) at the previous meal.

- Difficulty concentrating: they find it tough to focus or have a foggy brain.

- Weight gain: especially around the middle; the aptly named 'muffin top' can be a sign.

- Dark skin patches/skin tags: these are often found on the neck, armpits, elbows, knees and knuckles.

- Frequent urination: if they are rushing to the bathroom more often than usual, it could be because their body is trying to get rid of excess sugar.

Do remember, these symptoms are not exclusive to blood glucose regulation and might be related to other conditions, or even just the stresses of everyday life, but if you're noticing any of these signs, especially if they are new, it's important to check in with your doctor for advice and tests to check for insulin resistance and pre-diabetes.

BRILLIANT STORY OF HOPE – BLOOD SUGAR BALANCE

I met Ollie and Jack as delightful 6-year-old twins. Both had been flagged up as on the Dyslexia pathway; they were in the bottom set in Maths and English and found it very hard to concentrate. I suggested to their mum to switch their breakfast from cereal (carbohydrate) to eggs (protein). This made such a huge difference to both boys that we didn't need to do much else. Quite quickly they were moved up to the middle set and continued to grow in self-confidence and both found academic work much easier. One of them was even appointed head boy at their school – and to this day, now aged 18, he still eats at least a couple of eggs for breakfast!

HOW TO HELP MANAGE BLOOD GLUCOSE

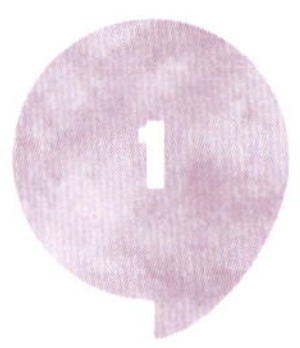

Start the day with a protein-based breakfast,[359] ideally a savoury one, which could include eggs, cheese, Greek yoghurt, nut butters, seeds, turkey, chicken or fish. Protein can help to stabilize blood sugar levels from the start, reducing cravings for sugary foods later in the day.

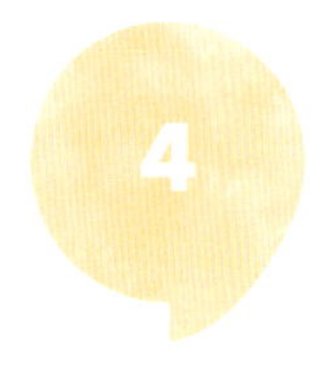

Serve protein and healthy fats with every meal and snack to help to balance their blood sugar levels by slowing the digestion and absorption of carbohydrates.[363] Why don't you try pairing an apple with cheese, crackers with nut butter and carrots with hummus?

Encourage your kids to eat their vegetables at the start of a meal, the protein in the middle and save their carbohydrate or sweet foods for the end of the meal. This can help to lower the overall glycaemic index of the meal, reducing blood sugar spikes.[360]

Get them into a habit of low-grade exercise after eating, like a gentle walk or a good stretch, to help to lower blood sugar levels after a meal.[364]

Include apple cider vinegar or lemon juice where possible in drinks and meals. These acids help to slow the absorption of sugars, again reducing blood sugar spikes.[361,362]

In terms of supplements, consider vitamin B1, vitamin B2, chromium, magnesium, zinc,[365] and biotin.[366] These minerals can all help to improve insulin sensitivity and regulate blood sugar levels.

CAN'T EAT, WON'T EAT

8

Having got this far in *Brain Brilliance*, you might be thinking this all sounds great in theory, but my child is such as fussy eater, and I cannot imagine them embracing any changes. You're certainly not alone. If you talk to most parents of neurodivergent children, a common theme will be that their kids are highly selective and very particular around what they will and won't eat. This is not just because they are being stubborn or oppositional – far from it. With neurodivergence, the old parenting style 'let them starve until they eat' usually does not work at all – it can in fact backfire badly and days may go by without any food passing their lips.

IDENTIFYING SENSORY PROBLEMS RELATED TO FOOD

Many feeding issues boil down to sensory issues surrounding the food, in terms of texture, smell and taste. This is not just about mouth feel and can stem from how the brain and the nervous system perceive the food. Sensory issues usually send kids into one of two camps: crunchy or smooth. If your child only eats food they can chomp and munch, such as crisps, crackers, breadsticks and toast, they may be in the crunchy camp. Similarly, kids who only choose 'slurpy' and blended foods, such as porridge, yoghurt and fruit pouches, are probably in the smooth camp.

Consider the following strategies to manage sensory food aversion and poor oral muscle tone in your child:

► Gradually introduce changes to the foods they already like and feel safe with. Make small but consistent changes to these so you can comfortably transition them to new foods. If they enjoy shop-bought waffles, try home-made ones. Add some red lentils to a tomato sauce or ground seeds to porridge.

► Brush their teeth using a vibrating toothbrush. Gently assist your child to brush the sides and top of the tongue, as well as inside the cheeks. This gets them used to different feelings in the mouth.

► Get them to drink using a curly wurly straw – this encourages oral tone.

► Encourage as many interactions with food as you can, even if initially it's just touching it, to familiarize them with different textures. This doesn't need to be in the kitchen – they may be more likely to touch, smell and taste a new food in the garden or on a walk.

► Involve your child in cooking as much as possible. This provides a stress-free environment and they might feel bold enough to try something new because they are in a more casual, fun setting.

► Engage them with shopping, not just at a super-market, but in farm shops, pick-your-own and farmers' markets, so they can experience other sensory input from food smells and textures.

FOOD CHAINING

Sometimes you need to take an even slower approach to change. This is known as 'chaining', which means one tiny step at a time. These are little gradual changes to a food they will accept to help broaden the diet and to introduce more nutrient-dense food versions. Here is the example of making chicken nuggets more nutritious. Many kids are hooked on chicken nuggets and this is how I would try and improve them to provide more overall nutrition (see also my recipe on page 138):

Step 1: upgrade to supermarket chicken nuggets with fewer additives – if these are accepted, then start to make your own.

Step 2: make your own chicken nuggets replicating the shop version as closely as you can, by using the same basic ingredients listed on the packaging. Use a combination of gram (chickpea) flour, rice flour and cornflour (corn starch) to make the crunchy coating at this stage, as well as blended up (ideally organic) chicken breast. This way you avoid the raising agents, flavourings, extra starches and added glucose.

Step 3: switch from chicken breast to thigh meat to add in more iron and other minerals.

Step 4: replace the first-stage flour coating on the chicken with chickpea flour.

Step 5: dip the floured chicken into whisked egg.

Step 6: make the crust out of ground lentils.

In a similar way, chaining can be used for smoothies, where you initially replicate the recipe of a shop-bought smoothie at home then slowly start supercharging it – maybe with a leaf or two of spinach or some yoghurt, ground seeds or nut butter.

MEDICAL AND PHYSICAL REASONS FOR SELECTIVE EATING

The other vitally important thing is to look for co-morbidities, meaning other medical or physical reasons that may be limiting your child's diet. Here are some to consider:

ORAL PROBLEMS

Always peek into your child's mouth if they are having difficulty eating.

Hypotonia, or low oral tone, which is discussed in chapter 12, can make it harder to chew and swallow food as well as delay speech development. If your child rejects chunks of meat, nuts and seeds they may not have the muscle strength to chew and swallow efficiently.

Tooth or gum infections can cause significant pain and overcrowded teeth, a high-arched palate, even tongue or lip-tie can make it hard to eat. Chronically swollen tonsils can also make swallowing uncomfortable, while painful mouth ulcers can put a child off their food. Wearing dental braces can be painful for teenagers and may be the cause of sudden selective eating at this stage.

GUT TROUBLE

From my clinical experience I have seen repeatedly that children prefer not to eat than to experience any kind of gastric pain. If your child only eats one or two mouthfuls and then stops abruptly, perhaps on some level they have made the connection between the food they are eating and the gut pain they are experiencing.

Acid reflux or the regurgitation of food or milk, is very common in babies, and it is often assumed that a child will simply grow out of it. However, throat and oesophageal pain from reflux and allergies can be troublesome throughout life and can affect both appetite and food choices. The pain from reflux can be so extreme that it becomes the root cause of many aggressive outbursts as well as agitation, anxiety, self-injury and sleep challenges, especially if the child is non-speaking and unable to express easily that they are in pain.[367]

If your child gets constipated regularly, you may well have seen a pattern of low appetite when they are bunged up and then a mighty appetite once they have emptied their bowels. If a child has a sore tummy, much of the time this is due to an impacted bowel, backed up with poo, which can affect how much a child eats as well as what they will and won't eat. Loose, stinky poo containing undigested food can also be signs there is trouble in the gut, and this may well go hand in hand with eating only a tiny amount or rigid eating patterns.

If your child complains of a sore tummy most days or it wakes them up at night, then it is likely that this gut pain is the underlying cause of their fussy eating. If your child has a habit of sleeping curled in a ball or they tend to lie with their tummy pressed against furniture or on the floor during the day, then this may be their way of telling you that they have a sore belly.

If you have a hunch that there is trouble in your child's tummy driving the picky eating, here are some tips you can try to help with the regurgitation, gut pain and slow bowel:

- Work on soothing any inflammation or gut pain by adding herbs like slippery elm, marshmallow root, or aloe vera to a little fruit purée or smoothie.

- Try cooked and blended fruit and vegetables that are easy to digest, such as apple purée, mashed root veggies and soup. Keep it simple with mashed banana or avocado.

- Smoosh up lots of goodies in smoothies and milkshakes (see pages 212–218).

- Encourage the production of gastric juices by adding a dash of apple cider vinegar to food such as bolognaise or to apple juice. Try squeezing lemon or lime juice over food or into drinks. Another option is to give digestive enzymes to aid food digestion. These are food supplements that can be added to water or chewed.

- A child's sense of smell and taste can be diminished if they are low in zinc. Start adding in some zinc drops to help encourage gastric juices and oral senses.

- Shortfalls in folate and B12 can affect a child's neurological system and in turn this can affect their sense of smell and taste. Supplements come in drops, which can easily be added to food or drinks.

- Try live bacteria supplements to help bolster the gut microbiome and help dial down any residual inflammation. Probiotic supplements come in drops and powders and are available tasteless, so they are easy to hide.

FOOD SENSITIVITIES?

One of the most common underlying drivers of picky eating is undetected low-grade food allergies and intolerances as well as other food-related gut reactions. Instead of the more classic (IgE) allergies triggering rashes and swelling of the lips and throat, there are other food sensitivities known as non-IgE allergies[368] or food intolerances which can irritate the gastric tract.

Many neurodivergent kids suffer from gut issues triggered by food, which can include Coeliac disease (wheat and gluten), Lactose intolerance (milk, yoghurt, cream and ice cream), Fructose intolerance (mainly fruits and honey), Eosinophilic Oesophagitis (often wheat, dairy, egg and soya), Food Protein-Induced Enterocolitis Syndrome (FPIES)[369] (again often wheat, dairy, egg and soya) or Histamine intolerance (tomato, citrus, spinach and avocado. All of these can be diagnosed by an allergy consultant or gastroenterologist.

All of the above food sensitivities can lead to gastric discomfort or distress, which can in turn lead to picky eating. And I generally find that kids with an out-of-sync gut restrict their diets to eating only the food that sits most comfortably in their tummy. Often, I find that when you remove the food that is irritating their gut, the child's appetite increases and their repertoire of other foods broadens beyond the parent's expectations. This is presumably because their tummy now feels a lot more comfortable.

IMMUNITY

If food fussiness sets in after a major illness or accompanying a longer series of milder infections, then a poor immune system may be part of the picture. Also, a course of antibiotics can affect the fine balance of gut flora; I sometimes find that a shortfall in beneficial gut bacteria can be the reason why fussy eating gets worse. Antibiotics may trigger a low-grade yeast infection that can result in oral thrush or *Candida albicans* in the gut and I find both of these can bring on carbohydrate fixation and sweet cravings (see chapter 4), which may explain why a child's good feeding habits can disappear rapidly in favour of eating the sweet stuff. Probiotics and fermented foods may be the answer, as they replace the lost beneficial bacteria that the gut needs to build immunity.

Scarlet fever or other *Streptococcus* infections such as 'strep throat' can make it far too painful to eat, leaving only certain foods feeling comfortable enough to swallow. In most cases, normal eating returns quickly once the infection has gone. However, if the food restriction continues beyond the duration of the infection and is accompanied by a sudden change in personality, anxiety, tics, obsessional thoughts, urinary frequency or a decline in schoolwork, it is important to consider whether the underlying cause is the condition called PANDAS[370] (see chapter 6).

NUTRIENT DEFICIENCIES

Chapter 2 highlighted that a zinc deficiency can be a cause of poor appetite, and that low zinc stores can alter the sense of taste and smell. Therefore, zinc supplements would be my first recommendation for any degree of selective or disordered eating. A sore tummy and poor appetite are symptoms of low iron levels (also covered in chapter 2) – another possible cause to consider. Finally, the B vitamins are key for the neurological system if texture or certain smells/tastes seem to be the problem.

ADDICTION TO GLUTEN AND MILK

Some neurodivergent kids have a very strong preference or even crave foods containing gluten and casein, the main proteins in wheat/gluten and milk products respectively – it's as if they are addicted to them and will often exclusively eat foods containing wheat and milk – this might look like milky cereal for breakfast, a cheese sandwich for lunch and pizza for supper – on repeat. This effect may be due to an 'opioid-like effect' of the peptides or mini proteins within these foods that can affect some sensitive people.[371] These peptides are specifically gluteomorphin (also known as gliadorphin) in gluten, and casomorphin in dairy products (except clarified butter, known as ghee). Research involving autistic kids suggests that when this opioid effect is active, there is less eye contact, poorer attention, reduced learning capacity, hyperactivity, a high pain threshold and self-harm, as well as more stereotypical and repetitive behaviours.[372,373]

I have seen this effect in several kids who are not autistic, and the peptides can make some children very wired and anxious and they can find it difficult to get to sleep. Some kids may experience vertigo or dizziness and disorientation as well as clumsiness. Other signs can include brain fog, feelings of unproductiveness, and difficulties with learning, working memory and processing.

This peptide theory means that some children do not produce enough of the right enzymes in their gut to break down the gluten and casein peptides, therefore these are only ever partially digested. If there is gut permeability (known as 'leaky gut'), the undigested peptides move from the gut into the bloodstream and then head to the brain, causing all the havoc.

When you take gluten and dairy foods out of a child's diet, very often the symptoms start to go away. If you are curious, try removing all foods containing gluten and casein for 4–6 weeks from their diet and avoid all traces of wheat or dairy during this time. If the change is working and your child is calmer and more engaged, then carry on for the longer term. If there are no positive changes, you can probably rule out gluten and casein as the primary issue and it is important to resume a normal diet.

If you are going to continue, it is important to work alongside a nutrition professional to ensure your child gets enough of the right nutrients, especially so if your child is a highly selective eater. At the very least you need to consider alternative food sources of key nutrients like calcium, iodine and B vitamins. Consuming nutrient-dense home-made foods is preferable to buying manufactured 'free-from' items if you want to ensure your youngster is getting enough nutrients when excluding gluten and dairy. This is where you need my range of delicious, healthy recipes up your sleeve!

A diet free from gluten and casein certainly does not make a difference to every neurodivergent child. However, it is worth noting that some parents have said this diet has been 'life-changing', even if meta studies can't suggest this as a blanket intervention. It should not need to be a permanent change, but cutting out gluten and dairy may help to some degree until the gut permeability is healed, and it is possible to help your child find it easier to digest and break down the gluten and dairy peptides over time, so you can reintroduce them.

THE STRUGGLES OF BINGE-EATING AND COMPULSIVE CRAVINGS

Binge-eating is a major problem for many neurodivergent tweens, teens and young people, and it is thought to be more common than *Anorexia nervosa* (restricted eating) and *Bulimia* (overeating and purging food) combined.[374,375] Often, binge-eating is linked to addictive behaviours associated with craving highly processed foods that combine fat, sugar and additives like glucose–fructose syrup.[376] These cravings can also be the body's way of crying out for more vitamins and minerals. I have found that cravings as well as binge-eating patterns reduce quite dramatically when a child is getting enough of the key vitamins and minerals.

If a child is obsessed with food and can't stop thinking about it, they are likely to be eating too many carbs and not enough protein and healthy fats. Binge-eating and cravings are often signs that a child's blood sugar is in disarray.[377] When their blood sugar drops quickly, they will be likely to munch on junk food to help get them out of the funk of feeling unfocused and irritable (see chapter 7).

Interestingly, a lot of kids and teens who binge-eat also have ADHD, an association which may be due to the impulsive nature of the ADHD. It may also be because they can experience a temporary dopamine boost from eating these 'blissful' foods high in salt as well as refined sugar and oils.

ADHD medications can suppress appetite during the day, making the child incredibly hungry and more likely to binge-eat at the end of the day or even at night. Eating a big breakfast and supper full of healthy proteins and fats can really help to ameliorate these cravings to graze incessantly if a child is taking stimulant medications for ADHD.

Stress is a key factor in the development of bingeing and craving. It can trigger both extremes – eating too much or too little. Stressors come in many forms and affect people differently and include the overwhelming demands of school, the intensity of over-exercising, or a lack of sleep.

Older kids can practise mindful eating by chewing every mouthful well and spending a moment reflecting on which foods keep their blood glucose stable and which ones keep them satiated.

BRILLIANT STORY OF HOPE – AUTISM AND SELECTIVE EATING

Sarah, at the age of 2, had been diagnosed with Autism. She exclusively only ate two foods: one type of sweet yoghurt and one type of cracker. She cried all day; she was very constipated; and she had never acknowledged or interacted with anyone except her parents. The doctors who diagnosed her suggested she would never speak or go to mainstream school.

I suspected Sarah had a problem with digesting dairy and gluten, both present in the only two foods she was eating at the time! I also discovered that her pancreas was not producing sufficient enzymes to allow her to digest the complex proteins in these foods. Her parents therefore switched her to dairy-free yoghurt and gluten-free crackers, which she accepted, and then they added enzymes by way of a supplement to her water. These interventions seemed to open up Sarah's world quite quickly and she soon started to eat full meals – even meat and three veg!

Sarah also started connecting with the world around her and began to speak, once her gut was working properly and her food intake was providing the nourishment her brain needed. She attended mainstream school throughout her educational journey and is now at college studying A levels – and she can't stop talking!

9 EMOTIONAL DYSREGULATION

We all know what it is like to become overwhelmed by day-to-day stresses and how easy it is to have a meltdown from ongoing tension and life's pressures. It is perfectly normal to experience this from time to time. Neurodivergent kids, however, seem to be much more sensitive when coping with day-to-day stresses and change, and emotional dysregulation can kick in much more easily.[378,379]

Dysregulation is the inability to control emotional responses, marked by bursts of what is termed emotional lability or volatile mood swings, that can switch in a split second. Mood dysregulation can mean that there is very poor natural control of feelings, such as sadness, irritability, anxiety or anger, and this can result in starting arguments, pacing, extreme meltdowns, rage, aggression or self-injury. It is important to identify the root cause of emotional dysregulation and work out ways to help neurodivergent kids to build resilience to inevitable everyday changes and disruptions.

Emotional dysregulation can sometimes be due to past trauma, pressures from social media or because a child's current school, therapies or their life situation is not meeting their needs adequately. These scenarios must not be overlooked. However, biochemical and hormonal processes can be part of the picture, which is what I am going to share in this chapter.

PYRROLE DISORDER

Pyrrole Disorder, or Kryptopyrrole (KPU), is a common inherited metabolic issue that means the child needs to consume much higher levels of zinc and Vitamin B6 than the average kid. The hallmarks are mood swings, social withdrawal, compulsive behaviour and emotional eating. See page 35 for more details.

CORTISOL IMBALANCE

Very often, neurodiverse kids live in a mild to moderate state of adrenal 'fight or flight' stress response; after all, it can be hard living in a neurotypical world when your brain is wired differently. Cortisol is a steroid hormone produced by the adrenal glands, two walnut-sized glands located just above the kidneys. Cortisol is what gets us up in the morning and keeps us awake during the day.

A cortisol imbalance is particularly marked in families who have experienced significant psychological or social adversity. Kids with a high degree of separation anxiety are also frequently in a high cortisol state. Too much cortisol can also affect blood glucose balance, increase blood pressure and affect sleep quality.

A HIGH CORTISOL STATE

A classic sleep pattern for anyone experiencing a chronic high cortisol state is to struggle to get to sleep, and to be awake around 4am for a couple of hours, then fall into a deep sleep just as the alarm is going off. So, this can mean your child ends up waking up late and feeling groggy and tired during the day.

Sugar (even naturally sweet fruit) and high-carb foods often make a child in a high cortisol state feel worse, while high-protein foods can make them feel better. Some teens tend to be very sensitive to the caffeine found in coffee, cocoa or chocolate, tea and green tea, as well as some energy drinks and supplements.

The hallmarks of a youngster in a high cortisol state include being snappy, unrelaxed, hyper, jittery, hypervigilant, overreactive and wired – the kind of kid whose mood can easily flip in an instant. You can sometimes spot if a child is in a high cortisol state as their pupils can be very dilated like 'Disney eyes'.[380]

To help reduce a high cortisol state, there are several natural remedies, including herbs such as chamomile, magnesium and omega-3, and then saffron, ashwagandha and reishi mushroom for older kids and teens.

A LOW CORTISOL STATE

After experiencing long periods of a high cortisol fight-or-flight state, neurodiverse kids, teens and young adults are more likely to reach an adrenal burnout stage where the cortisol levels crash and the release of cortisol from the adrenal glands is lower than optimal. Being stuck in a low cortisol state can also reflect post-traumatic stress disorder (PTSD), a mental health state triggered by experiencing or witnessing a terrifying event or prolonged distress or trauma.

Kids in a low cortisol state can experience feelings of exhaustion and burn-out and they might find it hard to fight infection. They can also have poor executive function with lowered working memory and cognitive flexibility.[381] A blunted cortisol stress response is also common in young people with behavioural challenges, including oppositional defiance disorder (see page 11).[382]

The hallmarks for a low cortisol state tend to be fatigue, low or flat mood, feeling zoned/spaced out, dizzy or lightheaded and can be perceived by outsiders as daydreaming. Kids and teens with low cortisol can easily become 'hangry' and irritable if a meal is delayed and need regular snacks to keep them on an even keel.

Anyone whose cortisol is low when they wake in the morning can feel quite cold, weak and wobbly and crave sugar and carbs as well as caffeine. This is because when cortisol is low, the body tends to default to a low blood sugar state called hypoglycaemia as well as low blood pressure. Studies have found that those diagnosed with the inattentive type of Attention Deficit Disorder (ADD) often have lower baseline cortisol levels during the day.[383,384]

Vitamin C, a vitamin B complex supplement as well as eating some salt, liquorice or grapefruit can temporarily lift cortisol levels.

THE MANY ROLES OF THE VAGUS NERVE

The vagus nerve acts as a 'super-highway', constantly sending information up and down from the gut to the brain, and helps us deal with stress, anxiety and fear. It is what causes the heart to race and why we get butterflies in our tummy when we are nervous or feel a sense of threat to our wellbeing.

Equally, the action of the vagus nerve is the reason why our breathing slows right down, and our body relaxes when friends or family give us a welcome hug and make us feel safe. This vital nerve helps your body to develop a healthy stress response and to become more resilient; it is our child's innate way of counteracting the fight-or-flight adrenal response.

Any time a child's brain perceives a threat, the sympathetic nervous system can trigger this fight-or-flight cortisol response. However, provided the vagus nerve is healthy and well-toned, it turns on the parasympathetic nervous system, which does the opposite: it calms them down. The vagus nerve can help a child to remain cool, calm and collected in a stressful situation, and also let them know when they are no longer in danger.

The tone of the vagus nerve is very important, because with low vagal tone the nervous system may struggle to adapt to change and has less flexibility. The higher the vagal tone, the greater a person's window of tolerance to adapt to change and stressful situations. Poor vagal tone can mean a child's window of tolerance is narrow and they can be tipped into an emotionally dysregulated state: either they can quickly become hyper-aroused, which can manifest in anger, anxiety and irritability, or they become hypo-aroused and their emotions freeze up, and they can feel numb and become dissociated.

Vagal tone can be tracked from a young age, even in babies, and it has been the subject of quite a bit of research. It seems that babies with stronger vagal tone tend to show more interest and more joy when meeting new people. Babies with low vagal tone tend to be more wary in social situations and have a preference for solitude when they are older.[385,386]

Higher vagal tone is also linked to greater feelings of compassion and empathy. Children with a healthier vagal nerve tone tend to be more sympathetic to other children, to comfort them when they are distressed, and are more likely to learn to share with others.[387] Interestingly, people with greater vagal tone flexibility find it easier to detect social and emotional cues from facial expressions[388,389] and can more easily remember people's faces.[390] Furthermore, a well-toned vagus nerve helps with digestion and our ability to rest, and aids sleep quality.[391] Poor vagal tone may even contribute to children having more nightmares.[392]

In summary, a healthy vagal tone means better emotional regulation, greater connection with other people and the environment as well as better physical health.

WAYS TO IMPROVE VAGAL TONE

The vagus nerve can be 'exercised' and strengthened in simple ways. Here are some you can try:

COLD EXPOSURE

Studies indicate that exposure to cold air or water on a regular basis can have a positive effect on the parasympathetic system through activation of the vagus nerve, while lowering the sympathetic fight-or-flight response. Try going for a walk on a chilly day with your child, swimming in the sea together, splashing their face with cold water or taking a brief cold shower.

DEEP, SLOW BREATHING

Practising deep, slow breathing has been shown to decrease anxiety and increase the activity of the parasympathetic system. Most people typically take between 10 and 14 breaths per minute. By reducing the number of breaths to about 6 per minute, your older child or teen can reduce stress levels and tone up the vagus nerve.

SINGING, HUMMING, CHANTING AND GARGLING

The vocal cords and muscles in the back of the throat are both linked to the vagus nerve. Singing, humming, chanting or gargling water exercises these muscles, stimulating the vagus nerve.

SOCIALIZING AND LAUGHING

Good social connections can influence vagal tone and promote positive emotions. Simply laughing more with friends can be beneficial.

YOGA AND MEDITATION

Yoga postures and breathing techniques are believed to increase vagal tone by stimulating the relaxation response in the body. Meditation is a proven way to calm the sympathetic nervous system and it too can be effective in stimulating the vagus nerve and increasing vagal tone.

EXERCISE

Exercise stimulates the vagus nerve, which may further contribute to its positive effects on the brain and mental health. This can be as simple as walking, running, kicking a ball, rock climbing or bouncing on a trampoline.

MASSAGE

Massage and reflexology can increase vagal activity and tone. Many neurodivergent kids benefit from a gentle foot massage before bed.

PROBIOTICS

Gut bacteria affect the vagus nerve and improve brain function. Studies show that taking the probiotics *Lactobacillus*[393] and *Bifidobacterium*[394] can reduce stress, anxiety and depression-like behaviour.

TAKE FOOD SUPPLEMENTS

A lack of vitamins B1, B6, B9 and B12 can cause the nervous system to 'misfire' and lead to lower vagal tone. Recent research has suggested that omega-3 fatty acids can bolster vagal tone and activity.[395]

AVOIDING AFTER-SCHOOL MELTDOWNS

Do you have a child who is a perfect angel at school and then very different when they get home?

Many kids find they really need to let off steam after school and usually parents and siblings get the brunt of it! Every child will occasionally go into meltdown when they are overtired, under too much pressure or unwell. But when this behaviour turns into a regular pattern, and becomes more profound, it can make family life very tough.

After-school explosive behaviour is more common in neurodivergent kids, who often try their best to mask their differences during the busy school day then let off steam when they can't bottle it up any longer. The dysregulated behaviour is common in kids with sensory issues who cope with all the noise and intensity of school, then afterwards they are overwhelmed.

Much of the time this boils down to a combination of a high cortisol fight-or-flight state with 'hanger' caused by very low blood sugar levels, especially if your child isn't very good at eating lunch at school. Meltdowns after school can be a red flag that the nervous system and adrenals need better support. Here are ways in which you can help:

▸ Give them a more substantial breakfast packed with protein and healthy fats – consider eggs, peanut butter, ground seeds, slices of turkey/ham or cheese – it helps to blunt 'hangry' outbursts at the end of the day.

▸ Supercharge after-school snacks – again ensure there is some protein and healthy fat in these, not just a carby/sugary offering – this will help the mood and focus during the latter part of the day.

▸ Allow proper downtime after school – perhaps by listening to an audio book or music, or wrap up in a heavy blanket with a calming cup of chamomile tea. Some kids respond well to a diffuser with soothing essential oils.

▸ Work on sleep – magnesium is very grounding and can help kids to get a deeper, more refreshing night's sleep. It also helps with blood sugar regulation. Magnesium is abundant in green veg, nuts, seeds and dark chocolate. Magnesium flakes can also be added to a bath because it can be absorbed through the skin.

▸ Herbal support – to help stop kids reaching that tipping point, calm down their fight-or-flight response – consider supplements containing theanine, passionflower and lemon balm.

10 ANXIETY, OCD & TICS

Anxiety, obsessive thoughts and compulsive rituals, as well as tics, often go hand in hand with neurodivergence. Anxiety is something that can affect anyone at some point in their lives, especially faced with new experiences. Neurodivergent kids often experience anxiety triggers differently, for instance, autistic children may have heightened sensitivities to sensory inputs like loud noises or bright lights, which can trigger anxiety. Similarly, kids with ADHD may experience heightened anxiety due to struggles with executive functioning, such as difficulty in organizing tasks or managing time, which again can lead to feelings of overwhelm and stress.

UNPACKING ANXIETY

Anxiety can lie behind many of the deep-seated traits and behaviours that neurodivergent kids experience. It can be the root cause of shyness, selective mutism, pathological demand avoidance and oppositional defiance (see page 11) as well as school refusal and meltdowns. When it grips hard and affects all areas of a child's life, anxiety can be very debilitating.

Interestingly, anxiety and excitement act in a very similar way in the body. Both emotions trigger a faster heartbeat and an adrenaline surge – and feelings of excitement can easily flip into anxiety. It can affect many systems in the body. These are some of the symptoms of anxiety:

- Feeling overwhelmed
- Phobias
- Irritability
- Trouble concentrating
- Gut issues, including pain, constipation or diarrhoea
- Dizziness
- Trouble breathing
- Persistent worrying
- Separation anxiety
- Obsessions and compulsions
- Self-harming
- Over-achievement
- Tics and involuntary movements
- Headaches
- Poor sleep patterns

WHAT IS OCD?

Obsessive Compulsive Disorder (OCD) often comes alongside anxiety. OCD manifests when someone becomes trapped in a pattern of obsessions and compulsions. Obsessions consist of unwanted, intrusive thoughts, images or impulses that bring on severe feelings of distress – and can repeat over and over in the brain. Compulsions, on the other hand, are actions or rituals performed to mitigate the distress of these obsessions. This might be tapping the feet a certain number of times before being able to go through a doorway, or handwashing until the skin on the hands goes red, raw and bleeds.

It is common for everyone to experience obsessive thoughts or engage in compulsive behaviours at some stage in their lives, especially when they are anxious. However, this does not mean that everyone has 'a bit of OCD'. For a formal diagnosis of OCD to be confirmed, this cycle of obsessions and compulsions must be so severe that it dominates a significant portion of time, incurs intense distress, or interferes with significant activities that the child normally loves to do. A psychologist or other mental health professional can successfully help to support both anxiety and OCD, but sometimes this is not enough, and at this point many people turn to nutrition and look for underlying metabolic causes and triggers.

TICS AND TOURETTE SYNDROME

Tics and twitches are involuntary repetitive movements that the person cannot control. These include eye blinking, throat clearing, shoulder shrugging or blurting out unusual sounds. Tourette Syndrome shares the same tics and twitches and is usually diagnosed when the tics have been frequent and continuous for at least 12 months.

WHAT CAN DRIVE THIS TRIO?

The reasons for developing these conditions may be genetic, or triggered by trauma, illness or deficiency. Here are some metabolic and nutritional imbalances that you may want to look into if you feel the anxiety, OCD, tics and twitches have become hard to manage and you need additional support:

PANDAS

PANDAS is an autoimmune neuropsychiatric disorder that occurs in children, typically triggered by a streptococcus infection such as tonsillitis, a sore throat or scarlet fever. Rather than the child's body appropriately combating the infection, the illness targets the basal ganglia in the brain, leading to symptoms that can come on almost overnight and include OCD, tics, anxiety, urinary incontinence and food restrictions, and other sudden behavioural changes (see chapter 6 for more information).

Gut out of balance?

We know that our gut and the bacteria that live in it play a pivotal role in how our brain functions. The equilibrium between beneficial and less desirable bacteria that make up our gut microbiome can get out of balance. Research is emerging that gut bacteria diversity can play a pivotal role in the development of anxiety and OCD. Chapter 4 explains how the gut microbiome can influence the brain in more detail.[396,397]

B vitamins or iron deficiency?

The B vitamins and iron are critical for supporting brain health – these are primary nutrients to optimize if anxiety and OCD become a key issue. Deficiencies in these vitamins and minerals are now very common due to modern-day eating habits, such as choosing white meats over red meats and dodging green vegetables. Refer to chapter 2 for more details.

Inositol

Inositol, or myo-inositol, is often referred to as vitamin B8, but it's not really a vitamin. It is a type of sugar that is abundant in the brain and is used as a food supplement to help support panic disorders, depression, and OCD.[398,399,400] Inositol is also an excellent female hormone balancer and is thought to help balance serotonin and dopamine. Despite being a form of sugar, it helps to regulate insulin response and in turn blood glucose levels in the body. Foods that naturally contain inositol include almonds, walnuts, Brazil nuts, oats, beans, peas, cantaloupe melon, oranges and limes. It is important to be aware that, because of its effect on serotonin, a child cannot take inositol as a supplement if they have been prescribed a Selective Serotonin Reuptake Inhibitor (SSRI) antidepressant medication.

FIVE SUPPLEMENTS FOR SUPPORTING THIS TRIO

1 Theanine in tea (black or green tea) contains excellent levels of the neurotransmitter GABA which helps us to keep calm and relaxed (see chapter 2). Theanine can also be given as a non-caffeinated supplement even for young kids and is helpful when someone is experiencing anxiety,[401] OCD[402] and tics.

2 Magnesium has been used for many years as a remedy for anxiety, OCD and tic disorders to promote calmness and aid sleep.[403,404,405,406] Studies have found that during periods of extreme stress, the body often depletes its magnesium levels.[407]

BRILLIANT STORY OF HOPE – TICS

Ethan, like most of his class at school, contracted scarlet fever. Although he recovered quite easily from the infection, shortly afterwards he developed some tics – blinking all the time with some facial grimacing. He started to be bullied at school because of these tics, which was devastating and knocked his self-esteem.

Ethan started to take some magnesium and theanine, which calmed down his tics, to the extent that no one noticed them, except his parents when he was very tired. Over time, the tics disappeared entirely, and did not return, so he was able to stop taking the magnesium and theanine. His confidence also increased immeasurably over this time period.

We all experience anxiety, but neurodivergent kids can find this a daily challenge, and this can manifest neurologically as tics as well as OCD. It can be hard to keep these in check all the time, but food, supplements and working on the underlying immune system can make all the difference and ease a child out of the difficult patches.

3 Vitamin B6 is often given in conjunction with magnesium or theanine[408] to calm the nervous system and can be used for people with generalized anxiety[409] and tic disorders[410] as well as OCD.[411] See chapter 2 for more information.

4 Having enough Vitamin D in the system is critical in supporting anxiety[412] and people with OCD and tic disorders have been found to have low levels of Vitamin D in their blood.[413,414] Known as the 'good mood' vitamin, a significant sign that your child needs more vitamin D is if the anxiety or OCD worsens with less sun exposure, for example during the winter.[415]

5 OCD or tics may be an early manifestation of a shortfall in Vitamin B12, which is an important vitamin that helps to make both serotonin and dopamine. If your child is plant-based or rarely eats animal products such as meat, fish and eggs, you may want to consider supplementing.[416,417,418]

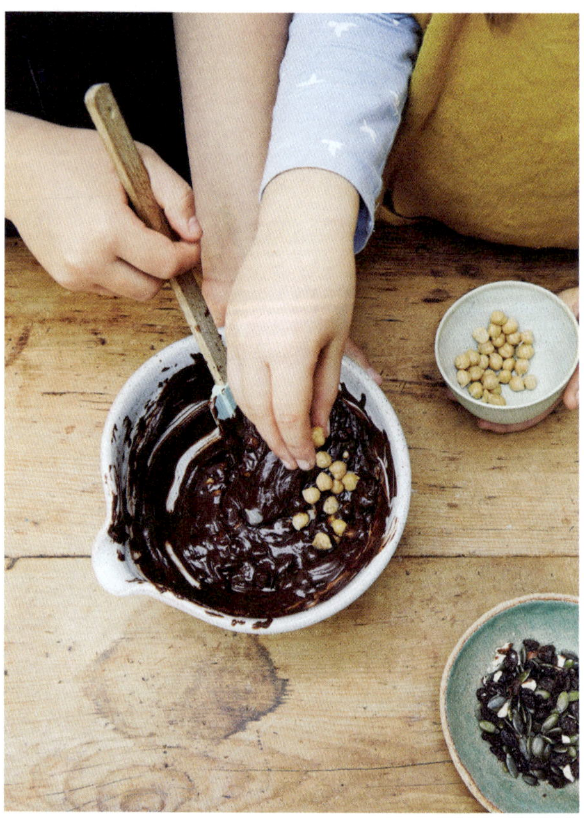

THE SLEEP THIEF 11

Achieving regular sleeping patterns and a refreshing night's sleep can be one of the greatest ongoing challenges for neurodivergent children. It is common for kids to take a very long time to wind down and get to sleep, while teens and young adults can easily become night owls. Often sleep can be light and fitful and some wake up super-early and cannot get back to sleep. In our NatureDoc clinic we commonly see kids who, despite being put to bed at 7pm, are still awake at 10 or 11pm, and many teens who find their brain only wakes up mid-evening, and then it can be 3am before they get to sleep.

We all know that we perform better the next day when we have had a good night's sleep and, equally, that we can feel tired, blurry and our blood glucose can be out of sorts if we don't have enough quality sleep.[419] I found my ADHD far worse when my kids were little, and I think this partly boiled down to having lots of broken nights and light sleep.

THE IMPORTANCE OF MELATONIN

One of the key reasons why neurodivergent kids struggle with their sleep is that they find it hard to make enough melatonin, a hormone that helps us get to sleep. Melatonin synthesis and release are stimulated by darkness and suppressed by light, hence it is often called the 'hormone of darkness'. Melatonin is one of the only medications doctors in the UK can prescribe to autistic children, and this is also available over the counter in other countries.

Melatonin plays a crucial role in regulating the body's circadian rhythms, which are natural behaviour patterns that respond to light and dark on a repeating 24-hour cycle. The circadian rhythms are our internal body clock, regulating our daily habits – dictating when we feel alert or sleepy, when we feel hungry – and even our body temperature. Melatonin also influences the stages of sleep, particularly the REM (rapid eye movement) stage, when we are dreaming, and the deep-sleep stage, both of which are crucial for cognitive and physical health.

Melatonin kicks in when the sun sets and during the first few hours of darkness. In the morning, as the sun rises and light levels increase, melatonin production drops, signalling that it is time to wake up. By the time you're fully awake, levels are barely detectable. Melatonin is primarily made in the body, and there are also small amounts of melatonin found in some foods like cherries. Here are my tips to help your child produce more melatonin in the evening:

► Get plenty of natural morning light. Expose them to natural light during the day (especially at the start of the day), which can help regulate melatonin production and improve your sleep–wake cycle.

► Dim the lights in the evening. Lower the intensity of artificial lights in your home to signal to their body that it's time for bed.

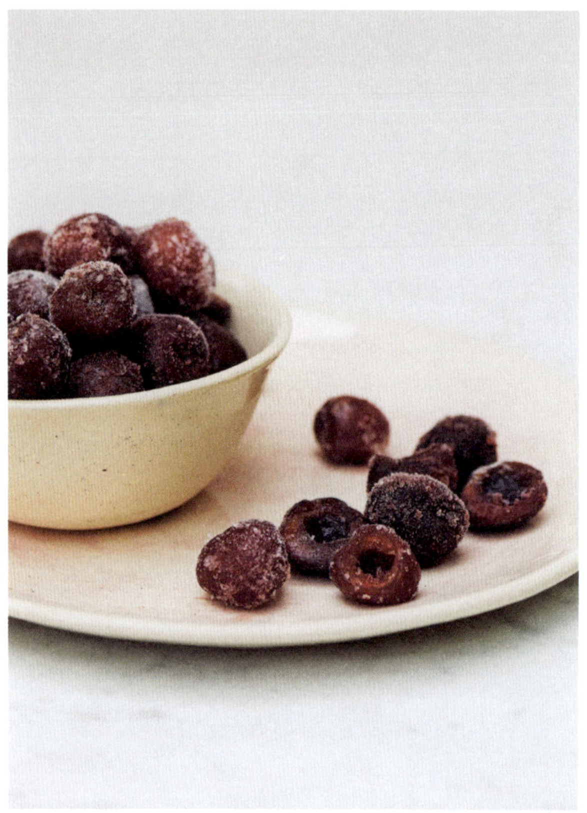

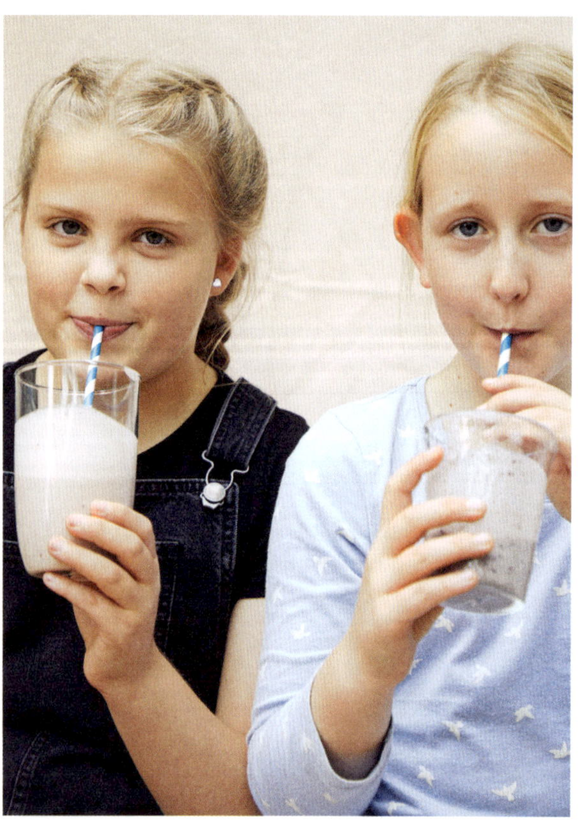

► Encourage foods rich in tryptophan, including turkey, chicken, bananas, avocados and cashew nuts, which is then turned into serotonin. As darkness falls this serotonin is converted into melatonin.

► Increase their magnesium intake,[420] especially via Epsom salt baths (magnesium is absorbed through the skin) and magnesium-rich foods or supplements.

► Feed them plenty of cherries,[421] cherry juice or supplements with the sour cherry variety Montmorency, in the evening.

SLEEPY GABA

GABA is another neurotransmitter that helps kids to sleep well. It's known for its calming effect on the body's central nervous system, slowing things down and helping them to relax. During sleep, GABA is important for enabling the body and mind to rest and recover from the day. It affects the deeper stages of sleep, particularly the REM stage, which is essential for restful, restorative sleep. Here are my top sleep tips:

► Establish a bedtime routine. Develop a calming pre-sleep routine that signals to the body and mind that it's time for bed. This could include taking a warm bath and then reading them a book.

► Avoid feeding them refined sugar, from biscuits (cookies) and sweets (candy) to chocolate/cocoa, during the late afternoon and the evening.

► Rub in magnesium skin lotion. This is soothing as well as being beneficial for magnesium intake.

► Turn off electronic devices at least an hour before bedtime to help them transition into sleep mode. Suggest listening to some music or a podcast if they find it hard to wind down in silence. But make sure this isn't just an excuse for more gadget time.

► Create a sleep-friendly environment. Make sure their bedroom is dark, quiet and cool. Consider using blackout curtains, a white noise machine (see chapter 13), or a fan to create a comfortable sleep setting. Some children rely on a weighted blanket if they seek sensory input at night.

▶ Encourage regular exercise but not too late in the day. Regular physical activity during the day can help improve sleep quality. However, exercising late into the evening can be overstimulating for some kids.

▶ Practise relaxation techniques. Deep breathing, yoga or meditation can help calm the mind and prepare the body for sleep.

▶ Avoid lie-ins in the morning. The longer they are resting in bed in the morning, the more their circadian rhythm shifts to a later schedule.

SLEEPY BEDTIME SNACKS

A dip in blood glucose levels can cause a jolt of adrenaline, which can disrupt sleep around 2 to 4am. One way to help prevent this dip is to give your child a balanced bedtime snack, one that contains both complex carbohydrates and protein to promote slow and steady digestion and absorption, keeping their blood sugars stable while they sleep.

Examples of bedtime snacks include frozen cherries with oats and milk or oatcakes with cream cheese, nut butter or fish pâté. Or try my Chamomile & Cherry Sleepy Smoothie (page 218).

If the waking time is as early as 4 or 4.30am then it may well be caused by a cortisol spike (see chapter 9). Passionflower or lemon balm tea and capsules have been used for their calming and sleep-promoting effects. They may help with anxiety and sleep issues, thereby promoting longer and more restful sleep. Saffron has similar effects. Ashwagandha is another good supplement that can be beneficial for early risers and can be given to teens and tweens.

A note for teens and young adults: caffeine and alcohol consumption can disrupt sleep – even in small amounts. It's particularly important to avoid caffeine in the afternoon and evening because it can be overstimulating. Alcohol, on the other hand, may initially make them feel sleepy, but even one drink can reduce the quality of their sleep. Their brain may be much foggier the day after drinking alcohol.

BRILLIANT STORY OF HOPE – GETTING TO SLEEP

Emilia, aged 9 years old, has a diagnosis of ADHD and Dyslexia and has always found it hard to get to sleep – her parents would put her to bed at 8pm and most nights she would still be wide awake until 11pm. This meant she was crabby and tired in the morning and her parents felt the lack of sleep was affecting her learning and focus during the day.

Emilia agreed to stop looking at all screens an hour before bed and instead to listen to an audiobook. She also adopted the habit of taking an Epsom salt bath before bed, which she loved, and this helped her wind down and start to feel soporific. Because her ADHD medication suppressed her appetite in the daytime, we also built in a filling smoothie to drink each evening containing cherry and chamomile to help stimulate some natural melatonin. Soon Emilia was dropping off to sleep by 9pm most nights and this made a huge difference to her focus and performance at school.

12 HYPERMOBILITY, LOW MUSCLE TONE & PAIN

Hypermobility (very bendy joints), hypotonia (low muscle tone) and chronic pain often go hand in hand with neurodivergence. It is estimated that neurodivergent folk are more than twice as likely to have unusually flexible joints and associated symptoms.[422 423] Teens and young people may also be more likely to experience chronic pain such as deep muscle pain (fibromyalgia).[424 425]

Although the exact reasons for the higher prevalence of hypermobility, hypotonia and pain in the neurodivergent population are not yet clear, theories suggest that they include shared genetics as well as overlapping neurological, metabolic and inflammatory pathways within the body.

HYPERMOBILITY

Hypermobility can give your child great joint flexibility, and this can be described as double-jointed. It can be easy for them to do the splits and their party trick may be being able to bend their thumb so it can touch their forearm. In young children, hypermobility can be identified easily and may include bendy long and slim 'piano fingers', floppy legs or arms. Many hypermobile kids sit most comfortably with their legs in a W shape. Hypermobility can be one of the reasons why your child was a 'bum shuffler' and never crawled, or that they hated tummy time when they were tiny.

There are some real positives to having a bendy body, and such innate flexibility helps kids to be great at gymnastics and dance. However, hypermobility or hyperflexible joints can sometimes set a child up for a wide range of health difficulties, such as increased risk of sports injuries, dislocations, long-term pain, and even wider-reaching associated problems such as gut issues and fatigue. Nutrition can play a role in helping to prevent the difficulties associated with hypermobility.

Apart from hyperflexible joints, hypermobility can also mean a higher likelihood of delicate blood vessels or soft or stretchy skin and a child may well bruise easily. Poor wound healing and easy scarring can also be linked with this condition. It is thought that this is due to genetic variations in the way collagen, elastin and fibrillin are produced as they knit skin, joints, cartilage and muscles together. Think of these as the scaffolding that provides structure within the body and gives the skin strength and elasticity.

Ehlers-Danlos Syndromes (EDS) are a group of inherited disorders primarily affecting the connective tissues.[426] Symptoms of EDS are similar to hypermobility but usually more systemic and affect more than the joints. Common symptoms include exhaustion, gastric issues,[427] such as gastroparesis, constipation[428] and acid reflux, as well as heart valve issues,[429] urinary incontinence and prolapse. Postural Tachycardia Syndrome (PoTS) – dizziness or faster heart rate upon standing – is also common in people with EDS.

HYPOTONIA

Have you ever been told your child has hypotonia or low muscle tone? Many neurodivergent people find that they have generalized low muscle tone, which can make it harder to chew, swallow and speak, as well as hop, skip, walk and run. It can also affect gut motility, leading to slow digestion and constipation. Sometimes hypotonia is caused by problems with the mitochondria[430] – the group of 'batteries' inside every cell that controls energy and cell renewal. Mitochondrial dysfunction does need to be checked out by a paediatrician or nutrition professional and may well be supported with food supplements, such as carnitine, co-enzyme Q10 and B vitamins, which, over time, can improve muscle tone and strength.[431,432] Also, being aware of this is the first step to addressing the issues with specialist exercises and eating more protein.

NUTRITIONAL SUPPORT FOR HYPERMOBILITY AND PAIN

Besides medical intervention and physical therapies, dietary changes and supplements can support youngsters with hypermobility or EDS to help manage pain, inflammation and mobility.[434,435] Here are the key nutrients you need to consider – build them in one at a time until things improve:

- Vitamin C is a primary nutrient and is essential for the production of collagen, a protein that helps maintain the integrity of skin, blood vessels and connective tissues.[436] Think of oranges, lemons, limes, strawberries and parsley.

- Magnesium can assist with muscle and nerve function. It is one of the key supplements for people with pain and hypermobility.[437] Feed your child plenty of nuts, seeds and green leafy veg, and consider topping up with a supplement.

- Palmitoylethanolamide (PEA) is a naturally occurring fatty acid compound that has been shown to have anti-inflammatory effects and may help with pain management.[438,439] You can find it in eggs, soya beans, peanuts and milk.

A WEAK CORE AND PINCER GRIP

The inner core muscles located in the abdominal area keep our backs nice and straight. Signs that these muscles are strong include a good posture and a well-functioning pelvic floor! A weak core can affect coordination as well as back health. It can reduce the tone of the shoulder muscles, which in turn affects the pincer grip, which is key for fine motor skills such as good handwriting, drawing, using scissors and doing up laces and buttons.[433] This is common among kids with developmental coordination disorders such as Dyspraxia.

Occupational therapy exercises can help to support core strength – many people start by exercising on a trampoline, or by sitting on a Swiss exercise ball (or, more practically, a flat version called a wobble cushion) during classes and at home while eating or watching TV. My husband swears by his mini trampoline. Rain or lack of time is never an excuse for exercise when it's right there in your home.

▶ Quercetin, a plant pigment with potent antioxidant and anti-inflammatory effects,[440,441] can also support the health of delicate blood vessels. Eat plenty of apples, red onions and red peppers.

▶ Turmeric's active ingredient, curcumin, has well-documented anti-inflammatory properties and can help to manage pain.[442] Add ground turmeric or freshly grated root to curries and dhals or make turmeric lattes.

▶ Omega-3 fatty acids can help with joint health and reduce inflammation as well as muscle damage.[443,444] The best sources are oily fish such as salmon, mackerel and sardines.

BRILLIANT STORY OF HOPE – PAIN

Tabitha is 16 years old and was diagnosed as autistic during her time at primary school. She developed some significant mental health challenges in her early teens, which resulted in self-harm and at one point she was hospitalized. She tested positive for Kryptopyrrole and has been more mentally stable since taking zinc and vitamin B6 (see chapter 2 for more details).

More recently, Tabitha has also been experiencing deep muscle pain and fatigue, which has been diagnosed as fibromyalgia. She was keen to learn how to manage the pain and has adopted a Mediterranean-style diet. She is now also taking magnesium, turmeric, PEA and omega-3 and feels so much better: she is more vibrant, in much less pain and feels empowered to manage her symptoms going forward.

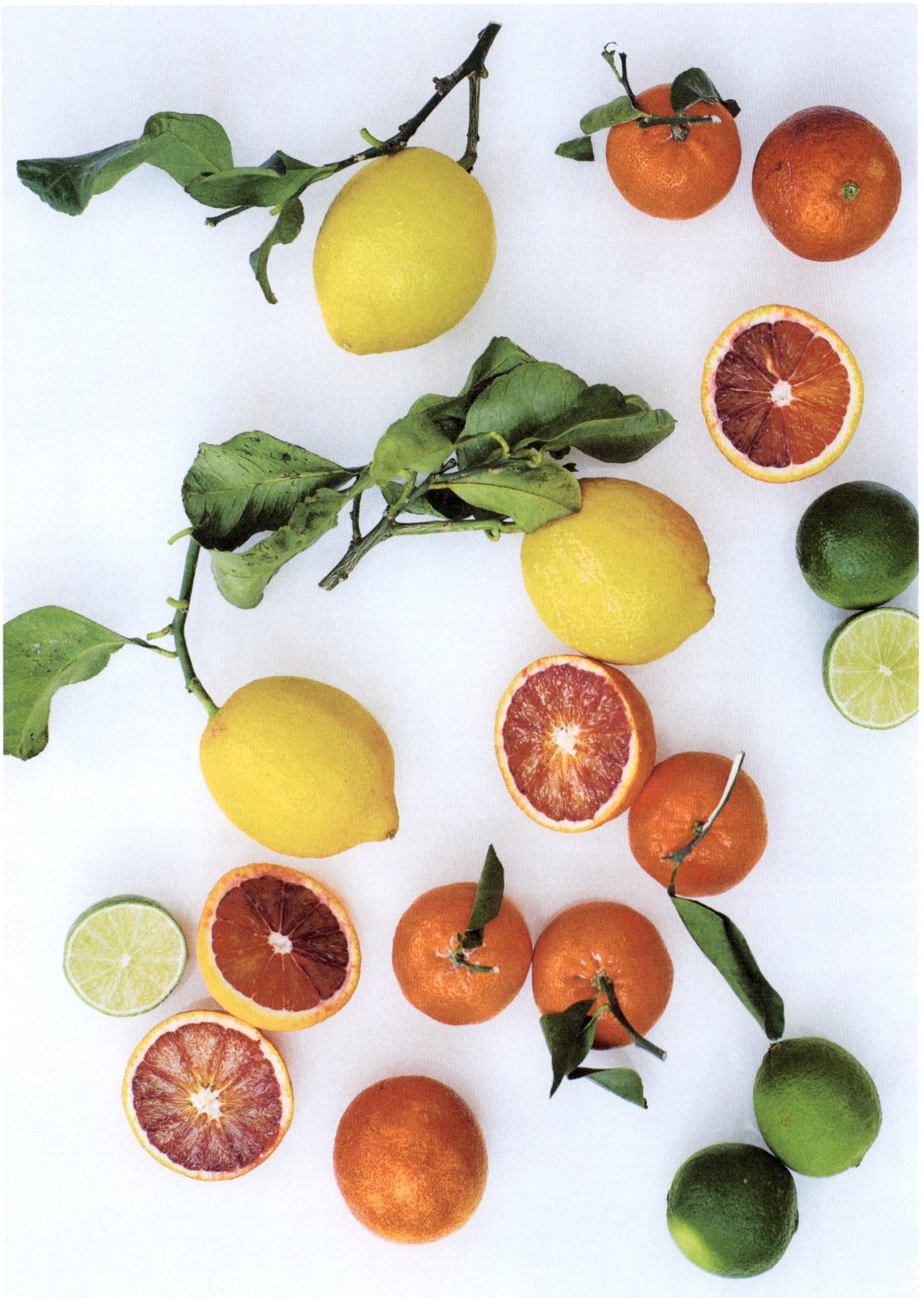

13 DIAL DOWN NOISE SENSITIVITY

If loud noises, such as fire alarms, hair dryers, vacuum cleaners, lawn mowers or the clamour of lots of people talking at once, really bother your child – they are not alone. Noise sensitivity is a common issue for many neurodivergent kids, and some sounds can be very overwhelming or distracting, causing them to feel really upset and uncomfortable, and making it hard for them to continue with normal activities like schoolwork or hanging out with their friends.

Kids who are non-speaking or find it hard to express their emotions through words, might react to noises that are too loud by covering their ears, fidgeting, becoming irritable, angry or over-excited, or by shutting down or no longer concentrating. Some of these responses may be down to other reasons, but if they stop when they wear headphones or move to somewhere quiet, then it is likely that they are displaying noise sensitivity.

Many kids with noise sensitivity find that living in a peaceful home, staying away from busy public places and wearing ear defenders when out and about can help to keep them calm. Discreet specialist ear plugs and loops are also available to block out distracting or dysregulating sounds.

Many neurodivergent kids feel calmer when they listen to soft sounds such as white noise, which is the type of noise produced by combining sounds of all different frequencies to create a calm, comforting noise. It provides a steady, consistent sound environment that can help mask other, more distracting, noises. Examples of white noise include appliances such as electric fans, air conditioning and washing machines, as well as the natural sound of rainfall, waterfalls and the rustling of trees. White noise devices are commonly used to aid sleep, help concentration or provide a calming atmosphere. Another way to address noise sensitivity is through Auditory Integration Therapy, a therapy that introduces special musical sounds via earphones to help rebalance the auditory circuits.

ASPECTS OF NOISE SENSITIVITY

Different types of sound sensitivity are commonly experienced by many kids and can cause distress and high anxiety. They include:

- Phonophobia – this describes when normal sounds, such as cars on the street, a kettle boiling or a door closing, become frightening.

- Hyperacusis – when they cannot handle regular noise like talking. Sounds can feel loud and hurt their ears. Hyperacusis can be worse in busy places like classrooms or parties.

- Misophonia – some kids get really upset by ordinary sounds, such as other people chewing their food or yawning.

▶ Tinnitus – this is a ringing or buzzing sound in the ears. At the same time kids might also feel dizzy or as if the room is spinning, or even nauseous. It is a condition that can wax and wane.

▶ 'Glue ear' or frequent ear infections can disturb hearing and make loud sounds seem even worse.

▶ Illness can also worsen noise sensitivity. Contracting Covid 19 has increased hearing loss and tinnitus in some people, even if they didn't get that unwell from the virus.[445]

As well as practical lifestyle changes to help manage noise sensitivity, there may be nutritional factors that can exacerbate how noises are perceived. Here are some things to consider if sound sensitivity is part of a broader overreactive nervous system response:

▶ Magnesium aids nerve function, controls blood pressure and even helps the brain to understand what our senses are communicating. A shortfall in magnesium may mean that certain medications are more likely to cause an imbalance in the ear, leading to poor hearing and tinnitus.[446,447]

▶ Vitamin B6 may also play a role in noise sensitivity when given with magnesium.[448,449]

▶ The mushroom lion's mane, taken as a supplement, has been indicated to prevent hearing deterioration and improve speech recognition.[450,451,452]

BRILLIANT STORY OF HOPE – NOISE SENSITIVITY

Noah, aged 6, was developing neurotypically, except his parents noticed that he got quite distressed at family gatherings or parties. He was also frightened of the vacuum cleaner and hand dryers. It was when he started school that things started to go downhill. He really struggled in the classroom and kept holding his ears and having meltdowns. It turned out he was very sensitive to the noise of a busy classroom.

He started wearing ear loops while he was at school which helped to block out any overwhelming noises. He also started to take magnesium and Vitamin B6 supplements to augment his diet. Quite quickly he was able to stay in the classroom most of the time and found it easier to learn because he could hear the teacher so much better.

14 EYESIGHT, READING & WRITING SUPPORT

A world with partial, distorted or no vision at all is a reality for many neurodivergent children. There are also genetic conditions which can predispose people's eyesight to deteriorate over time; and this can happen during childhood and the teenage years.

Sometimes visual impairment is picked up at a new baby check, but quite often vision difficulties are found later down the line. If a parent suspects their child is developing differently, one of the first steps to take is to have their eyes checked by an optometrist or an ophthalmologist. If any vision irregularities are identified, glasses may be prescribed to correct the vision, or eye patches and eye operations may be needed to help the child to see better. Some children with Dyslexia and any child with reading difficulties or visual problems also benefit from being assessed by a behavioural optometrist who looks for other irregularities that may hamper their ability to read and learn through visual prompts.

Not all visual differences are due to physical or mechanical eyesight problems. Some are caused by neurological brain differences as well as the strength and tone of the optic nerve, which connects the eye with the brain. Optic-nerve problems can present as headaches, colour blindness, visual snow and eye pain, as well as visual impairment. These may be congenital or acquired through inflammation or damage from viruses and other infections. Nutrition can play an important role in eye development, vision, the neurological system and immunity, and how the brain processes visual cues.

Many youngsters with Dyslexia and other slices of neurodivergence can have problems with clearly seeing letters and their order – some say the words jump around the page. This may be caused by an abnormal development of the visual 'magnocellular' nerve cells that enable us to detect the orientation and position of objects in space.[453] They help to rapidly identify letters and their order because they control our natural visual guidance. Research has found that these cells can become better developed over time when children consume plenty of omega-3 intake. I will elaborate more on this below.

As well as visual issues, people with Dyslexia, Dyspraxia and ADHD can also have issues with working memory, which can affect reading and writing.[454,455] Working memory is the ability to hold bites of information in the brain long enough to process them. A child with poor working memory can find it hard to follow more than one instruction at a time or easily lose track of what they are meant to do.

Dyslexia is highly heritable, which means multiple family members across different generations are likely to exhibit signs of the condition. Several genes have been identified as contributing to Dyslexia and primarily affecting reading and language-based skills. However, the origins of Dyslexia are complex, with various genetic, nutritional and environmental factors contributing.

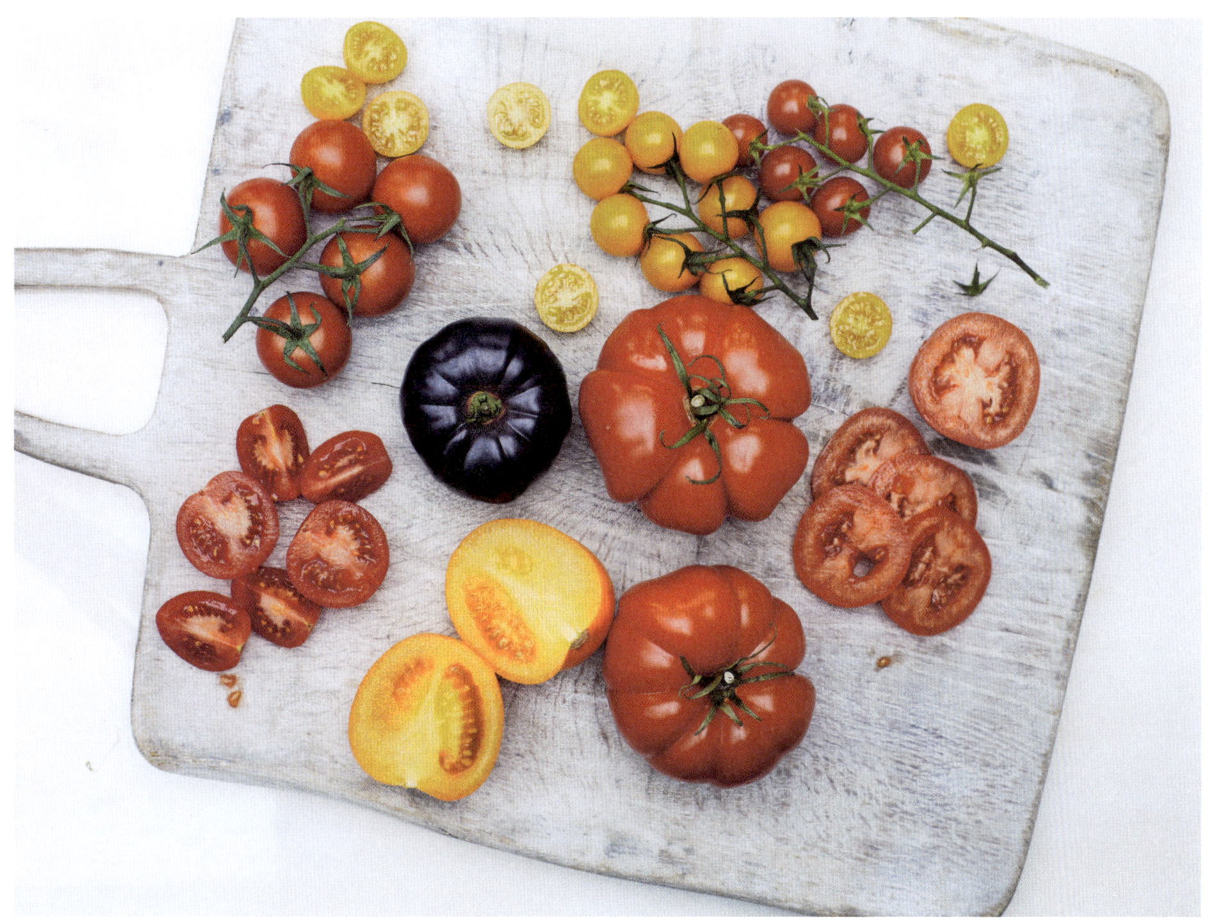

KEEP MINERALS IN BALANCE

One of the interesting patterns that has emerged from research into Dyslexia is the link with imbalances in certain nutrients. Studies have found that kids who struggle with their schoolwork are often sensitive to even mild imbalances in their copper and zinc levels, where typically copper is too high, and zinc is too low.[456,457,458,459]

Other research has suggested that exposure to environmental toxins such as lead (usually from paint chips) and cadmium (usually from passive smoking or the burning of fossil fuels) could also be associated with the development of signs of Dyslexia.[460] Interestingly, lead and cadmium exposure has also been found in conjunction with low zinc levels, so the effect of these together could be compounding the situation.[461]

Iron is another key mineral for brain function, and it seems that kids with Dyslexia might not be getting enough. Research has found that many dyslexics are either anaemic or have low iron levels,[462] which may be attributed to selective eating or not eating enough iron-rich foods.

THE RIGHT FATS

I listed quite a few healthy fats and oils in chapter 2 and specifically highlighted a unique brain fat called docosahexaenoic acid (DHA), the most important omega-3 essential fatty acid for both eye and brain development. Even small shortfalls can affect a child's ability to read and to track words along a line of text.[463] Low levels of DHA can also affect working memory and the ability to process visual prompts.[464]

Lack of certain brain fats has been particularly observed in a form of Dyslexia called Meares-Irlen Syndrome,[465] where poor signals between the eye and the brain cause the misreading of words or difficulty tracking words along a line, as well as an intolerance of bright lights. As well as insufficient DHA, people with Meares-Irlen Syndrome often have

BRILLIANT STORY OF HOPE – DYSLEXIA AND READING

Lucas was a very active boy, who would never sit still with his mum to read books. He was the sort of kid who would prefer to play when she read. When he got to school, he did not jump into reading like his peers, and he seemed distracted when there were any activities involving words. When he was 7 years old he was assessed for Dyslexia and was found to have problems tracking words along a line as well as poor working memory.

His parents decided to step up his nutrition with plenty of oily fish, eggs, dairy and red meat. Because he had chicken skin (see page 23) on the tops of his arms and face, they also gave him a high-strength omega-3 fish oil supplement. By the following term Lucas had caught up by two reading stages and was able to remember spellings much more easily.

very low cholesterol levels.[466] And if cholesterol levels are too low, then the transport of omega-3 to the eye becomes less efficient. (See chapter 2 for the importance of enough cholesterol).

VITAMINS AND ANTIOXIDANTS

Certain vitamins are also super-important for eye health and visual processing. Research has found that optimizing levels of vitamins A, C, D and E can be very helpful in supporting optical health.[467] Deficiencies in these key vitamins can lead to sensitivity to bright lights and poor sight.

Specific antioxidants called carotenoids have been identified to help with eye health and cognitive performance, working in unison together. Carotenoids are pigments that have antioxidant properties and are found in the red, yellow and orange colours in fruit and veg such as tomatoes, carrots, peppers, oranges and mangoes.

Additional antioxidants that can help with eye health include Lutein[468] and Zeaxanthin[469,470] and therefore may be helpful in supporting people who live with Dyslexia. They are believed to provide protection against damage caused by blue light from screens.[471] You can find them in foods like spinach, kale, peas and broccoli as well as egg yolks.

THE NUTRITIONAL APPROACH TO UNLOCKING SPEECH & LANGUAGE DELAY 15

Many children are reaching school age with either no speech or with significant speech delay, with current statistics showing that speech, language and communication support has become the most common type of Special Educational Needs (SEN) required, and the numbers are growing all the time.

Various factors can influence speech development, including mechanical causes of speech delay such as tongue-tie, lip-tie and cleft palate. Breastfeeding is thought to aid speech development as it encourages better oral motor skills. The ability to chew food well is a key motor skill that helps develop oral tone, which in turn helps with speech – this is one of the reasons why it is important to give children a variety of foods rather than only soft purée and melt-in-the-mouth snacks. Non-food exercises to help with oral muscle tone include blowing whistles, pipes and balloons and using a straw to drink.

Ear infections and glue ear are common childhood conditions that can hugely affect hearing and speech intelligibility and lead to speech delay.[472] Improving a child's underlying immunity can prevent such infections, and so too can identifying food allergies.

There are also rare medical co-morbidities that should be checked out by a neurologist, such as seizure activity. It is also important to check for cerebral folate deficiency (not enough folic acid getting to the brain) and mitochondrial dysfunction (mitochondria are the 'batteries' in all the cells in our body that control energy, speech and swallowing.)[473]

NUTRIENTS FOR GAINING SPEECH, LANGUAGE AND COMMUNICATION

Gaining speech is a very complex task and the reality is that a child with a delayed speech or a regression in speech will need a great deal of input both from speech and language therapists as well as nutrition input. It can take longer than anticipated and I always say that making improvements in this part of a child's development needs to be taken on like a marathon, not a sprint! The most important thing is to celebrate the little milestone wins – one new word at a time.

The gluten-free/casein-free diet can be transformative for some children and sometimes a child's voice will emerge once they are well established on this diet (see chapter 8).

Here are some key nutrients to consider, all of which have been found to help stimulate speech in autistic children[474] and would be worth exploring if your child has any kind of speech, communication or language delay:

► Omega-3 is well-documented for aiding development of verbal and non-verbal communication[475,476] (see chapter 2 for more details).

► B vitamins – especially B6, folate and B12 – are crucial in supporting speech and communication. A trial giving autistic children a combination of folate and vitamin B12 twice weekly over a three-month period led to improved expressive language and an average gain of overall skills of 7.7 months' development.[477] Vitamin B12 has also been found to help improve Gestalt Language Processing known as 'scripting', or 'echolalia', in autistic children, which is when a child speaks with memorized phrases, songs or words.[478]

► Vitamin D can help support speech, language and communication delay if a child is deficient, which may be due to its anti-inflammatory effect.[479,480]

► Palmitoylethanolamide (PEA) is an anti-inflammatory fatty acid and may help specifically with supporting expressive language.[481] Foods rich in PEA include eggs, soya beans, peanuts and milk.

► The flavonoids within extra virgin olive oil, as well as other flavonoids called luteolin, quercetin and rutin, all have antioxidant and anti-inflammatory properties that can potentially support speech and communication – for instance a four-month study of kids taking taking a mixture of these flavonoids found that 10 per cent of the children with regressive Autism restored the level of speech they had lost.[482] Foods such as celery, parsley, thyme and green (bell) peppers are good sources of luteolin. Quercetin is found in red onions, red (bell) peppers and apples, while rutin is naturally present in buckwheat, citrus fruits and figs as well as apples. A glug of extra virgin olive oil poured over food is an easy win when you are starting out!

FOCUS ON STUTTERING

Stuttering is another common childhood speech issue, which often starts around preschool age. Developmental stuttering, the most prevalent type in children, can happen when a child's speech and language development lags, or when their brain is functioning faster than their mouth can articulate. Sometimes, it can also be stress- or anxiety-induced.

Stuttering can also be triggered by *Streptococcus* infections.[483,484] Therefore, if stuttering begins abruptly after a throat infection or scarlet fever, it is crucial to consult with a medical professional to assess whether a 'strep' infection has triggered a neuroinflammatory autoimmune response. Strep is not the only infection that can lead to stuttering; one of the symptoms reported in active Covid 19[485] and Long Covid cases has been the onset of stuttering[486] and other neurological changes,[487] presumably due to the chronic inflammation and oxidative stress that the virus causes.

Nutritionally, studies have found that children who stutter often have lower levels of core minerals such as calcium, magnesium, zinc, potassium, chromium and molybdenum.[488,489] Low levels of vitamin B1 (thiamine), which is another essential nutrient, have also been associated with it.[490,491]

BRILLIANT STORY OF HOPE – STUTTERING

Matteo spoke relatively early, but around the time his baby brother was born and he started nursery, he developed a stutter. Initially, his parents assumed this was an emotional response to change. However, Matteo's stutter persisted for a long time. His parents had read how magnesium and vitamin B1 could make a positive difference to a child's development, and they started off by applying a magnesium lotion to the soles of Matteo's feet, supercharging his diet with magnesium and vitamin B1-rich foods and supplementing with both. Matteo's stutter became much less pronounced quite quickly and by the following school term it was no longer obvious to his teachers anymore.

HOW TO ENHANCE FOCUS, CONCENTRATION & IQ

16

Focus and concentration can be challenging for us all at the best of times. Our kids live in a world where distraction is all around, and they are now exposed to information overload and are rarely away from screens. For many kids with ADHD as well as other neurodivergence, focus and concentration can be really testing. Distractions from everyday tasks such as getting dressed or making breakfast can set them off on tangents. This can make every single day exhausting, unrewarding and frustrating, as tasks are left unfinished or done in a scattered way.

Teachers and parents can be very frustrated by their students, as they can see that they are super-clever inside and if only they could concentrate and focus, they would excel at school. A lack of focus and concentration is also deeply frustrating for the students themselves (even if they won't always admit it) and can be the key reason why they are held back from performing at their best.

DOPAMINE IS KEY

One of the key reasons why children cannot focus or concentrate is because they don't make enough of the neurotransmitter dopamine or find it hard to keep their dopamine levels in balance. Dopamine not only helps with focus and concentration but also gives us the motivation to begin tasks and helps generates that feeling of pleasure when a task is completed. Here are the key nutrients needed to create and synthesize dopamine well:

- Tyrosine is an amino acid and the building block of dopamine. Kids get it primarily from eating protein, which is abundant in poultry and other meat, fish, seafood, eggs, pulses, nuts and seeds.

- Iron is one of the key nutrient buddies to support the conversion of tyrosine to dopamine. Low levels of iron can be one reason why your kids can feel unfocused, unmotivated and impulsive. See chapter 2 for a deep dive into the importance of iron.

- Vitamin D is another buddy needed to create and maintain enough dopamine. During winter, when there is relatively little sunshine, it has been found that taking a Vitamin D supplement can help with inattention and poor focus.[492,493]

- Magnesium and zinc do not make dopamine directly, but they help to regulate dopamine, and both are often found to be low in the ADHD population. They are also helpful to take in supplement form alongside prescribed ADHD medications such as methylphenidate, as they seem to enhance its effectiveness.[494,495]

NATURAL DOPAMINE HIGHS

Dopamine can be made in all sorts of surprising ways, usually through pleasurable activities and experiences. These include the following:

▶ Natural light is important for making dopamine, especially spending time outdoors in the early morning.[496,497] When the light hits the retina in the eye, it affects pupil dilation, and this triggers more dopamine production. And – even better – the effect seems to be cumulative if your child is exposed to good levels of light over several days. This can be achieved by as little as 20 minutes outside each morning. That's one good reason for walking at least part of the way to school every day!

▶ Physical exercise is one of the best things anyone can do to raise dopamine levels. Children with ADHD are often better focused and less impulsive after exercise.[498] The link between exercise and better focus and improved mood regulation continues through adulthood[499] and could well be why many people find exercise such an important part of their daily life.

▶ Equally, listening to music is enjoyable and rewarding. Music can also be intensely motivational,[500] and it is thought that listening to music, singing or playing an instrument can bolster your child's dopamine levels.[501]

▶ As well as reducing stress, a relaxing meditation session can also help to stimulate dopamine in the brain, leading to feelings of pleasure and wellbeing.[502] Teaching your child meditation and mindfulness skills can be very helpful if you feel they will be receptive.

▶ ADHDers usually find change uplifting, and this is because new experiences and visiting new places can help to stimulate the creation and release of dopamine. So, change things around if your kid is in a funk!

BRILLIANT STORY OF HOPE – ADHD

Lily is a clever 14-year-old who was recently diagnosed with ADHD as she was really struggling to focus on her studies at school and was underperforming. She had sailed through primary school, so this diagnosis came as quite a surprise to her and her parents. In the year leading up to the diagnosis, she had chosen to adopt a mainly plant-based diet and she had also started her periods, which were very heavy each month. She was getting very tired, looked paler than usual and had developed acne, which was bothering her.

This seemed like a low-iron and low-zinc scenario, and that was confirmed by blood tests. Lily agreed to eat more foods containing these minerals and to take some supplements. She experienced an almost immediate increase in energy levels, and it was much easier to focus and keep on task. Her skin also improved, which she was delighted about.

WHAT HELPS AND HINDERS IQ AND LEARNING?

Intelligence Quotient (IQ) is a measure of relative ability in various mental skills. There has long been debate over whether IQ is down to nature, nurture, or a mixture of both. Even small differences in IQ can make a huge difference to grades and performance at school as well as accessing and understanding more intellectual matters.

A generalized increase in global IQs was achieved during the twentieth century, but since 1975 this increase has actually reversed in some countries. The IQ increase was researched by an American-born New Zealander, James R. Flynn, who attributed it to better nutrition.[503] The year 1975 marked the peak of IQ, which is what became known as the 'Flynn effect'. Since then, overall IQ has been declining. We do not know exactly why, but it is not thought to be

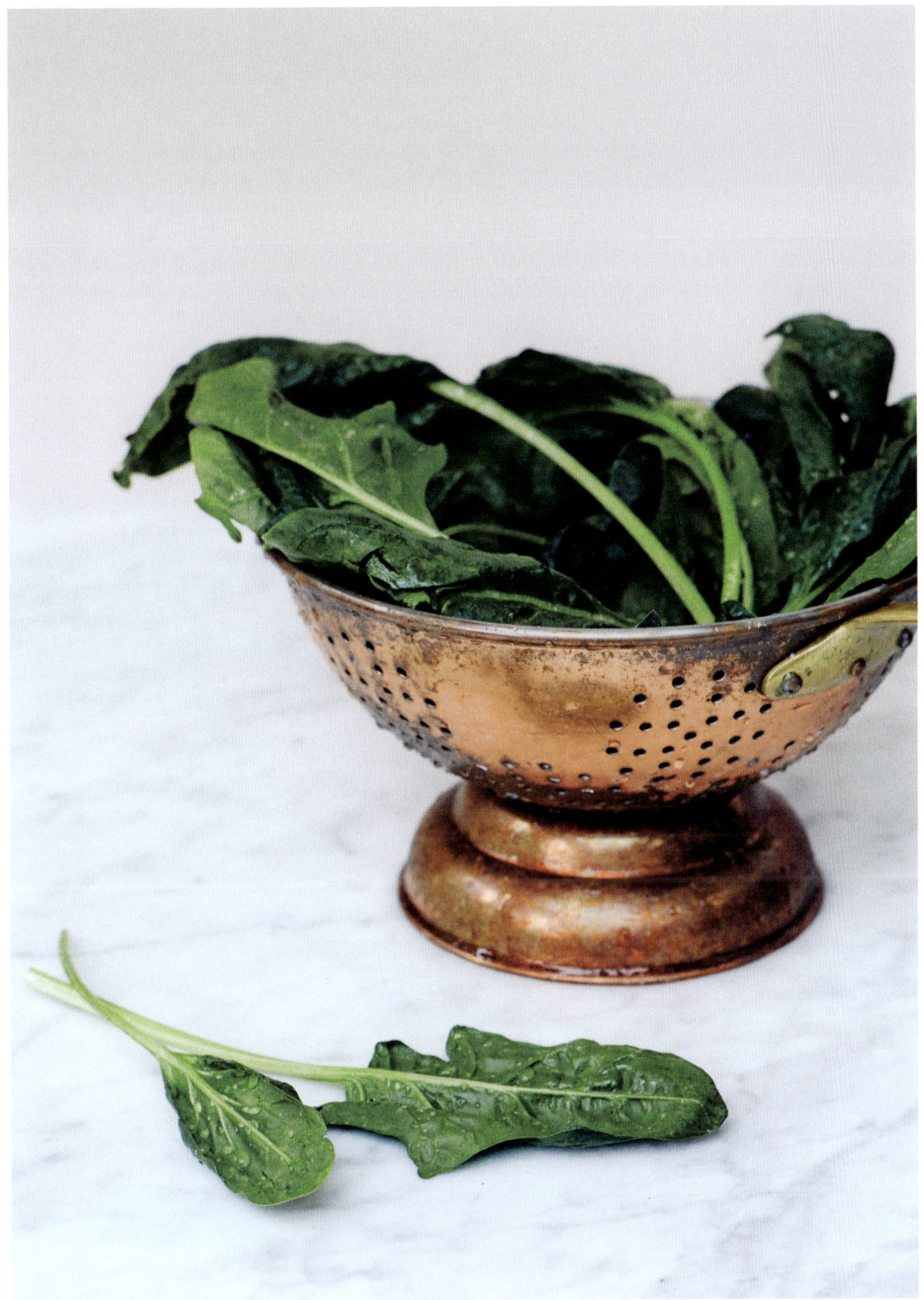

due to genetics. That mostly leaves nutritional and environmental factors in the frame to consider.

ENOUGH MINERALS

During pregnancy it is important that a woman consumes enough iron from red meat, green veg or pulses and iodine from fish or seaweed – two minerals that are key for building IQ in the unborn child. For this reason, nutritional advice for parents weaning a baby onto solids is that they are given iron-rich foods twice daily at the age of 6 months old. This is the point when blood iron levels start dropping off, especially if a baby has been entirely breastfed. This is because breast milk only contains tiny traces of iron or none at all.

ULTRA-PROCESSED FOODS

A study of 7,000 UK-based children linked eating too many processed foods at a young age with a slightly lower IQ and, conversely, that eating more fruit, vegetables and home-cooked foods seemed to increase IQ slightly by the time a child is 8 years old.[504,505] So upping the good-quality nutrient-dense foods really counts!

ENVIRONMENTAL TOXINS

A rise in air pollution may in part explain the decrease in IQ. One study found that installing a portable HEPA (high efficiency particulate air) filter in the home during pregnancy resulted in babies with a higher IQ even if the expectant mother was not taking pregnancy vitamins, was highly stressed and was less well-educated.[506,507]

Lead is a well-known and extremely common neurotoxin[508] that can affect both cognition and IQ[509] even when exposure is relatively low.[510] It is now thought that there is no safe level of lead in the blood[511] and that we need to take every precaution to prevent exposure.

Houses built before the 1970s often have old layers of paint on their walls, doors and skirting boards that contain lead. If these layers chip or particles from the paint accumulate on the floor in dust, and a child inadvertently puts these into their mouth, their brain is exposed to this toxic heavy metal. In the US and Europe all homes need to have a lead inspection certificate, but this is not the case in the UK; nor is lead toxicity routinely tested in kids with lower IQ.

The best way to reduce lead exposure, is to clean frequently using a HEPA vacuum and to regularly wipe floors, windows and windowsills with a damp cloth. Also, traditional children's toys may contain some lead.[512,513]

A child with a full stomach is less likely to absorb lead, and a child who consumes enough foods containing iron, calcium, vitamin C and protein will also absorb less lead.[514] If you think you or your child have been exposed to lead, it is important for them to consume plenty of foods containing pectin, such as apples, pears and citrus fruits.[515,516] Lead displaces calcium in the bones, so I also recommend consuming plenty of calcium-rich foods to prevent the lead from damaging the bones.[517,518]

MOVE FROM PROCRASTINATION & APATHY TO TAKING ACTION

17

I took a long time to write this chapter, as I can be quite a procrastinator myself! If you tend to procrastinate or your youngster has lost their sparkle and feels disinterested in life or lacking in motivation, then this chapter will probably resonate with you.

THE ART OF PROCRASTINATION

Procrastination is, at its core, a natural attempt to escape discomfort – both physical and emotional. This shying away from or delaying doing tasks often lies deep in our child's desire to stay within their comfort zone. Procrastination can prevent them from following through with their intentions and accomplishing their goals. Most procrastination is a way to escape from uncomfortable internal emotions, such as fear, the embarrassment of getting something wrong or not understanding the task enough to perform it.[519] It can happen when there is frustration, despair, boredom, or not enough mental stamina in the frame. It can equally be due to anger and resentment or anxiety. It is also where you prefer the instant tiny dopamine hit of something exciting to the discomfort of making an effort to get the task started – and the bigger dopamine reward from completion is too far off to be attractive.

By dividing tasks into smaller, more manageable chunks and identifying and developing strategies to regulate these emotional triggers and help your kids feel better about themselves, we can help them to ditch these internal distractions, increase traction and, ultimately, overcome their habit of procrastination.

APATHY AND LACK OF MOTIVATION

Apathy is a lack of interest, enthusiasm or motivation towards daily activities,[520] and is becoming increasingly common, especially among neurodivergent kids. This may present as indifference towards schoolwork, socialization, hobbies or even routine tasks such as personal hygiene and getting dressed. Who is used to hearing from their kids: 'I just don't care! It's soooooo boring...'?

This often leads to a lack of motivation to finish tasks or to achieve. When our kids feel apathetic, they may eventually complete a task, but it is often done grudgingly with little enthusiasm. Several factors can cause apathy, including depression, anxiety and low self-esteem.

Apathy can also be part of some neurodivergence such as Dyslexia, dyspraxia or ADHD, all of which can in themselves make it more challenging to start tasks and see them through to completion, as this requires the ability to focus and filter out distractions – skills that many youngsters find hard to master.

Apathy is associated with inactivity in both the frontal cortex and the basal ganglia areas of the brain, the parts of the brain that also assist with skills associated with learning, memory and behaviour, as well as movement, planning, organizing and decision making.[521,522,523,524]

KEY NUTRIENTS FOR INCREASED MOTIVATION AND PERFORMANCE

Nutrients that support areas of the brain that help with mental stamina and motivation include:

- Omega-3 fatty acids are vital for brain development and function. Increased intake of oily fish and other omega-3 rich foods is key. Research indicates that supplements can enhance motivation.[525,526]

- Choline is essential for synthesizing neurotransmitters related to motivation and executive function.[527,528] Add in plenty of eggs, liver, sunflower seeds and peanuts.

- Zinc supplements can improve motivation and learning skills, and reduce apathy.[529] Also increase zinc-rich foods such as seafood, meat, dairy, nuts and seeds.

- Vitamin B12 supplements can reduce apathy, depression, brain fog and irritability.[530] Vitamin B12 foods include meat, fish and eggs.

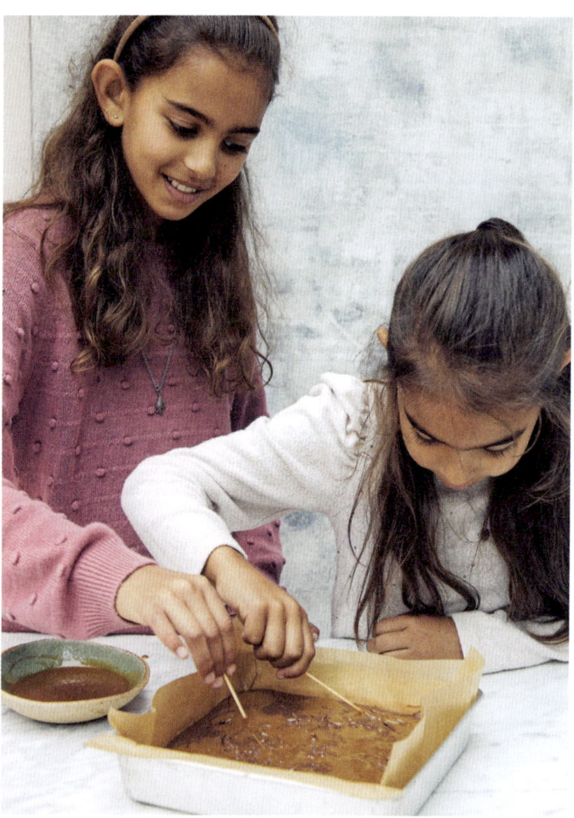

BRILLIANT STORY OF HOPE – MOTIVATION

Getting Billy, aged 14, out of bed in the morning was a huge struggle and he started to refuse to go to school. He seemed apathetic and unmotivated to do much in the day except to play computer games. It was even hard to get him to go for a walk or kick a ball. His parents assumed this was the beginnings of depression and were extremely worried.

His diet was a typical teen diet of ultra-processed foods and lots of sugar, so his parents decided to take a bold leap and stop buying any ultra-processed foods, and always ensured the fruit bowl was topped up. He was grumpy at first about not having his favourite snacks to hand, but he soon realized that this was a permanent change for the whole family.

His parents also gave him B vitamins and zinc as well as an omega-3 supplement. He started to wake up naturally at 7.30am and was soon saying that he would like to see friends and that he was prepared to give school another go – and once he was back at school, he loved it.

THE NUTRITION ROADMAP AND FOLLOWING MY RECIPES

As you have read so far, *Brain Brilliance* shares many of my clinical pearls and stories of hope from the wonderful families who have been under the care of NatureDoc clinic (names have been changed for anonymity). See this book as a nutrition toolkit to set the foundations for a healthier and happier life ahead, however your child's brain is wired. And as you have learned, a specific neurodivergent 'label' isn't necessary to benefit from a better diet and nutrition, and you can start nourishing your child's brain cells right away!

You have learned a nutrition roadmap to support the neurodivergent mind and now it is time to put everything into action and get busy in the kitchen! Whether you are cooking for one child or a tribe of kids, the most important thing is to have fun and enjoy your time cooking together.

I have created 60 delicious and nutritious recipes for you to build into your food repertoire. These all incorporate the principles of providing nutrient-dense brain foods in a way that is appealing and delicious for the neurodivergent child's palate. Some are super simple, using only a handful of ingredients which you don't even need to cook. Choose one new recipe a week and before you know it your kids will be eating plenty of yummy new foods stuffed full of nourishment.

You will see that I use less sugar than conventional recipes and try to use honey, maple syrup and coconut sugar as well as fruit, vanilla and cinnamon to ease the blood glucose highs and lows.

For the highly selective eaters you will find your fair share of crunchy beige recipes that are packed with goodness. I have also provided food allergy switches for the top 14 key allergens where possible, so no one misses out. And because we are all so busy, I've suggested the best way to store the food so you always have healthy options to hand.

Now is the time for you to make a big difference in your child's life and future. Many of you will recognize these traits in yourselves or your spouses, and the beauty of this approach is that you and the rest of the family can also benefit from these approaches.

So, make a plan of what steps you are going to take, and when you are going to take them. Go back over the chapters to highlight the things you think are 'lightbulbs' that shine brilliantly for you. Do set yourselves small milestones and celebrate the little wins. And then look back in a year's time on how much you have achieved.

Enjoy my recipes and enjoy nourishing your child's brilliant brain to become the best version of themselves – one mouthful at a time!

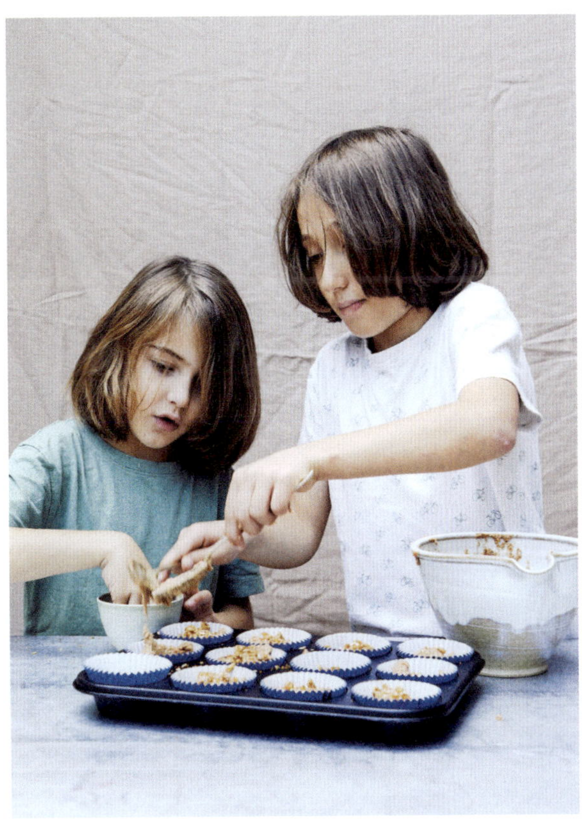

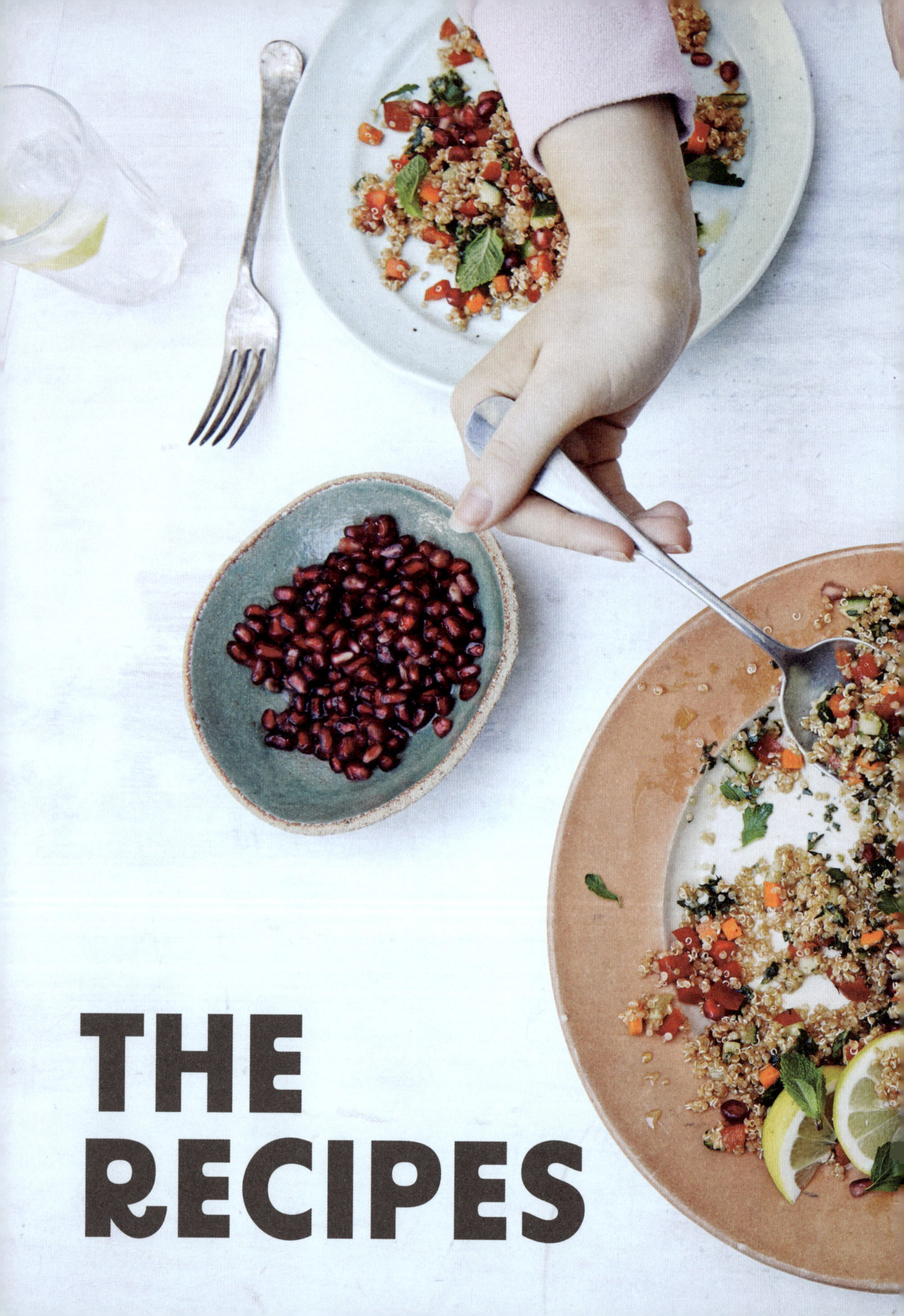

THE RECIPES

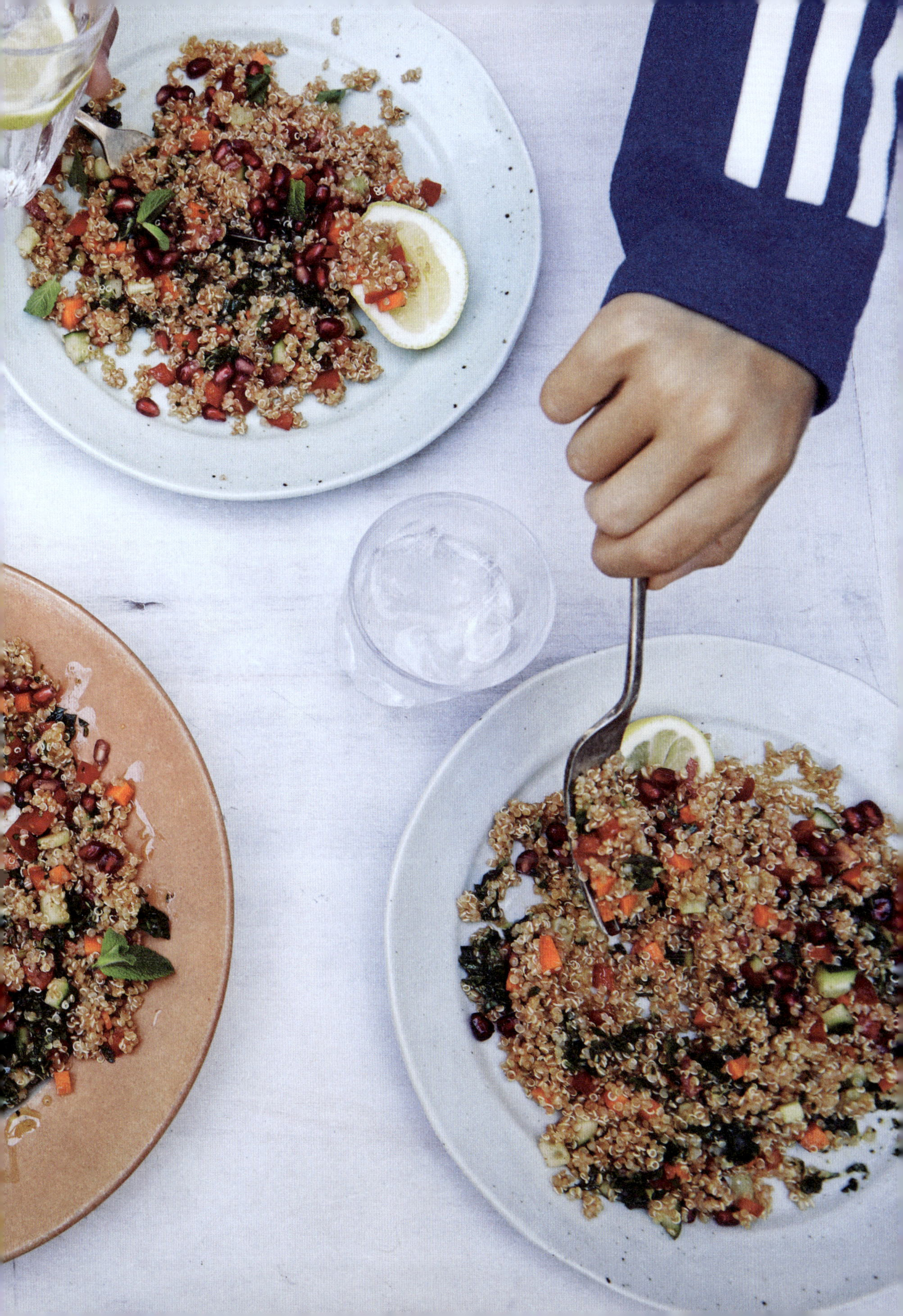

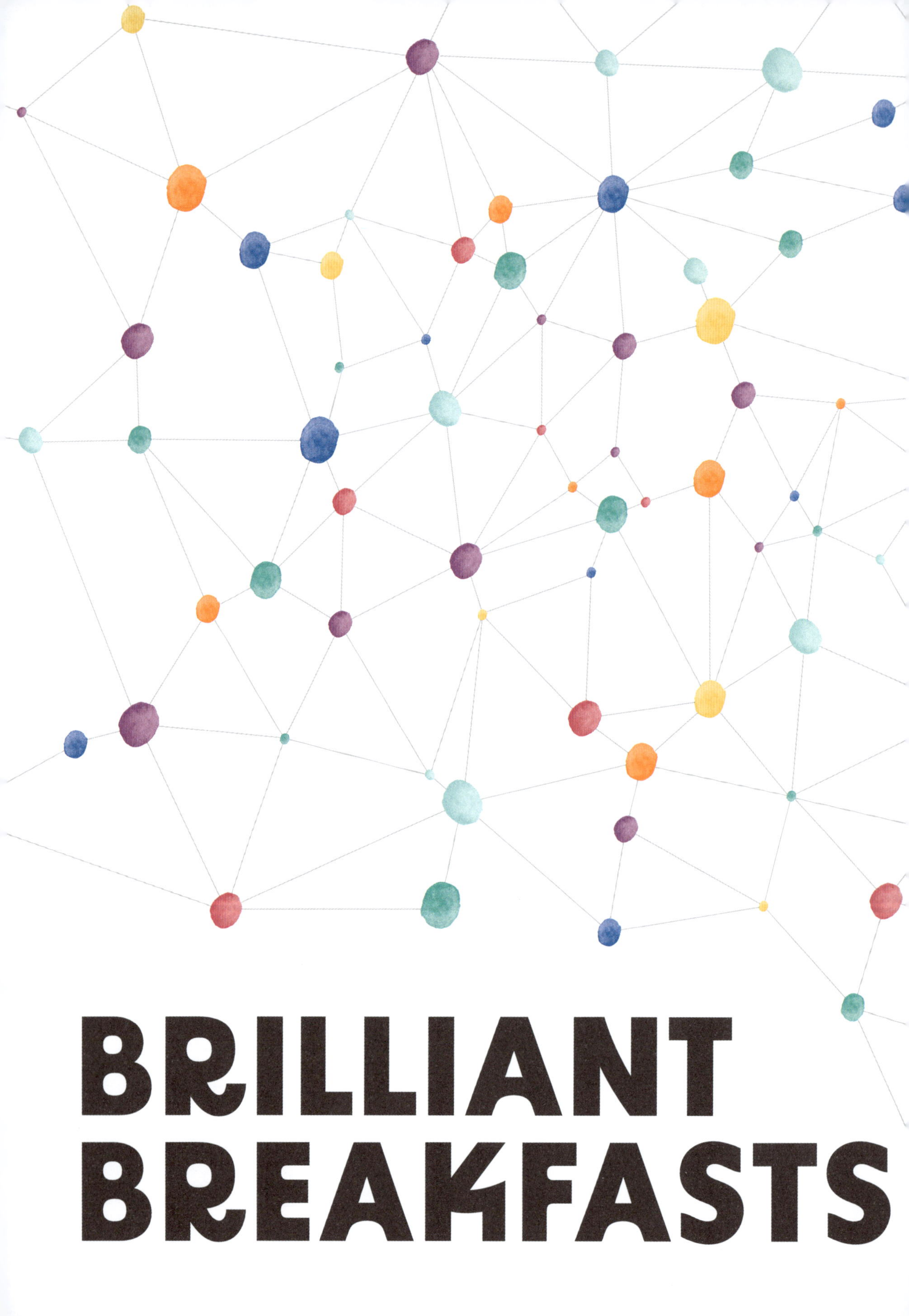

BRILLIANT BREAKFASTS

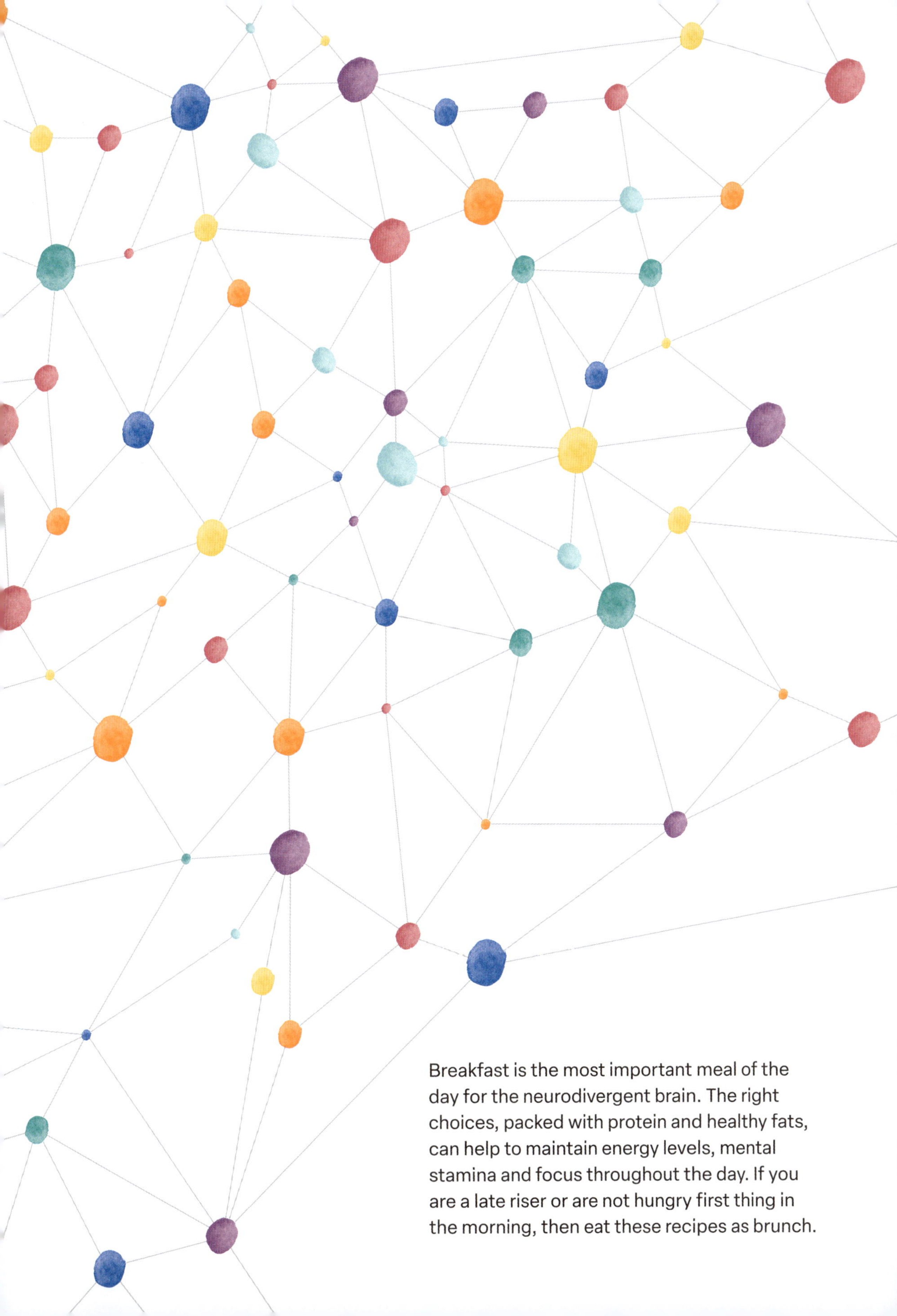

Breakfast is the most important meal of the day for the neurodivergent brain. The right choices, packed with protein and healthy fats, can help to maintain energy levels, mental stamina and focus throughout the day. If you are a late riser or are not hungry first thing in the morning, then eat these recipes as brunch.

CHOCOLATE ORANGE QUINOA PORRIDGE

Serves 2

40g (½ cup) quinoa flakes
240ml (1 cup) milk of choice, plus extra to serve
1 Tbsp tahini (sesame paste)
1 tsp chia seeds
2 tsp cacao or unsweetened cocoa powder
zest of 1 unwaxed orange
2 tsp maple syrup
raspberries, to garnish
dark chocolate drops (optional)

Chocolate and orange pair beautifully together and make a gloriously decadent morning porridge. Make this using protein-packed quinoa flakes, tahini and chia seeds – you are more likely to feel full until lunchtime and avoid a mid-morning energy crash. You can find quinoa flakes in your local health food shop or buy online.

Put all the ingredients except the raspberries and chocolate drops in a saucepan over a medium heat. Stir well to combine everything and cook for 6–8 minutes until the quinoa flakes are soft and cooked through.

Pour into two serving bowls and sprinkle over some raspberries, and a few dark chocolate drops and some orange zest if you wish, plus a little extra milk to help cool it down and for a nice consistency.

Cool and store in the refrigerator for up to 24 hours. Reheat gently, adding more milk as needed.

Swap the tahini for a nut butter (hazelnut, cashew or almond) or sunflower seed butter.

dairy-free
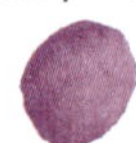
gluten-free
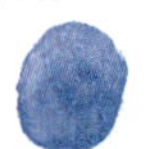
nut-free

sesame-free

egg-free

soy-free

vegetarian
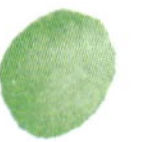

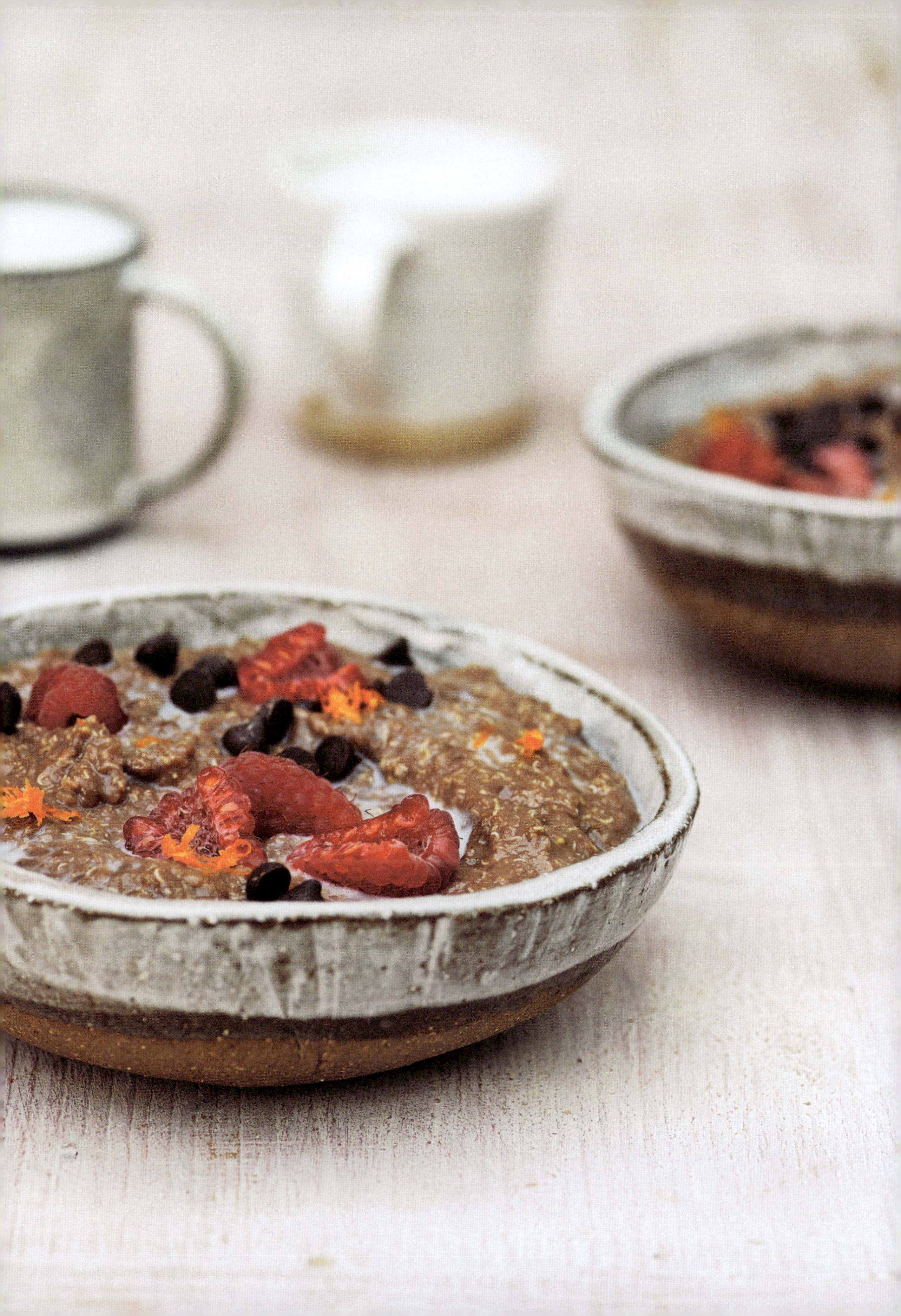

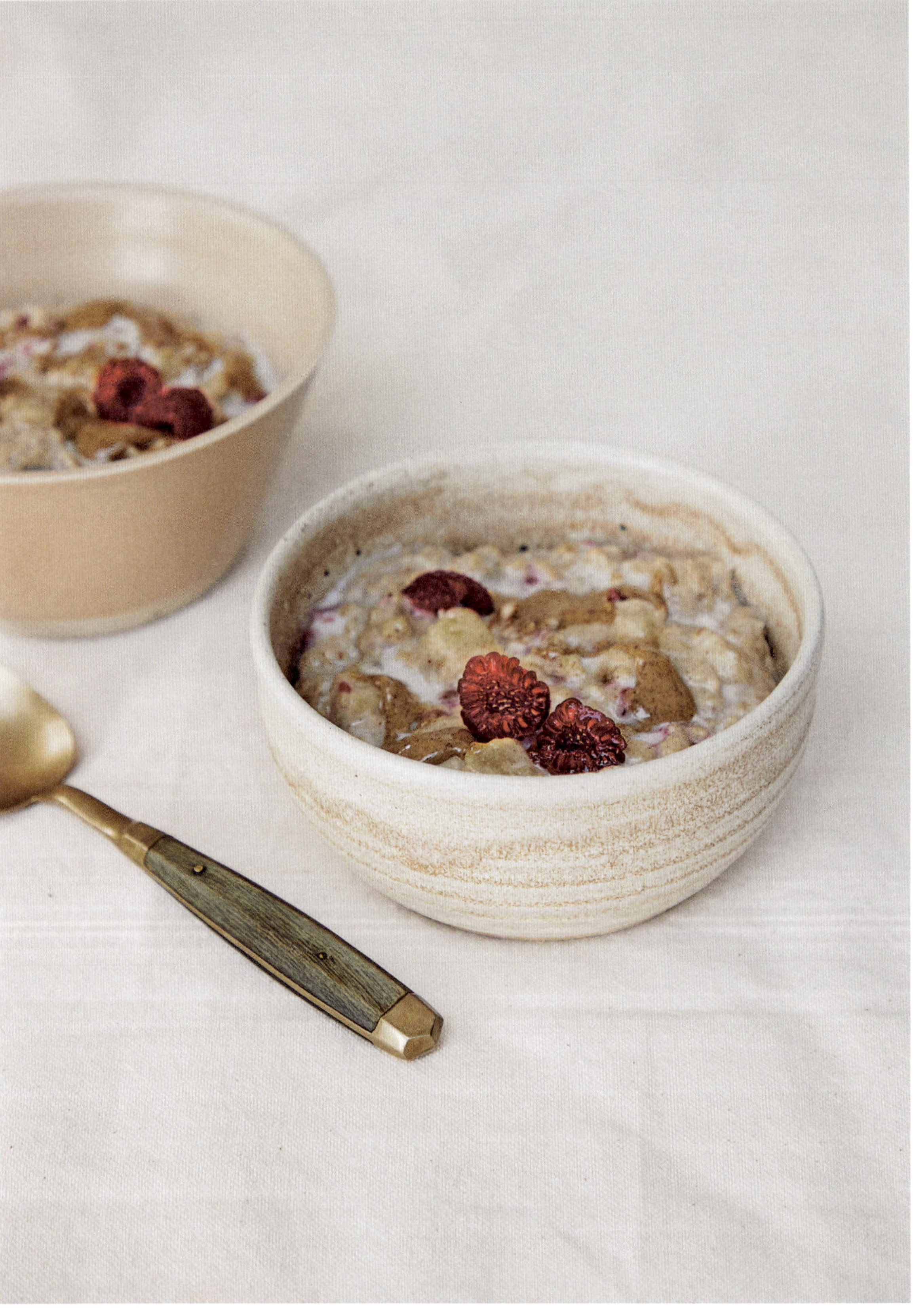

PEAR & RASPBERRY CINNAMON PORRIDGE

This is warming and comforting: creamy protein-dense porridge flavoured with lightly cooked fresh fruit and sweet cinnamon.

Cracking an egg into the oats as they cook is a brilliant idea; no one will taste the difference but you get the lovely benefits of the protein, iron and choline that eggs contain. This is one of my key hacks for my neurodivergent clients who need to eat more protein at breakfast but are not keen on eating an egg served on its own.

Serves 2

10g (scant 1 Tbsp) butter
1 pear, peeled, cored and diced
1 tsp ground cinnamon
8 raspberries (fresh or frozen)
50g (½ cup) rolled oats
240ml (1 cup) milk of choice, plus extra to serve
1 Tbsp almond butter
1 egg, preferably free-range
2 tsp maple syrup (optional)

Melt the butter in a saucepan and lightly fry the diced pear with the cinnamon for about 4–5 minutes or until soft. Stir in the raspberries.

Add the rolled oats, milk and almond butter and then crack the egg into the mixture, stirring well to combine all the ingredients. Cook over a gentle heat for 4–5 minutes until thick and creamy, stirring well every minute or so.

Pour into two serving bowls, drizzle over a little extra milk to cool it and for a better consistency; add some maple syrup if you like a little extra sweetness.

Cool and store in the refrigerator for up to 24 hours and reheat gently, adding more milk as needed.

Swap the butter for coconut oil or olive oil and use dairy-free milk.

dairy-free

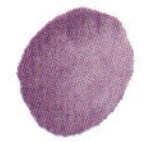

Use gluten-free oats, quinoa flakes, millet flakes or buckwheat flakes.

gluten-free

Switch the almond butter to tahini (sesame paste) or sunflower seed butter.

nut-free

sesame-free

Omit the egg.

egg-free

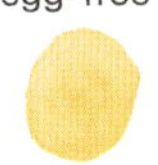

soy-free

vegetarian

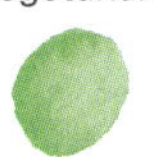

CRISPY FETA & CHICKPEA OMELETTE

Serves 1–2

1 Tbsp olive oil
2 eggs, preferably free-range
4 Tbsp gram (chickpea) flour (or 4 Tbsp dried chickpeas (garbanzo beans) ground to a coarse powder)
1 Tbsp crumbled feta cheese
1 tsp fresh parsley or ½ tsp dried (optional)
1 tsp fresh dill or ½ tsp dried

To serve (optional)
chilli sauce
avocado slices

This is the perfect savoury breakfast to set your brain up to be brilliant all day. It is the breakfast I have eaten most days while writing this book and it's given me great brain stamina! The combination of eggs, gram (chickpea) flour and feta is divine. Both crispy and cheesy, this is perfect for people who 'don't like eggs' – you are sure to be hooked!

For the more adventurous, you can gently fry some grated courgette (zucchini), chopped onion and red (bell) pepper or spinach before pouring the eggy batter into the pan, or just add some peas – frozen or fresh – with the mixture itself.

Heat the oil over a high heat in a small frying pan (skillet).

Crack the eggs into a small bowl, then add the gram flour, feta and herbs. Mix well with a fork so all the ingredients are combined. (Alternatively, blend the ingredients in a mini food processor if you prefer the consistency super-smooth.)

Pour the batter into the hot frying pan, tilting the pan so that the mixture is evenly spread.

Cook for 3–4 minutes until the omelette is browned and crispy on the bottom and then flip and cook the other side for a further 3–4 minutes. (For a crispier experience, cook for a further minute or two on each side.)

Transfer to a plate and serve with chilli sauce and sliced avocado if you wish. Serve immediately.

Swap the feta for 1 tablespoon of yeast flakes plus a pinch of salt.

Instead of the eggs, you can use 3 tablespoons of chickpea (garbanzo bean) water, known as aquafaba, stirred in straight from the can to help bind the chickpea flour.

dairy-free
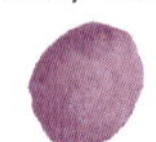
gluten-free

nut-free
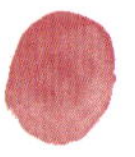
sesame-free

egg-free

soy-free
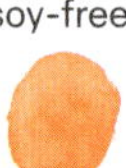
vegetarian
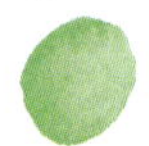

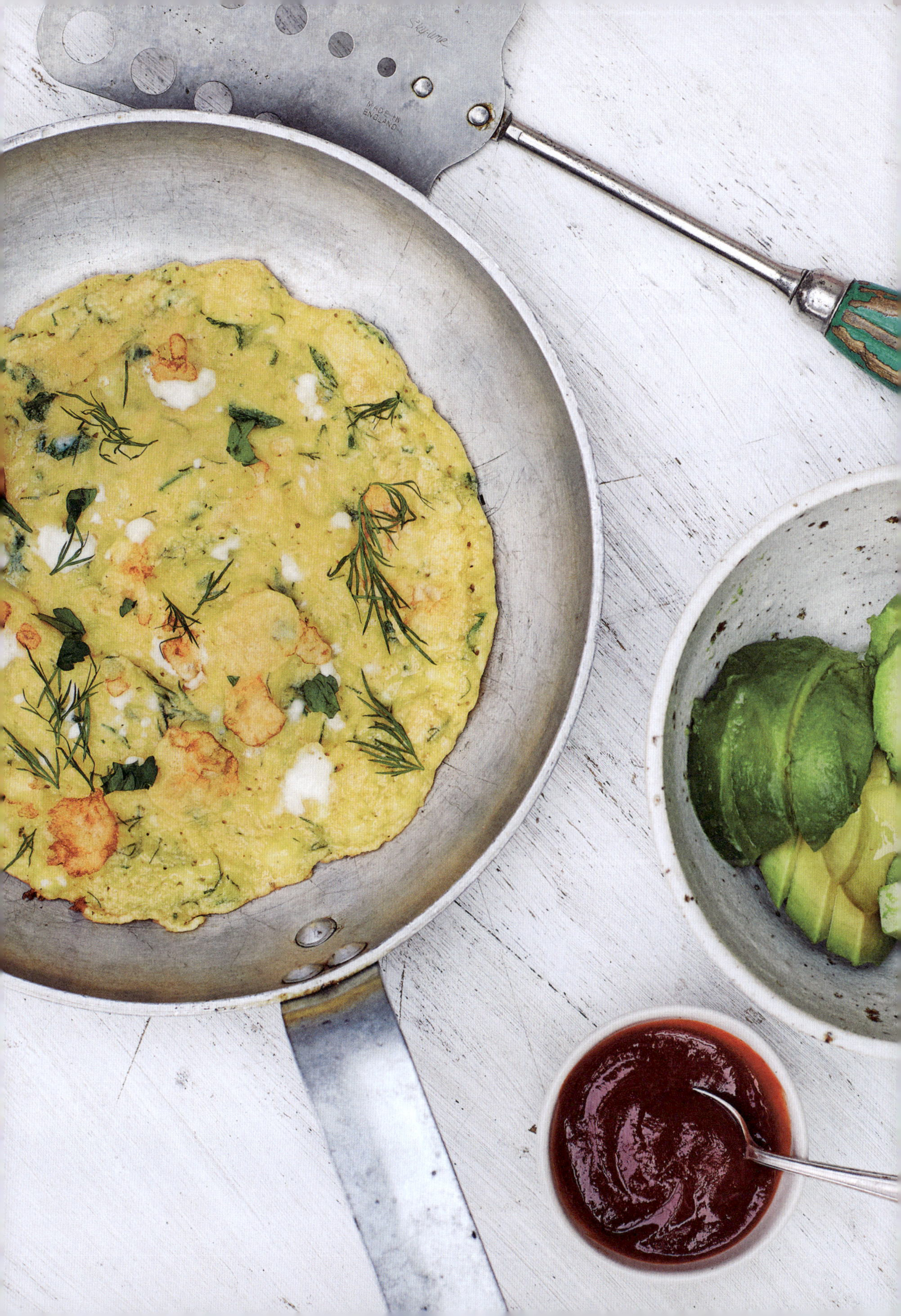
Sky-line
MADE IN
ENGLAND

CHOCCY HAZELNUT WAFFLES

These waffles will ensure you start the day with a touch of joy in your step! You can easily prepare them the day before or batch-cook at the weekend. Chocolate and hazelnuts are a winning combo, plus there is sweet potato hidden in the mix, which gives a little extra natural sweetness.

Dark chocolate, hazelnuts and sweet potato all contain magnesium and other key minerals that help keep the brain calm and focused. Eggs add a boost of protein and choline, both key nutrients for a brilliant brain, and this is a perfect way to get reluctant egg-eaters to enjoy a protein-rich breakfast.

These waffles also make a brilliant snack, and they freeze beautifully – just pop in the toaster straight from the freezer to defrost them and make them nice and crunchy.

Makes 6–7

150g (generous 1 cup) whole hazelnuts
100g (1 cup) rolled oats
3 Tbsp cacao or unsweetened cocoa powder
2 Tbsp coconut sugar or light muscovado sugar
1 small sweet potato, peeled and finely grated (shredded)
3 eggs, preferably free-range
1 tsp vanilla extract
2 Tbsp maple syrup
6 Tbsp milk of choice
50g (about ¼ cup) dark chocolate drops
A few sprigs of mint, ricotta, maple syrup and mixed berries, to serve (optional)

Turn on your waffle-maker and set to the highest heat.

Put the hazelnuts and oats into a food processor and blitz for about a minute, or until the hazelnuts are ground into a coarse flour.

Add in the cacao powder and coconut sugar, and blitz again for a few seconds. Add the sweet potato, then the eggs, vanilla extract, maple syrup and milk. Blitz again for another minute or two until the mixture is a cake-like batter. There may still be some hazelnuts and oats visible – this is OK! Stir the chocolate drops into the mixture.

When the waffle-maker is hot, spoon in enough batter just to fill each waffle iron (you can usually cook two waffles at a time); try not to overfill them or the batter will spill and make a mess. Cook the waffles for 5 minutes, checking them after around 4 minutes and turn them over. They should be ready once the steam has stopped coming out of the waffle-maker. Place on a wire rack to cool slightly while you make the rest.

Serve as they are or with ricotta, a drizzle of maple syrup and mixed berries and some mint leaves for garnish, if liked. Store in an airtight tin for up to 3 days or in the freezer for up to 3 months.

Use gluten-free oats, quinoa flakes, millet flakes or buckwheat flakes.

dairy-free

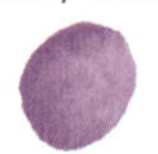

gluten-free

sesame-free

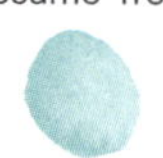

soy-free

vegetarian

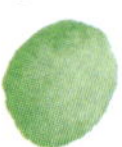

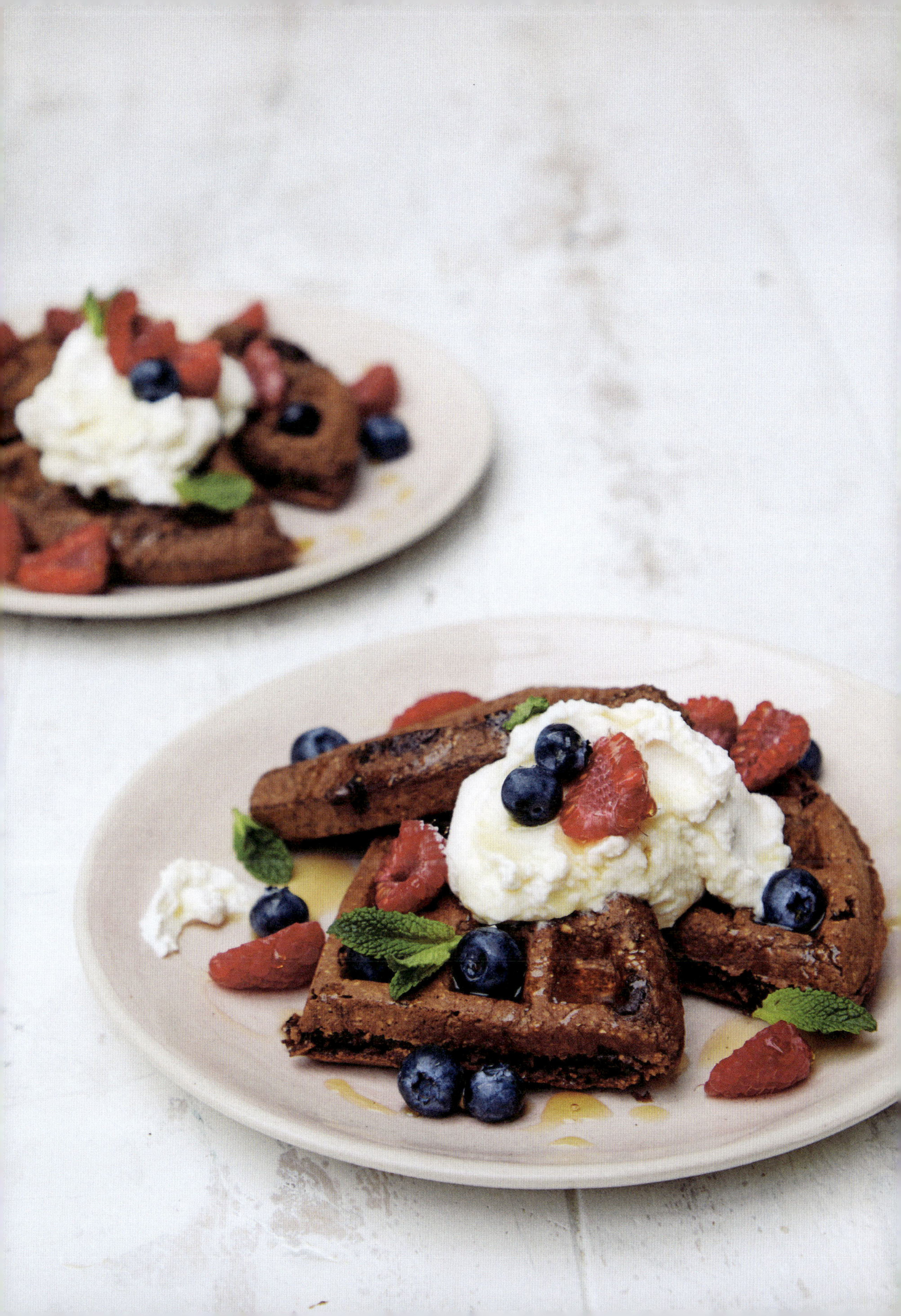

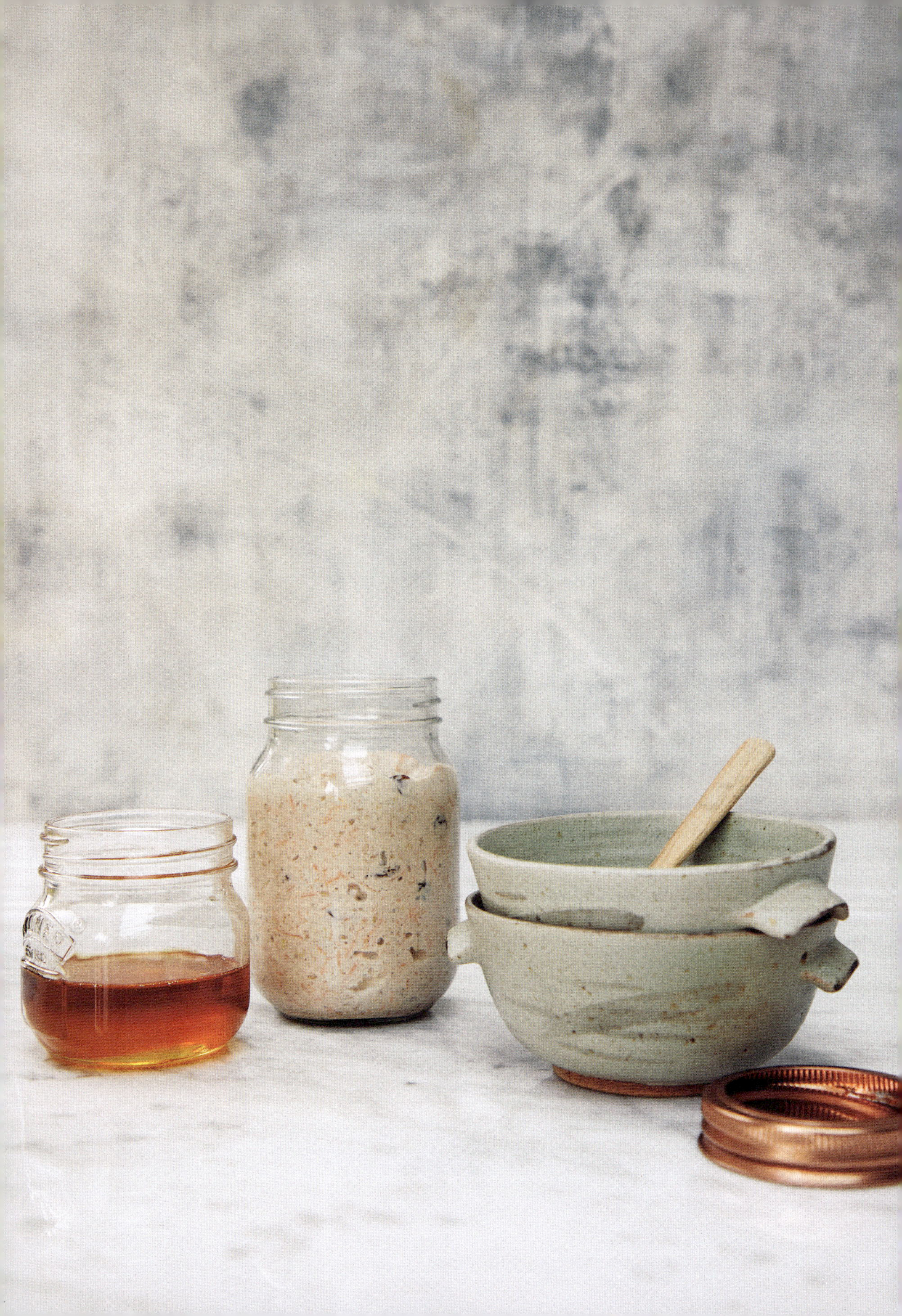

CARROT CAKE OVERNIGHT OATS

Serves 2

200g (1 cup) full-fat plain yoghurt or kefir
2 tsp vanilla extract (optional)
60g (scant ½ cup) rolled oats
2 small apples, finely grated (shredded)
1 small carrot, finely grated (shredded)
2 tsp mixed spice
4 tsp raisins
4 tsp pecan nuts, quartered
4 tsp flaxseed (ground or whole)
4 Tbsp milk of choice
runny honey or maple syrup, to drizzle

A dreamy creamy oaty breakfast, carrot-cake style!

Overnight oats are one of the most gut-friendly foods you can eat. Soaked rather than cooked, the oats are easier to digest. They retain more resistant starch, which acts as a prebiotic to nourish the good bacteria in your gut. The original recipe was developed by a Swiss physician who used raw food to help his patients recover from illness. This makes a brilliant speedy breakfast that you prepare the night before, so you can just grab it in the morning when you are in a rush.

Mix the yoghurt with the vanilla in a bowl, then stir in all the ingredients except the milk and the honey. Cover and place in the refrigerator overnight.

In the morning, stir in the milk and serve with a drizzle of honey or maple syrup. On cold mornings, warm up the milk before stirring it in, so that the oat mixture is less chilly.

Store, covered, in the refrigerator for up to 3 days. You may need a little extra milk if you leave it longer than overnight.

Use plain coconut yoghurt and coconut milk.

Use gluten-free oats, quinoa flakes, millet flakes or buckwheat flakes.

Swap the pecan nuts for a mix of sunflower seeds and pumpkin seeds or hulled hemp seeds.

dairy-free
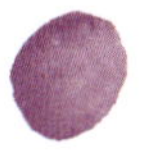

gluten-free

nut-free

sesame-free

egg-free

soy-free

vegetarian
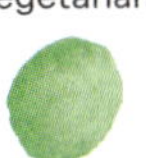

TURKEY & APPLE EGGY BREAD

Serves 2

butter, for spreading, plus an extra pat for frying (or use a little olive oil)
2 slices of wholemeal sourdough bread
1 slice of cooked turkey breast
¼ apple, cored and grated (shredded)
1 slice of Gouda cheese
1 egg, preferably free-range

This is a fantastic version of classic eggy bread. Turkey is a meat that is rich in tryptophan, an amino acid we can only obtain from food, which is super-important for making the mood-boosting neurotransmitter serotonin. Gouda, a cheese low in lactose and high in protein, is a source of relaxing GABA (gamma-aminobutyric acid), another neurotransmitter in the brain that reduces stress and anxiety, while the egg provides the key nutrient choline.

Butter both slices of bread on one side. Place the turkey on one slice, then the apple and then the Gouda. Press the second bread slice on top to make a sandwich.

Crack the egg onto a saucer and mix it with a fork. Dip the sandwich into the egg, ensuring both sides are evenly coated.

Melt the pat of butter in a frying pan (skillet) over a medium heat. Fry the eggy sandwich for 3–4 minutes on each side or until golden brown. Enjoy this hot.

Use a dairy-free spread. Omit the cheese.
Use gluten-free sourdough.

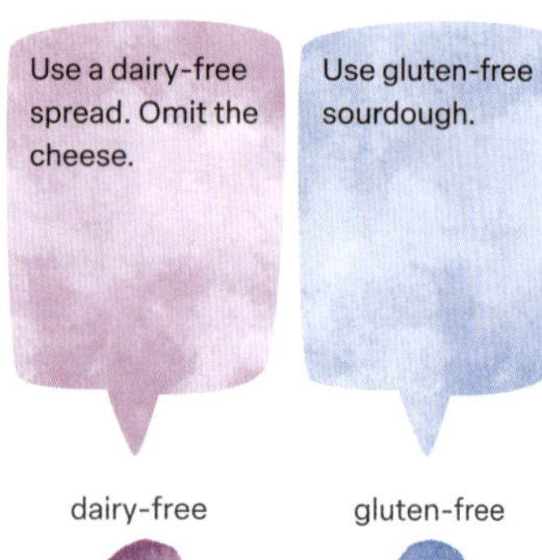

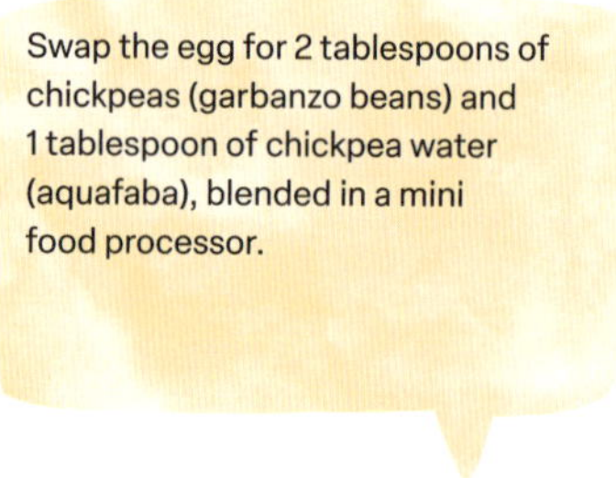

dairy-free · gluten-free · nut-free · sesame-free · egg-free · soy-free

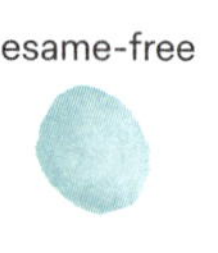

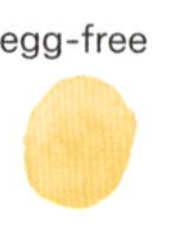

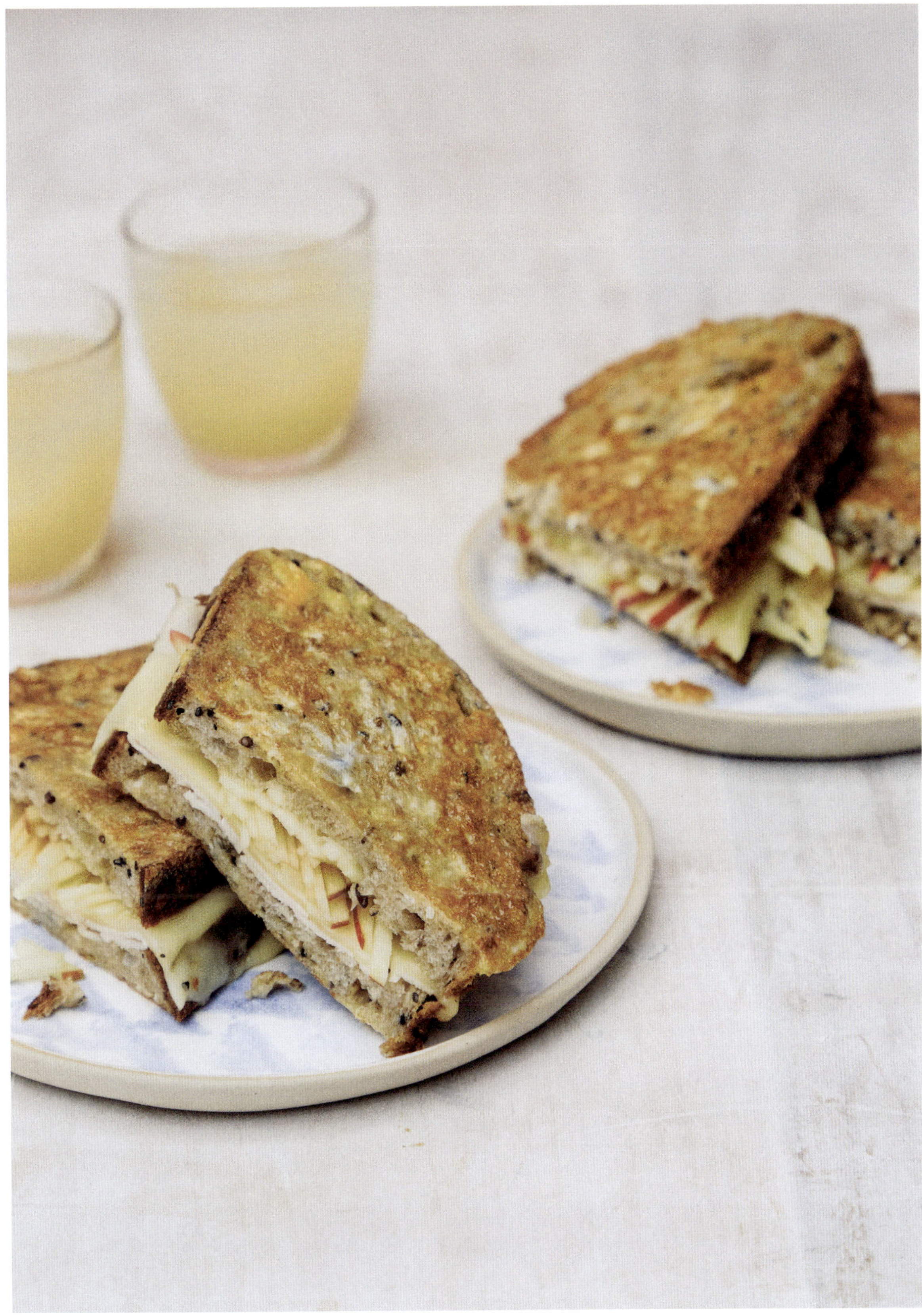

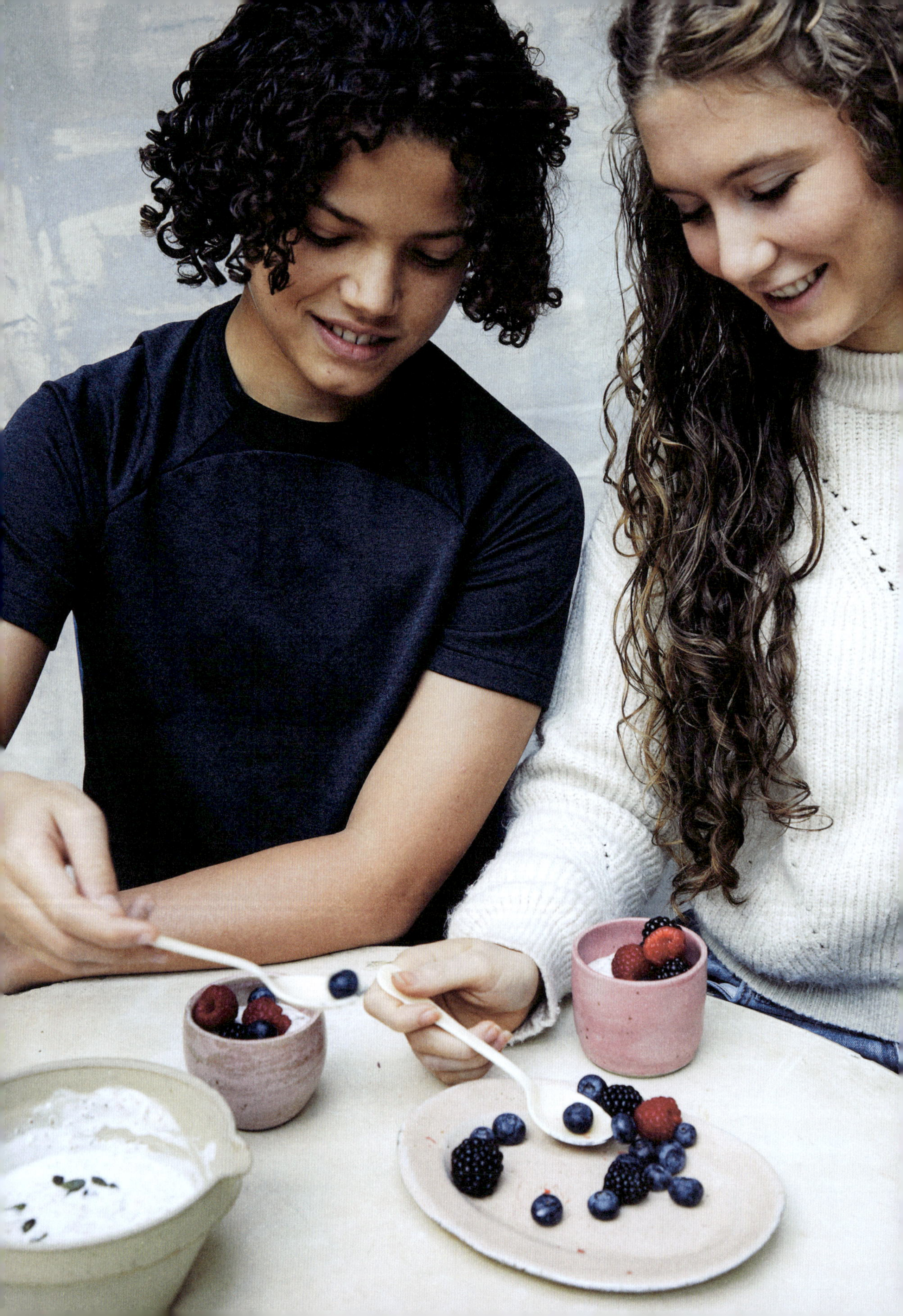

OMEGA BERRY GREEK YOGHURT

Serves 2

8 Tbsp full-fat plain Greek yoghurt
1 tsp vanilla extract
2 generous tsp honey (runny or set)
2 heaped tsp hulled hemp seeds
2 heaped tsp chia seeds
2 heaped tsp ground flaxseed
2 heaped tsp pumpkin seeds
mixed berries, fresh or frozen

This is another very simple breakfast that you can prepare the night before to make your morning easier. Overnight soaking allows the seeds to soften and become more digestible.

Greek yoghurt is a great source of protein and calcium and also helps to bolster the diversity of the gut microbiome. Berries contain important brain-supporting flavonoids, and seeds are rich in zinc and omega-3. If you intend to eat this regularly, make up a jarful with this seed mix to have on hand.

Mix the yoghurt, vanilla, honey and seeds together in a bowl and leave for 15 minutes or overnight.

Sprinkle on the berries and store in the refrigerator until you are ready to eat.

Store in a jar in the refrigerator for up to 3 days.

TIP
It is totally OK to eat this mixture without soaking the seeds, but those who are sensitive to textures will want to let the seeds soak. You can also blitz it – berries and all – in a blender to make it extra smooth. Alternatively, if you prefer a crunchy texture, sprinkle on some granola and add your choice of extra nuts and seeds.

Swap the Greek yoghurt for 4 tablespoons of coconut yoghurt, 2 tablespoons of plant-based milk and 2 tablespoons of dairy-free vanilla protein powder.

dairy-free
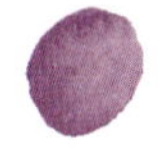
gluten-free

nut-free
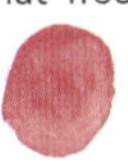
sesame-free

egg-free

soy-free
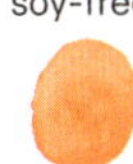
vegetarian
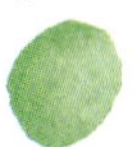

BROCCOLI BREAKFAST CLUB

Serves 2

2 slices of rye bread
4 broccoli florets, chopped into tiny florets
2 Tbsp Turmeric Hummus (page 176)
½ avocado, stoned, peeled and smashed with a fork
2 Tbsp Tamari Toasted Seeds (page 180)
microgreens, alfalfa sprouts or broccoli sprouts (optional)
wedge of fresh lime

Once you join the 'Broccoli Breakfast Club' there will be no looking back! This open toasted sandwich ticks all the boxes for goodness and taste. It's beautifully savoury and simple to assemble and stack high.

If you are in a rush, use cooked broccoli florets left over from the night before and shop-bought hummus. To add extra protein, serve with a poached egg, cooked flaked salmon or a slice of smoked salmon.

Toast the rye bread and meanwhile blanch the broccoli florets in a pan of boiling water for a minute, then drain.

Spread the hummus on the bread, and layer on the avocado, broccoli and toasted seeds. Top with microgreens if you have some handy. Finally give it a big squeeze of lime juice.

Once assembled, tuck in immediately. You can keep it in the refrigerator for up to 2 hours but be aware the avocado will start to discolour.

Use gluten-free bread.

Use tahini-free hummus.

Use toasted seeds without tamari.

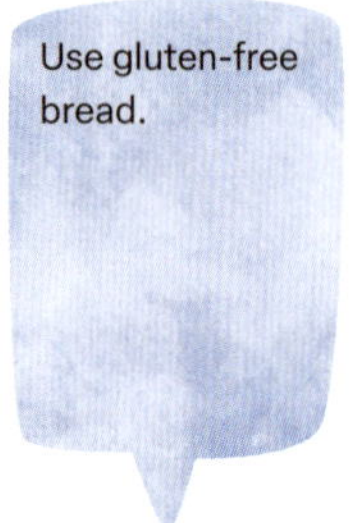

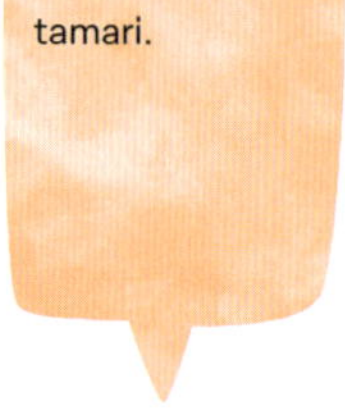

dairy-free

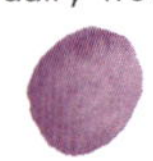

gluten-free

nut-free

sesame-free

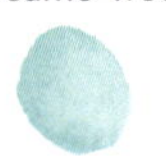

egg-free

soy-free

vegetarian

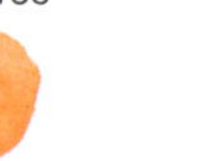

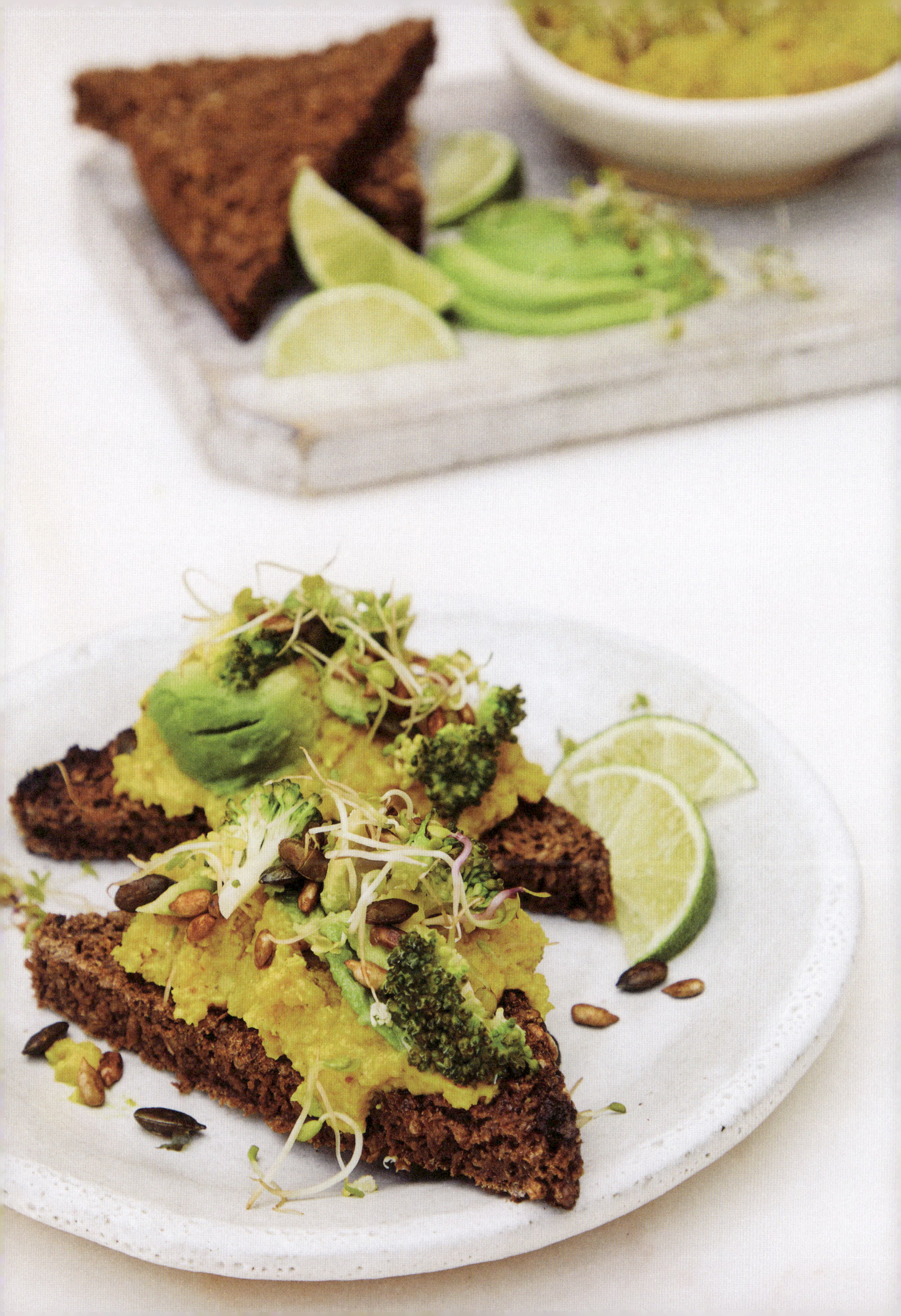

PEANUT BUTTER & RASPBERRY SOURDOUGH

Lots of people love peanut butter and jam (jelly) sandwiches, so this is my healthier version that is better for the blood glucose and the brain.

Use best-quality sourdough bread and peanut butter. Sourdough gives the blood glucose less of a spike than standard bread, especially when paired with protein and healthy fat from the peanut butter. Fresh fruit adds a nice touch of sweetness.

Serves 1

1 slice of sourdough bread
2 generous tsp peanut butter
½ small banana, peeled and thinly sliced
5 raspberries

Toast the sourdough and quickly spread on the peanut butter nice and thickly.

Add a layer of thinly sliced banana and top with raspberries – you can leave them whole or squish down.

Eat quickly while it is still warm.

Use gluten-free sourdough.
Swap peanut butter for cream cheese or tahini (sesame paste).

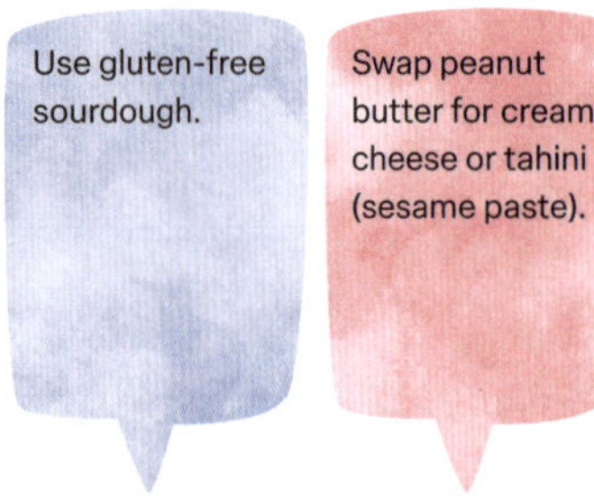

dairy-free
gluten-free
nut-free
sesame-free
egg-free
soy-free
vegetarian

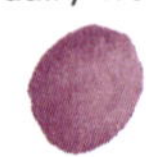

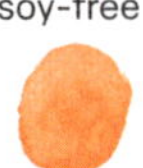

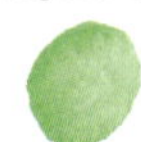

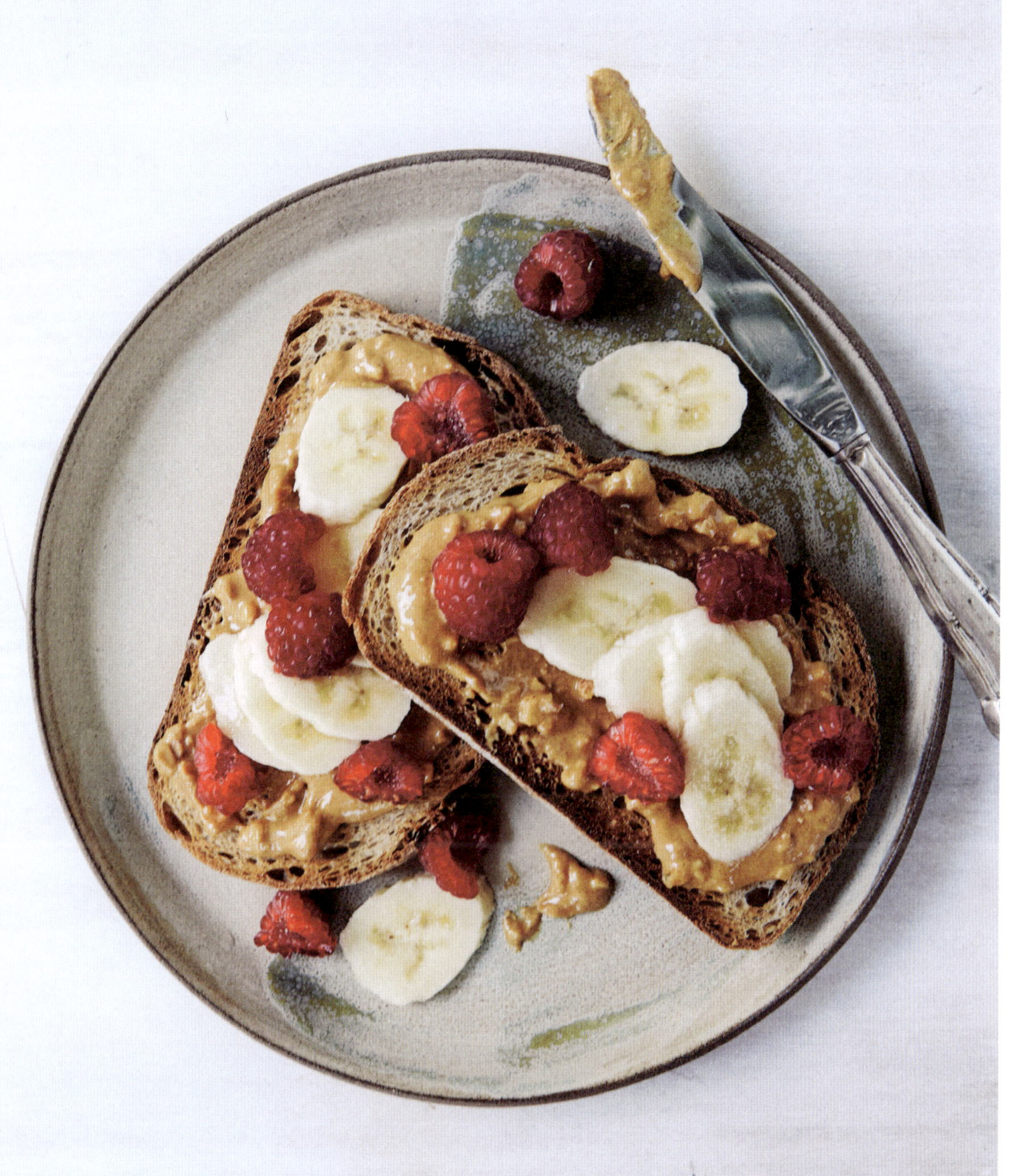

SWEET POTATO & WALNUT MUFFINS

These muffins are packed with protein and fibre in the form of sweet potato, oats and walnuts and flavoured with blood-glucose-balancing spices. Made ahead they are great if your day starts early, and you need to take breakfast with you. They are also perfect as an afternoon snack. What's more, the muffins freeze well and are quick to defrost.

Makes 6 large muffins

140g (5oz) sweet potato, peeled and roughly chopped
125g (1¼ cups) rolled oats
1 tsp baking powder
½ tsp bicarbonate of soda (baking soda)
½ tsp salt
½ tsp mixed spice
¼ tsp grated nutmeg
30g (scant ⅓ cup) chopped walnuts
40ml (scant 3 Tbsp) light olive oil
2 Tbsp almond butter
50g (¼ cup) coconut sugar or light muscovado sugar
1 egg, preferably free-range
1 tsp vanilla extract
2 Tbsp milk of choice
plain yoghurt, to serve (optional)

Topping
2 Tbsp chopped walnuts
1 Tbsp oats
1 Tbsp coconut sugar or light muscovado sugar
2 tsp light olive oil

Cook the sweet potato pieces in a pan of boiling water for about 15 minutes, until cooked through. Drain, mash and set aside to cool.

Meanwhile, whizz the oats in a blender for about 30 seconds to make a fine flour. Tip into a mixing bowl and combine with the baking powder, bicarbonate of soda, salt, mixed spice, nutmeg and chopped walnuts.

Put the cooled mashed sweet potato, olive oil, almond butter, coconut sugar, egg, vanilla extract and milk in a second mixing bowl and whisk until smooth. Add the dry ingredients and mix gently to make a batter.

Line a large, 6-hole muffin tray with paper cases and divide the batter between them. Put the tray into the refrigerator to rest for 20 minutes.

Preheat the oven to 220°C/200°C fan/425°F/Gas mark 7. Meanwhile, combine the topping ingredients in a small bowl.

When the muffins have rested, sprinkle with the topping and place in the preheated oven. Bake for 10 minutes, then reduce the temperature to 180°C/160°C fan/325°F/Gas mark 3 and bake for a further 10 minutes until they are risen, golden and cooked through (test with a skewer).

Remove from the oven, leave the muffins in the tray for 5 minutes, then transfer to a wire rack to cool. Serve the muffins just as they are or enjoy with a dollop of plain yoghurt.

Use gluten-free oats.

Swap the almond butter for tahini (sesame paste) or sunflower seed butter. Omit the walnuts and use a mixture of sunflower seeds and pumpkin seeds.

Swap the egg for 2 tablespoons of ground flaxseed mixed with 2 tablespoons of warm water. Soak for 10 minutes before adding to the mixture.

dairy-free
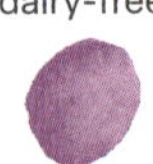
gluten-free

nut-free

sesame-free

egg-free

soy-free
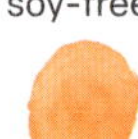
vegetarian

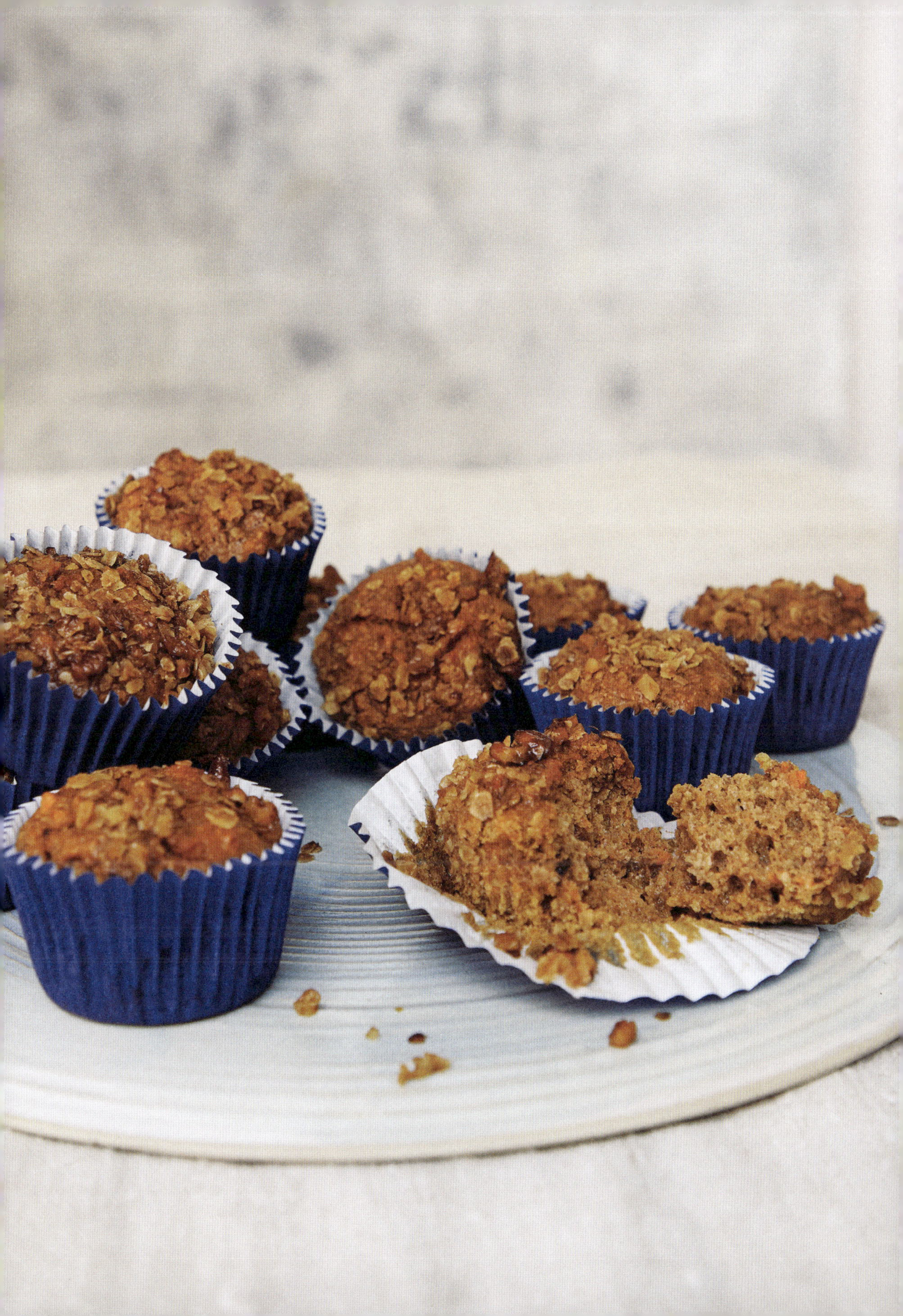

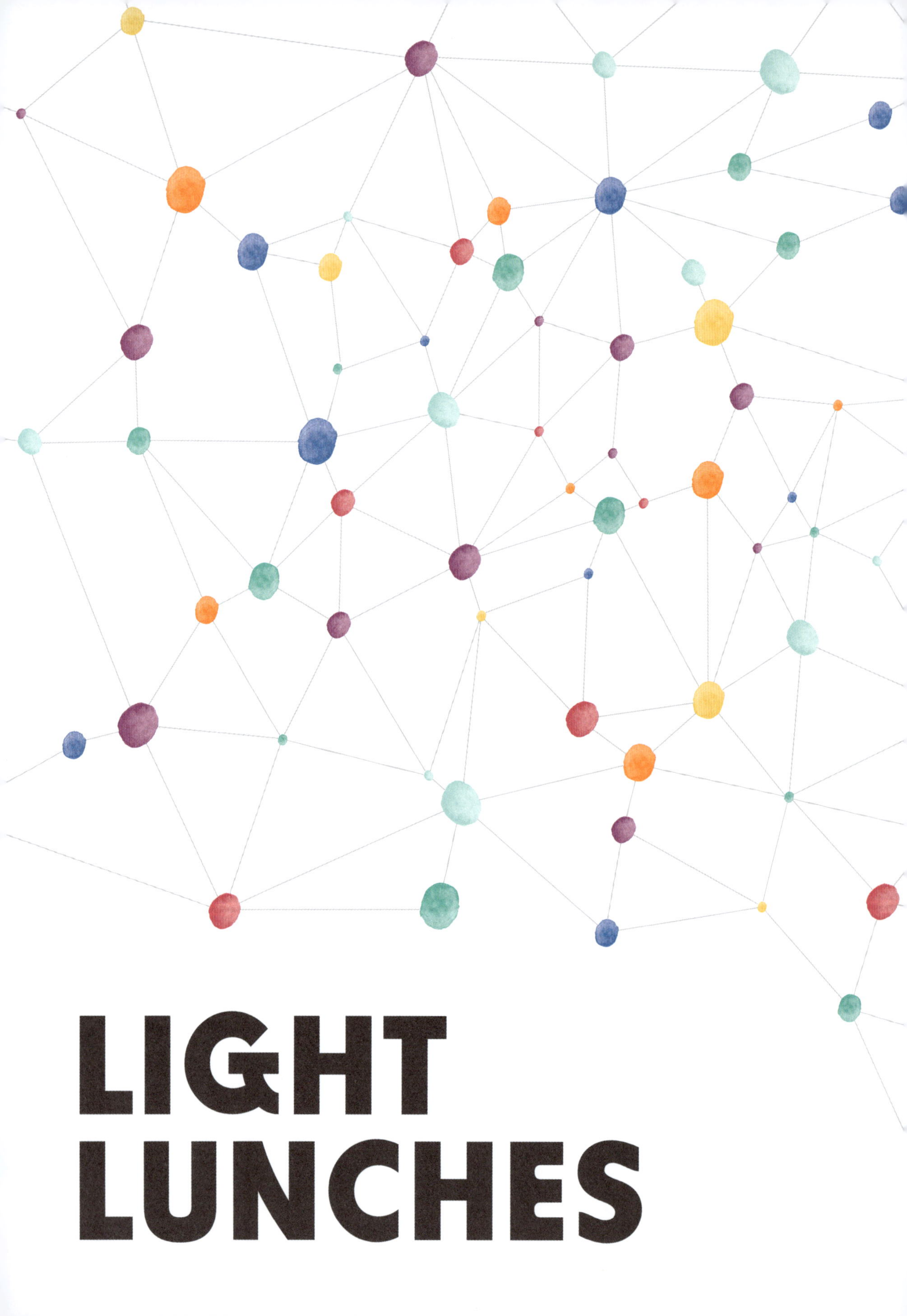

LIGHT LUNCHES

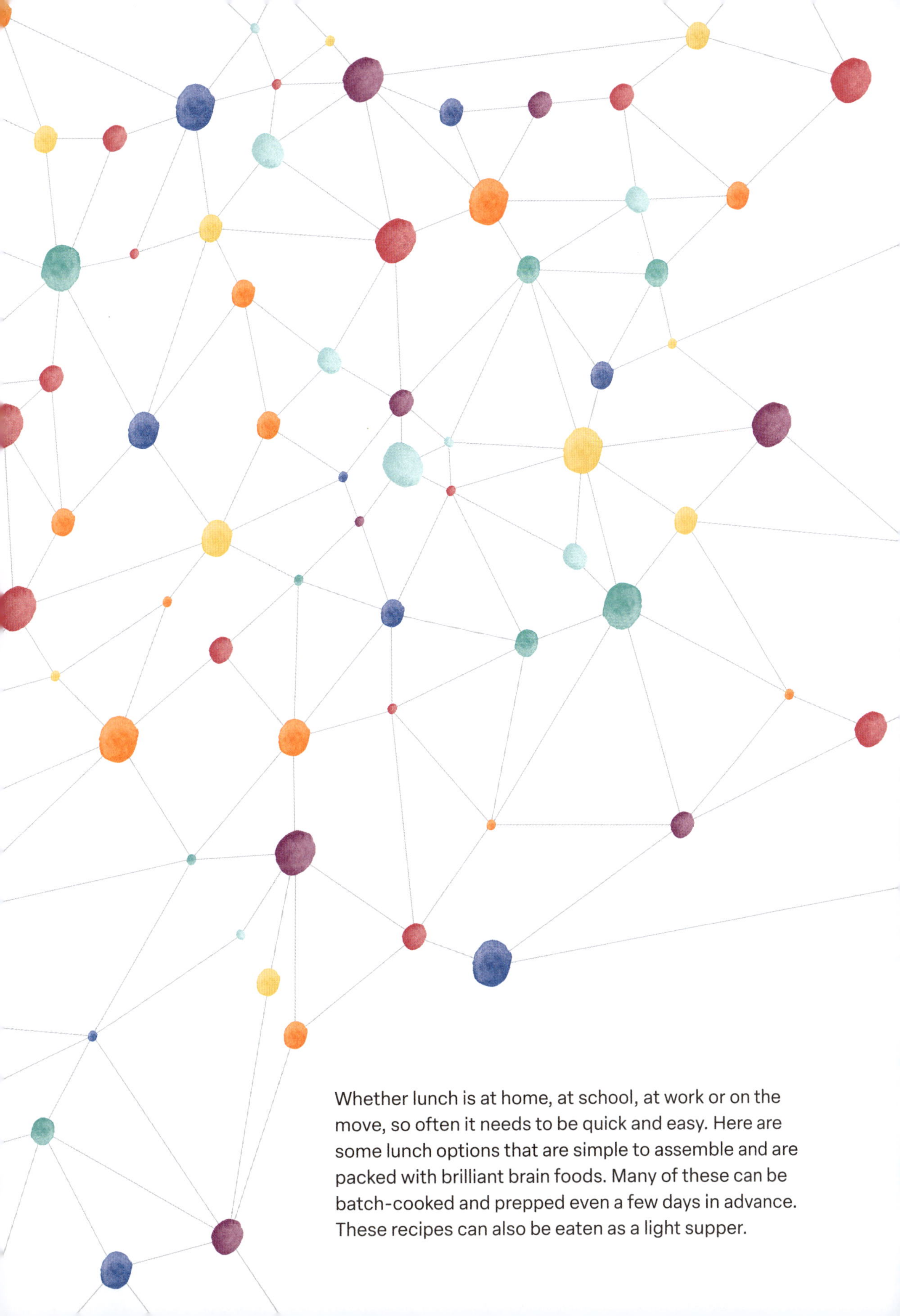

Whether lunch is at home, at school, at work or on the move, so often it needs to be quick and easy. Here are some lunch options that are simple to assemble and are packed with brilliant brain foods. Many of these can be batch-cooked and prepped even a few days in advance. These recipes can also be eaten as a light supper.

SALMON POKE BOWL

Serves 2

Bowl
150g (about ¾ cup) brown rice
1 Tbsp sesame oil
240g (8½oz) or 2 skinless salmon fillets, wild or organic if possible
75g (½ cup) shelled edamame beans, fresh or frozen
2–3 stems tenderstem broccoli
1 small carrot, grated (shredded)
½ avocado, stoned, peeled and sliced
¼ red (bell) pepper, sliced
2 radishes, thinly sliced
½ mango, cubed
4 tsp sesame seeds, toasted

Sauce
60ml (4 Tbsp) tamari soy sauce
35ml (2 Tbsp plus 1 tsp) apple juice
1½ Tbsp honey or maple syrup
½ Tbsp rice wine vinegar
½ Tbsp sesame oil
½ tsp minced ginger root (fresh or frozen)
½ tsp ground arrowroot
½ tsp water

A poke bowl is a great way to 'eat the rainbow' and enjoy a wide range of fruit and vegetables all in one meal. This poke is a super-tasty combination of salmon, rice and crunchy fresh goodies with a lovely tamari-based sauce that brings together all the flavours.

I have used brown rice, which contains more thiamine (vitamin B1) and fibre than white rice, but you can also use red rice, wild rice or a combination. To make it a bit more special, use prawns (shrimp) in place of the salmon, or, if you don't eat fish, try marinated diced firm tofu (beancurd) or chicken.

Rinse the rice and cook as per the packet instructions. Set aside.

Meanwhile for the sauce, combine the tamari soy sauce, apple juice, honey, rice wine vinegar and sesame oil in a small saucepan and gently warm through. Add the minced ginger and stir to combine.

Mix the arrowroot with the ½ teaspoon of water, then pour it into the sauce. Bring to a simmer, stirring all the time, until the sauce is thick and glossy. Pour into a jug and set aside to cool a little.

Heat a frying pan (skillet) and add the sesame oil, a splash of water and the salmon fillets, then brush the salmon steaks with some of the sauce. Cover with a lid and simmer gently until the salmon is fully cooked through and the flesh is completely opaque, about 8–12 minutes.

While the salmon cooks, steam the edamame beans and broccoli for a couple of minutes until al dente, then set aside. Ensure all the other ingredients are prepared.

Build the poke in two bowls (or lunchboxes for a meal on the go) by layering half the rice, the cooked and fresh vegetables and mango into each bowl. Flake the salmon on top, drizzle over the remaining sauce and sprinkle with the toasted sesame seeds. Eat immediately or allow to cool then store in the refrigerator if making ahead for lunch. A poke is great eaten hot or cold on the day it is made.

Replace the sesame oil with light olive oil or avocado oil and omit the seeds.

dairy-free
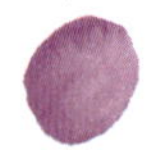
gluten-free

nut-free
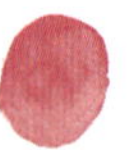
sesame-free
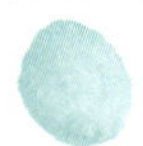
egg-free

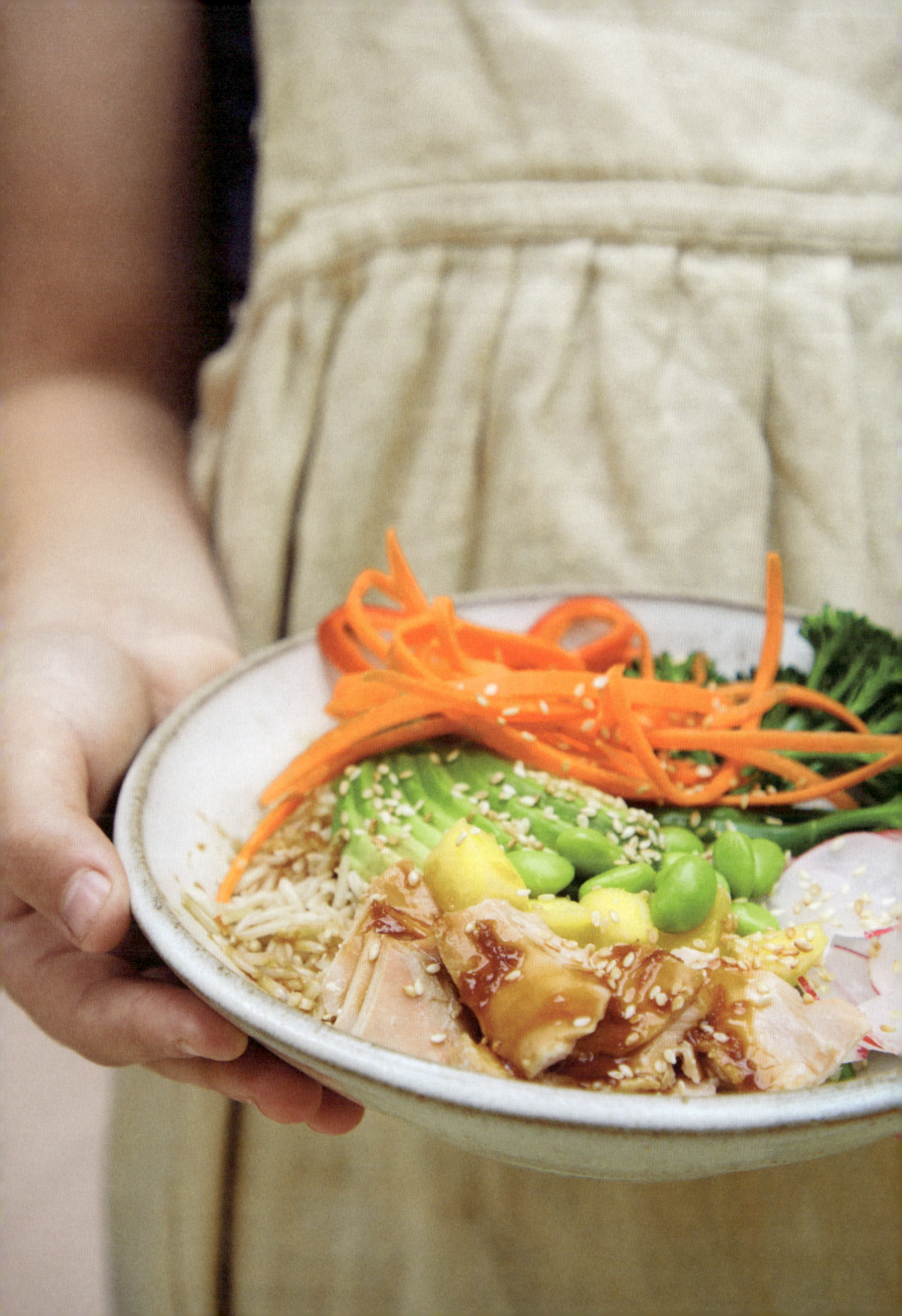

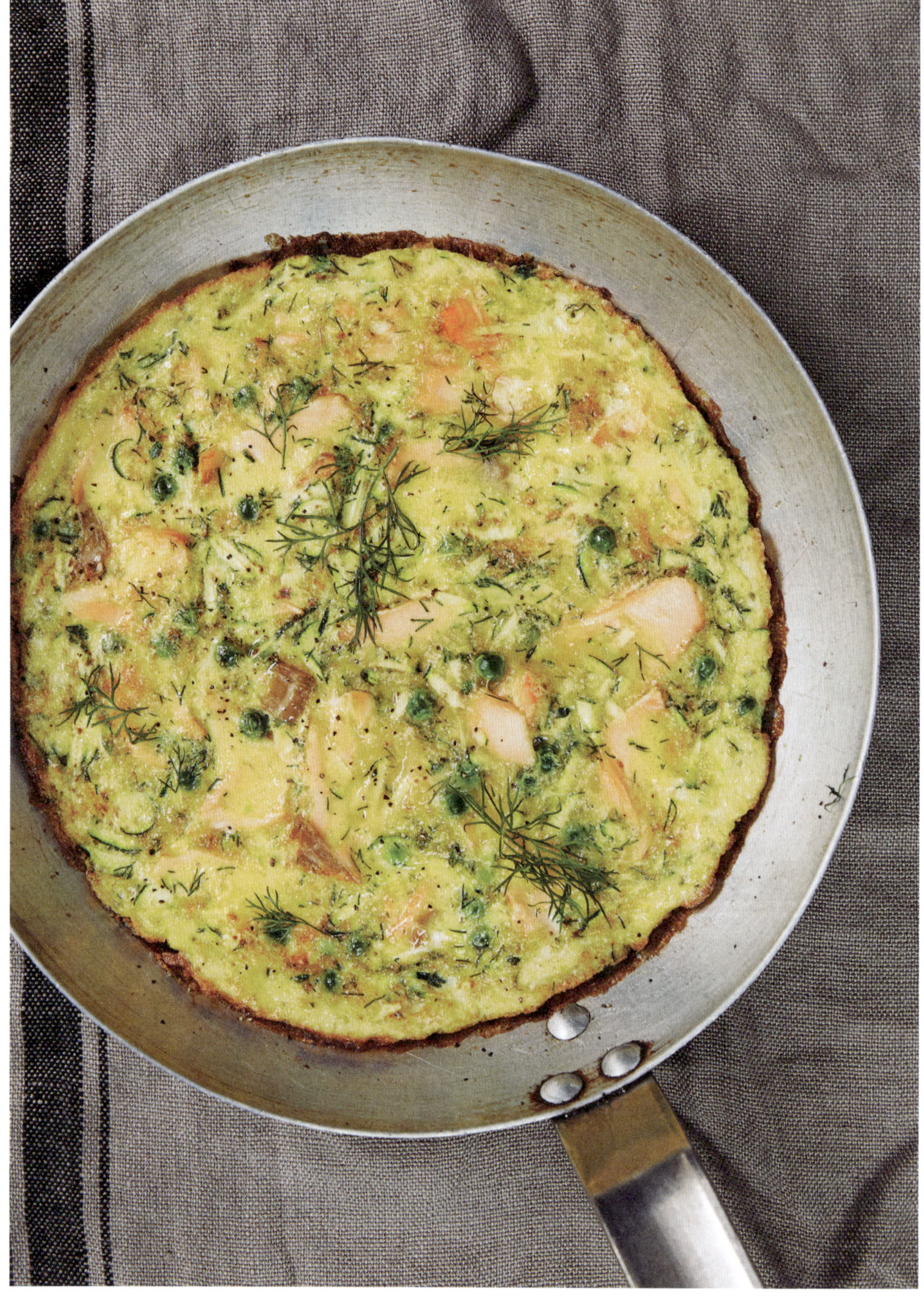

SALMON & PEA FRITTATA

Serves 2

½ courgette (zucchini), grated (shredded)
4 eggs, preferably free-range, beaten
1 cooked salmon steak, skin removed, and flaked
handful of peas, fresh or frozen
2 tsp fresh dill or 1 tsp dried
1 Tbsp olive oil, for frying
salt and black pepper

Salmon, peas and eggs are one of my favourite taste combinations and this recipe gives me a quick fix of omega-3, choline and folate, nutrients that make me mentally strong. Frittata is an easy and delicious lunch or light supper; you could even eat it for breakfast if you enjoy savoury food first thing in the morning. You can use fresh or frozen salmon – just ensure it's fully cooked before adding to the eggs, or use canned if you're in a hurry.

Squeeze out any excess liquid from the courgette using paper towels.

Mix together all the ingredients except the olive oil in a bowl and season with salt and pepper.

Preheat the oven grill (broiler) to its highest setting.

Heat the oil in a small ovenproof frying pan (skillet) over a medium heat. When it is hot, pour in the mixture. Cook for 3–4 minutes until the frittata is set on the bottom, then pop the pan under the grill to brown on top. The frittata will fluff up, developing a lovely light texture.

Serve immediately if you want it to remain light and fluffy as, over time, the frittata will sink a little.

If making ahead, store in the refrigerator for up to 48 hours and enjoy cold.

Replace the eggs with 50g (scant ½ cup) of gram (chickpea flour) and 160ml (⅔ cup) of water, mixed well together before adding the other ingredients. However, you'll need to treat this as an omelette and flip it in the pan, rather than put it under the grill.

dairy-free
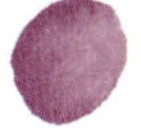

gluten-free
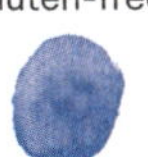

nut-free

sesame-free
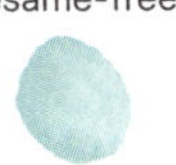

egg-free

soy-free

SMASHED CHICKPEA & AVOCADO SOURDOUGH TOAST

A crunchy and moreish lunch or breakfast toast recipe with a lovely combination of chickpeas (garbanzo beans) and avocado, with pickled dill cucumbers (dill pickles) to help nourish the gut microbiome.

If you don't eat bread, use the chickpeas as a filling for a baked sweet potato or make this tasty mix into a larger salad with lettuce, carrot, cherry tomatoes and alfalfa or mung bean sprouts to eat on its own or alongside a fried egg.

Serves 2

400g (14oz) can chickpeas (garbanzo beans), drained
⅛ tsp ground turmeric
60g (2¼oz) pickled dill cucumbers (dill pickles), sliced
2 Tbsp mayonnaise
1 tsp grainy mustard
2 slices of sourdough bread
½ avocado, stoned, peeled and sliced
squeeze of lime juice
chilli sauce (optional)
salt and black pepper

Mix the chickpeas with the turmeric and some salt and pepper, then smash with a fork.

Mix the dill cucumbers with the mayonnaise and grainy mustard, then stir in the prepared chickpeas.

Toast the sourdough, then spread the mixture on each slice. Top with the avocado and finish with a squeeze of lime. Add a little chilli sauce if you like a fiery kick!

The smashed chickpeas will store in the refrigerator for up to 3 days, but the avocado does need to be eaten quickly after cutting.

Use dairy-free mayonnaise.
Source a good-quality gluten-free sourdough.

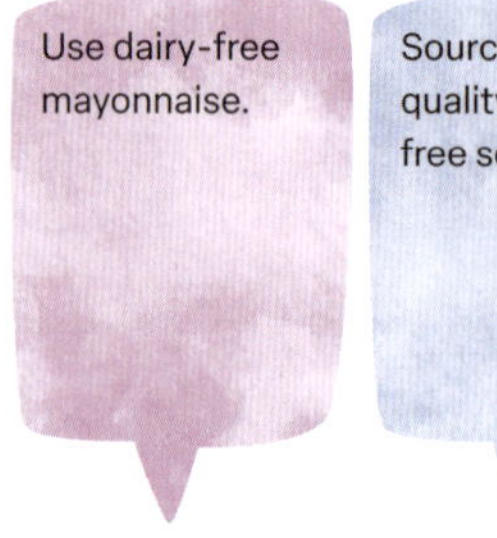

dairy-free

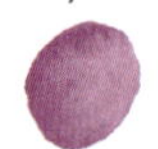

gluten-free

nut-free

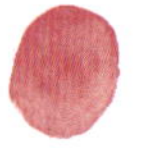

sesame-free

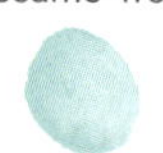

egg-free

soy-free

vegetarian

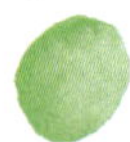

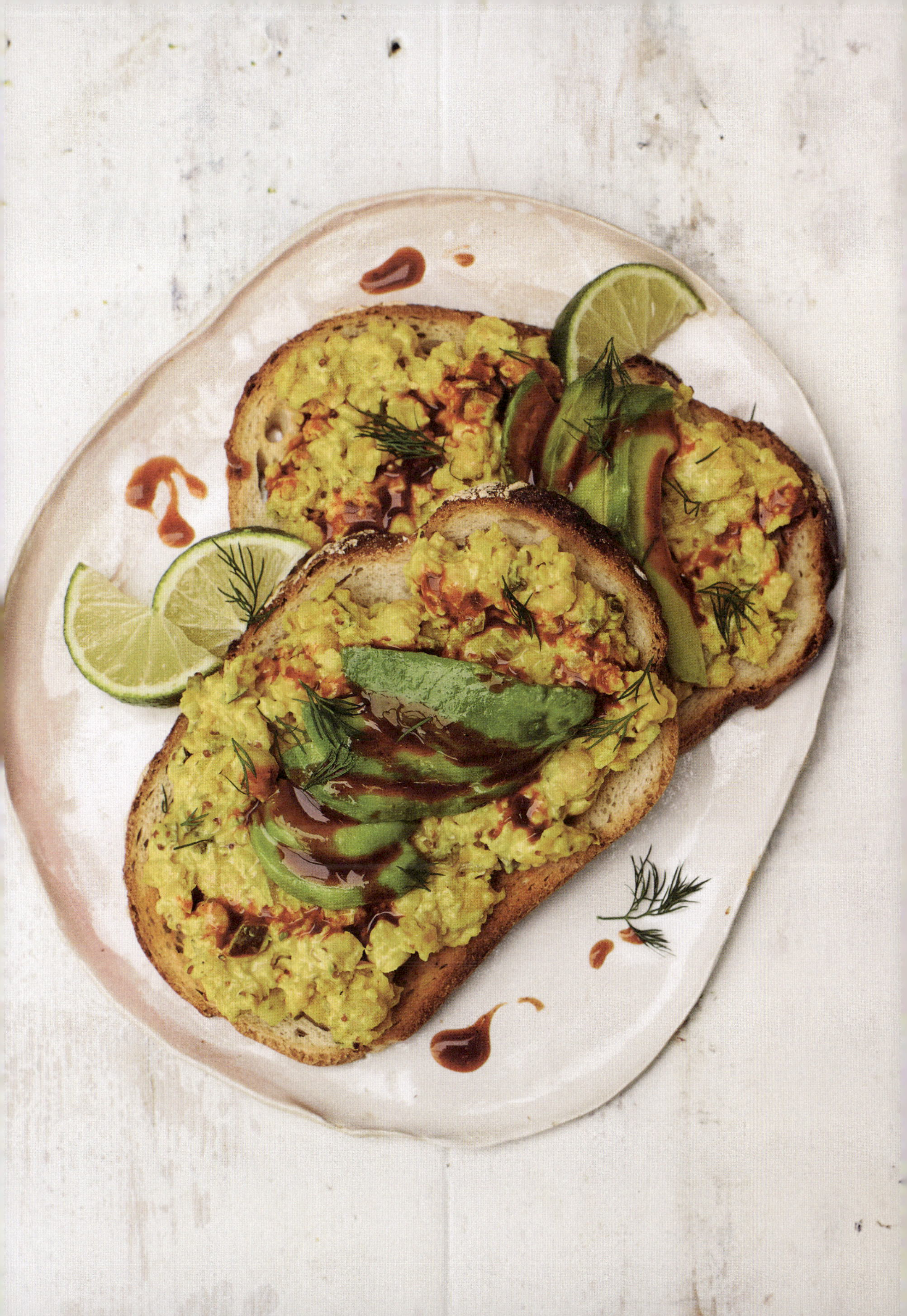

QUINOA & POMEGRANATE TABBOULEH

This protein-packed tabbouleh makes a perfect lunch or a side dish for something more substantial such as meat, chicken, tofu (beancurd) or fish. Unlike grains such as rice or wheat, quinoa seeds contain all eight essential amino acids found in protein. As the basis for this fresh and sweet salad with an array of wonderful polyphenol-rich ingredients, the quinoa will support a healthy gut microbiome and immune system – so you'll feel great.

Serves 4

¼ cucumber, peeled and finely diced
8 cherry or mini plum tomatoes, finely diced
200g (1 cup plus 3 Tbsp) quinoa
3 Tbsp olive oil
3 tsp baharat spice mix
3 Tbsp finely chopped fresh parsley
1 Tbsp finely chopped fresh mint
2 unwaxed lemons (zest of 1 and juice of 2)
1 small carrot, peeled and finely diced
½ red (bell) pepper, deseeded and finely diced
100g (about ½ cup) pomegranate seeds
sea salt flakes (kosher salt)

Put the diced cucumber and tomatoes into a small bowl, sprinkle with a pinch of salt and set aside to allow the salt to extract any excess liquid.

Meanwhile cook the quinoa as per the packet instructions. Once the water has been absorbed and the quinoa is soft, stir in 1 tablespoon of the olive oil, the baharat spice mix and a pinch of salt. Set aside to cool a little.

Put the parsley, mint, lemon zest and juice and the remaining olive oil into a mini food-processor. Pulse 10–12 times until the herbs are finely chopped, but stop before it turns into a sauce.

Drain any liquid from the diced cucumber and tomatoes.

Put all the ingredients except the pomegranate seeds into a large bowl and stir to combine, then sprinkle the pomegranate seeds on top to serve.

Store in the refrigerator for up to 3 days without the pomegranate and sprinkle the seeds on fresh each time you serve.

dairy-free

gluten-free

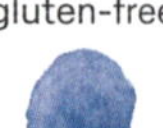

nut-free

sesame-free

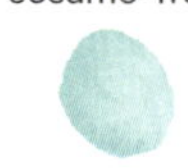

egg-free

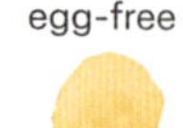

soy-free

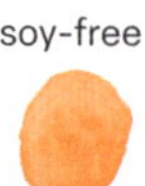

vegetarian

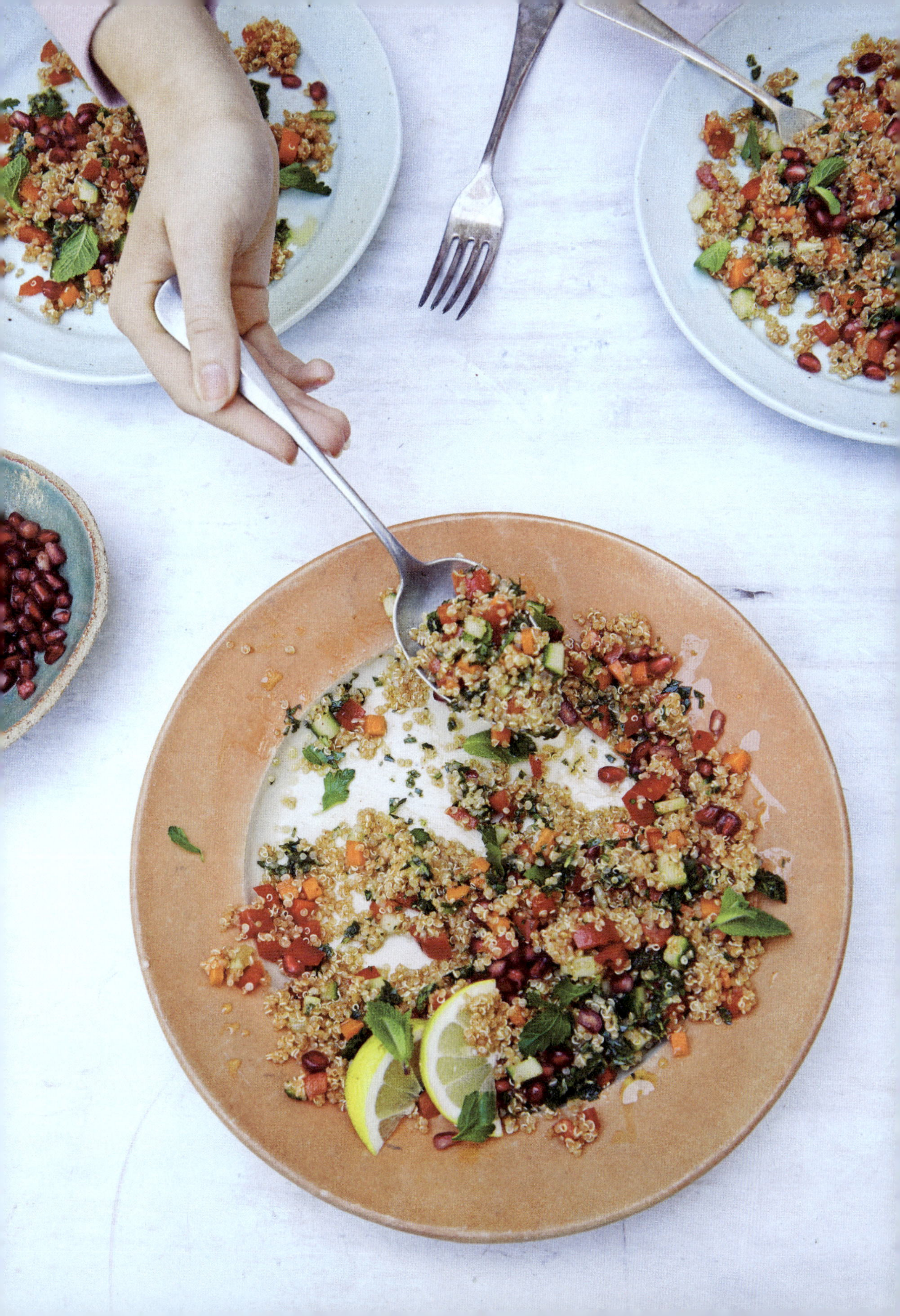

TZATZIKI & CHICKEN GYROS

Serves 2

1 tsp ground coriander
1 tsp ground cumin
1 tsp sweet paprika
1 tsp fresh oregano or ½ tsp dried
2 skinless, boneless chicken thighs
1 Tbsp olive oil
2 wholemeal pitta breads or wholemeal wraps
2 mini tomatoes, diced

Tzatziki
1 tsp olive oil
2 Tbsp full-fat plain Greek yoghurt (or plain kefir)
1 tsp chopped fresh mint or ½ tsp dried
1 thumb of cucumber, peeled and finely diced
¼ garlic clove, finely chopped or crushed (optional)
squeeze of lemon juice
salt and black pepper

Gyros is the Greek name for pitta breads stuffed with tasty rotisserie chicken and tzatziki. This recipe makes a delicious Mediterranean-style lunch with a speedy twist so that you can assemble it quickly. It is a protein-rich lunch to help the brain stay sharp throughout the afternoon – opt for wholemeal pitta for more fibre and protein. The Greek yoghurt helps to bolster the gut microbiome and, in turn, the brain's neurotransmitters.

First prepare the tzatziki. Mix together the ingredients and season with salt and pepper. Set aside.

Mix together the ground spices, oregano and some salt and pepper. Sprinkle this over the chicken thighs.

Place the thighs between two pieces of baking paper and use a rolling pin to bash them hard a few times to soften the flesh and flatten them.

Heat the olive oil in a frying pan (skillet) over a high heat and flash-fry the chicken until it is well browned on both sides and cooked through – this takes 8–12 minutes. Allow to cool a little, then slice with a sharp knife.

Warm the pitta breads and slit open on one side. Stuff with the chicken, diced tomatoes and the tzatziki. Serve immediately.

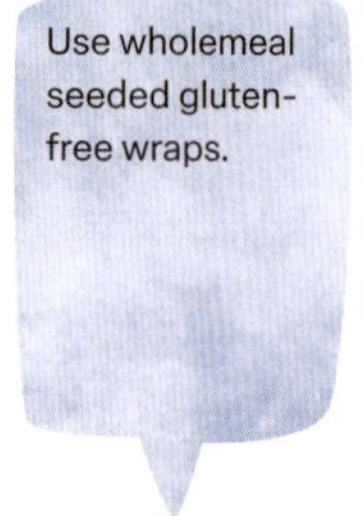

gluten-free

nut-free

sesame-free

egg-free

soy-free

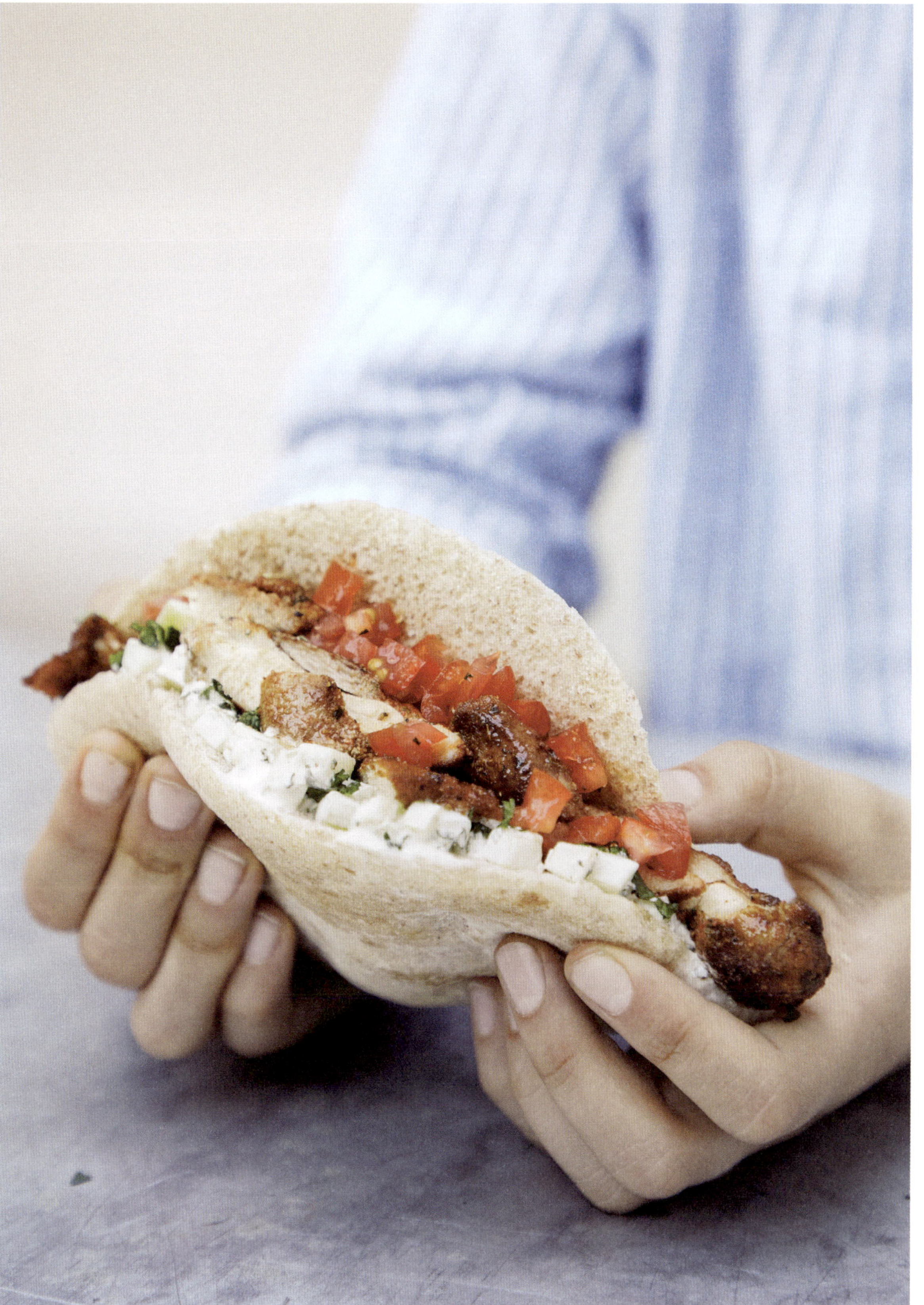

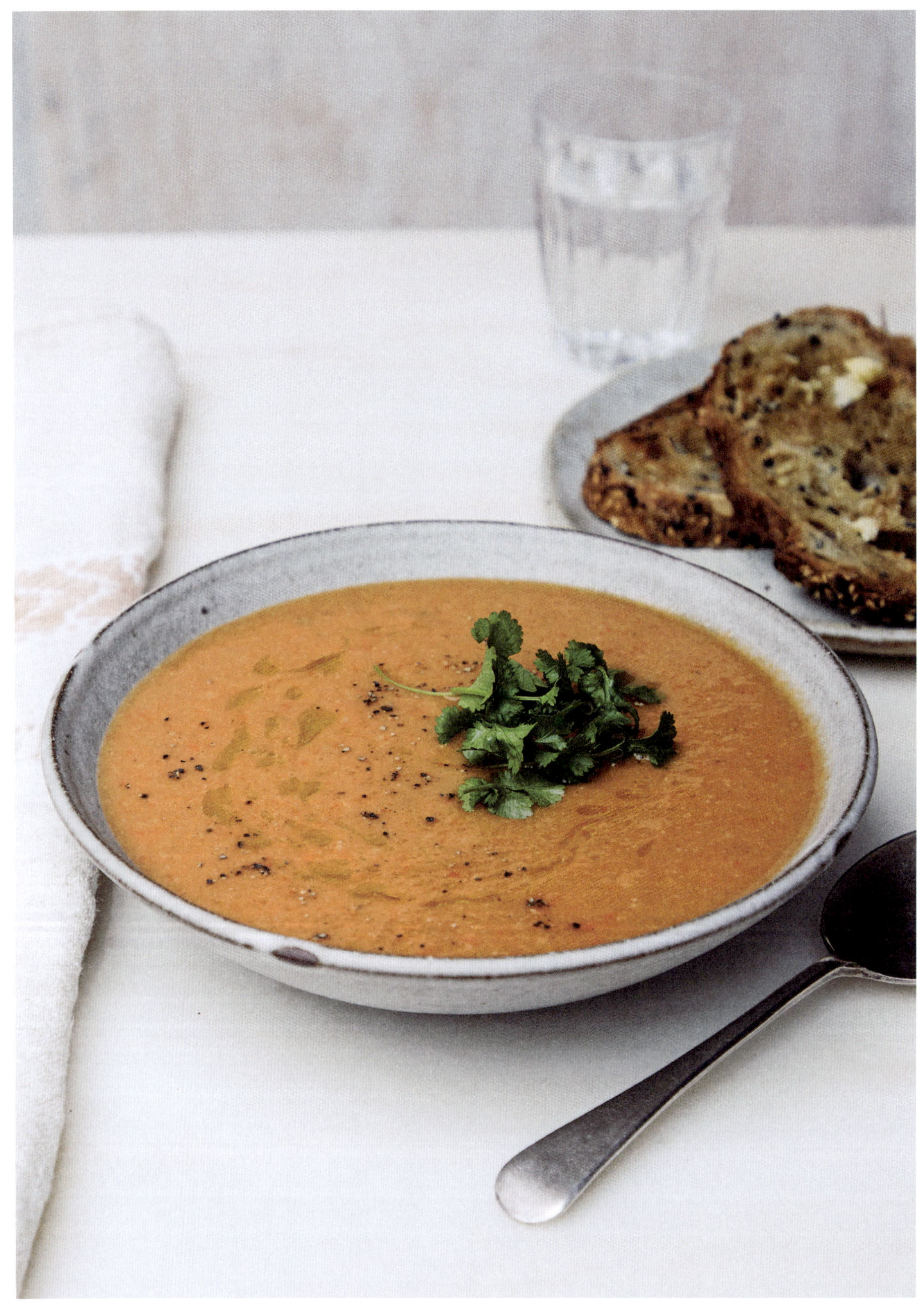

SWEET POTATO & CARDAMOM SOUP

This sweet and comforting soup is gentle on the tummy. It's packed with vegetables and beans and is both warming and filling – one to eat during the winter months – and perfect to batch-cook and freeze. I use chicken stock or bone broth, which benefits digestion and the immune system and strengthens bones, but you can also switch to a vegetable stock to make this entirely plant-based. Serve on its own or with crusty sourdough or seeded oatcakes.

Serves 2–4

2 Tbsp olive oil
1 pat of butter
1 red onion, finely diced
1 sweet potato, peeled and diced
3 carrots, peeled and diced
1 red (bell) pepper, deseeded and diced
400g (14oz) can white beans (haricot/navy or cannellini), drained
4 cardamom pods, lightly crushed
2 tsp ground cumin
2 tsp ground coriander
1 litre (4⅓ cups) chicken stock or bone broth
salt and black pepper
fresh coriander (cilantro) leaves, to garnish (optional)

Heat the olive oil and butter together in a large saucepan over a medium heat. Add the onion and fry for 3–5 minutes until soft and translucent.

Stir in the sweet potato, carrots, red (bell) pepper and the drained beans. Next add the crushed cardamom pods, the ground cumin and coriander along with the stock. Bring to the boil, then gently simmer for around 15 minutes until all the vegetables are soft.

Carefully remove the husks of the cardamom pods with a spoon (the seeds will have dispersed into the soup), then blend the soup until it is super-smooth. Season with salt and pepper as needed and garnish with coriander.

This can be stored in the refrigerator for 3 days or the freezer for up to 3 months.

Swap the butter for olive oil or a plant-based spread.

Use vegetable stock instead of chicken stock or bone broth.

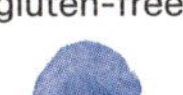

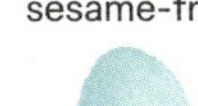

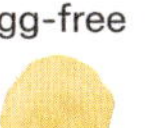

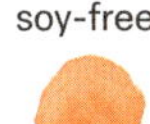

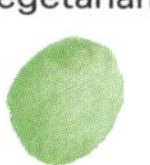

CRISPY GNOCCHI WITH BROCCOLI & ANCHOVY SAUCE

Gnocchi with a crunch! I like to serve these with lightly cooked broccoli florets and a wonderful polyphenol-rich sauce that has a deliciously moreish umami flavour from the rosemary, lemon juice and anchovies and is packed with omega-3 and calcium.

Serves 2

350g (12oz) pack of plain gnocchi
1 Tbsp olive oil
½ tsp salt
½ tsp garlic powder or granules
10 broccoli florets

Anchovy sauce
1 Tbsp fresh rosemary or ½ Tbsp dried
6 anchovies
2 Tbsp extra virgin olive oil
juice of 1 lemon

Drop the gnocchi into a pan of boiling water for 2 minutes, then drain. Toss the gnocchi in a bowl with the olive oil, salt and garlic powder until evenly coated and then fry in a large frying pan (skillet) for 11 minutes. Shake the pan every 3–4 minutes to ensure the gnocchi are crispy all over.

Meanwhile, steam the broccoli florets until al dente.

For the anchovy sauce, blitz the rosemary in a small food processor and then add the anchovies. With the motor still running, slowly add the olive oil and finally blend in the lemon juice to make a thick sauce.

Combine the broccoli and gnocchi and pour the anchovy sauce over or serve as a dipping sauce on the side.

Store in the refrigerator for 24 hours, keeping the gnocchi and broccoli separate from the sauce if you're not serving straight away, so they do not become soggy.

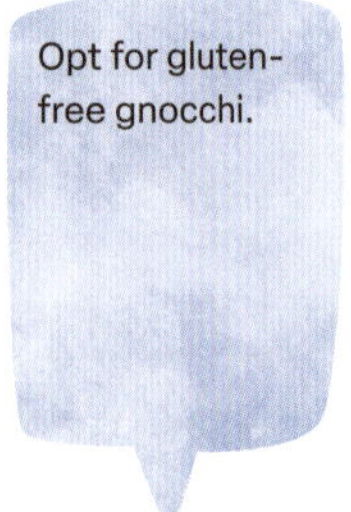

dairy-free
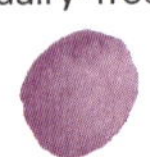
gluten-free

nut-free
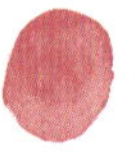
sesame-free

egg-free

soy-free

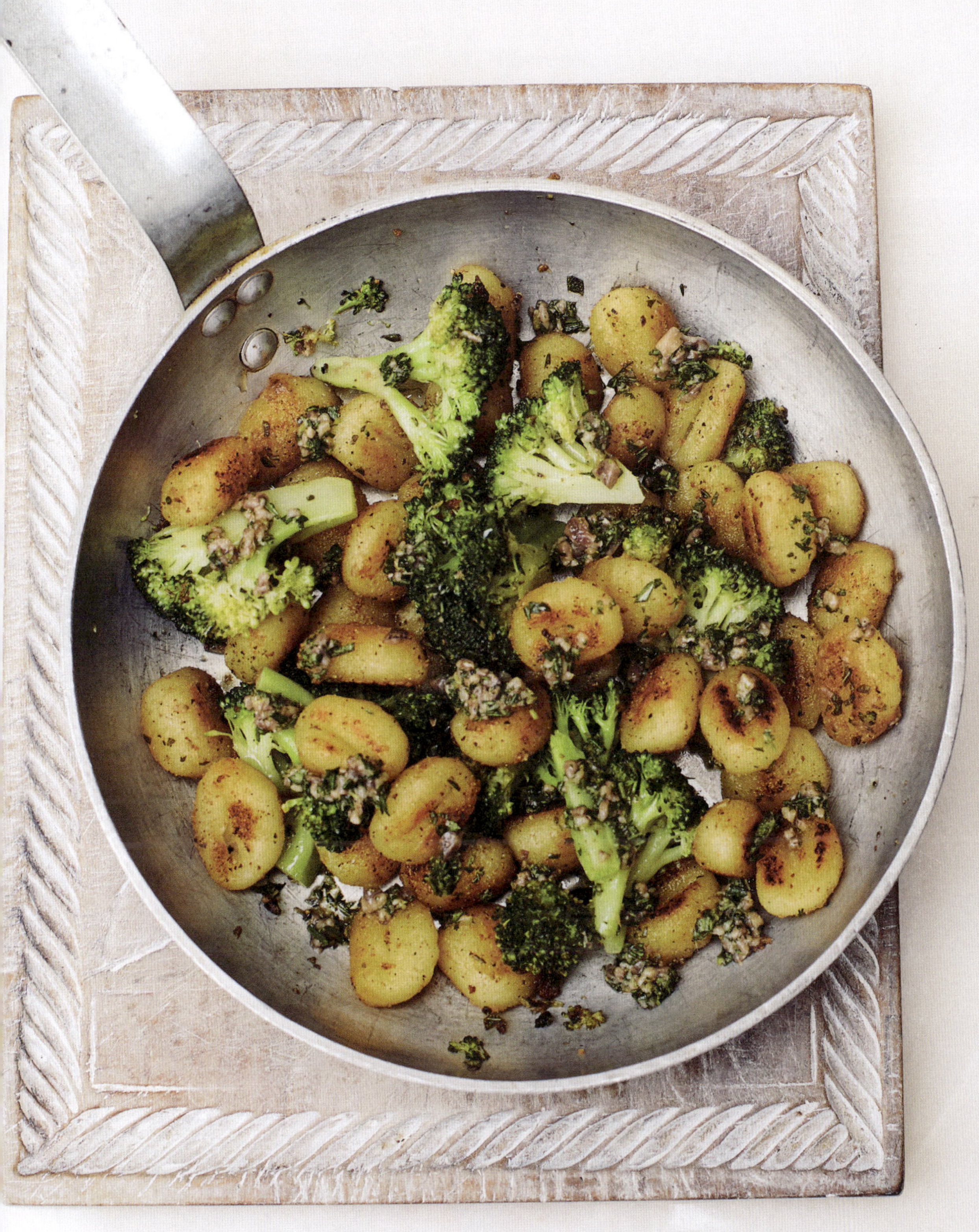

HOT-SMOKED SALMON & CREAM CHEESE WRAPS

Makes 2

1 hot-smoked salmon fillet
2 Tbsp cream cheese
1 tsp capers, rinsed and drained
1 tsp fresh dill or ½ tsp dried
squeeze of lemon juice
black pepper
2 wholemeal wraps
4 Little Gem (Boston) lettuce leaves

Hot-smoked salmon with capers, dill and cream cheese is a moreish combination. These wraps make a quick, easily assembled lunch that is packed with omega-3 and choline to keep the brain sharp all afternoon.

Break up the salmon fillet with a fork into small pieces and then stir in the cream cheese, capers, dill, lemon juice and a few grinds of black pepper.

Slather each wrap with the smoked salmon mixture and place two lettuce leaves on top.

Fold up the wraps carefully and cut into two.

The salmon mixture can be stored in the refrigerator for up to a week.

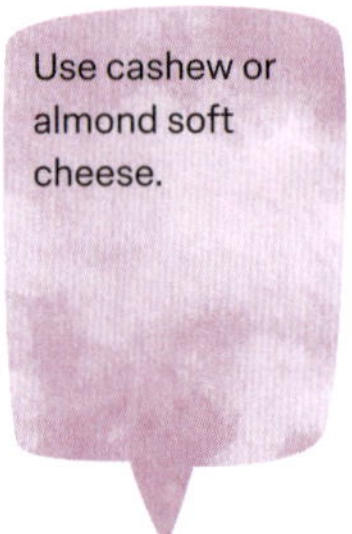

Use wholemeal seeded gluten-free wraps.

dairy-free

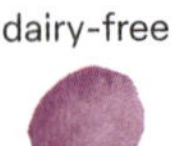

gluten-free

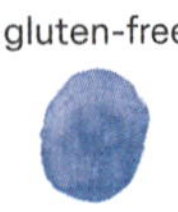

nut-free

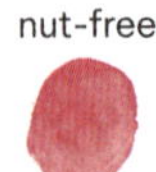

sesame-free

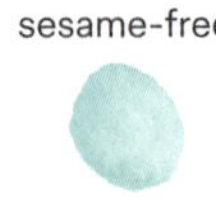

egg-free

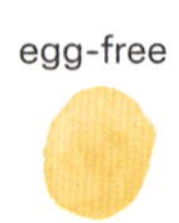

soy-free

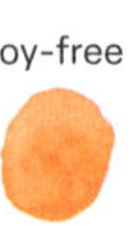

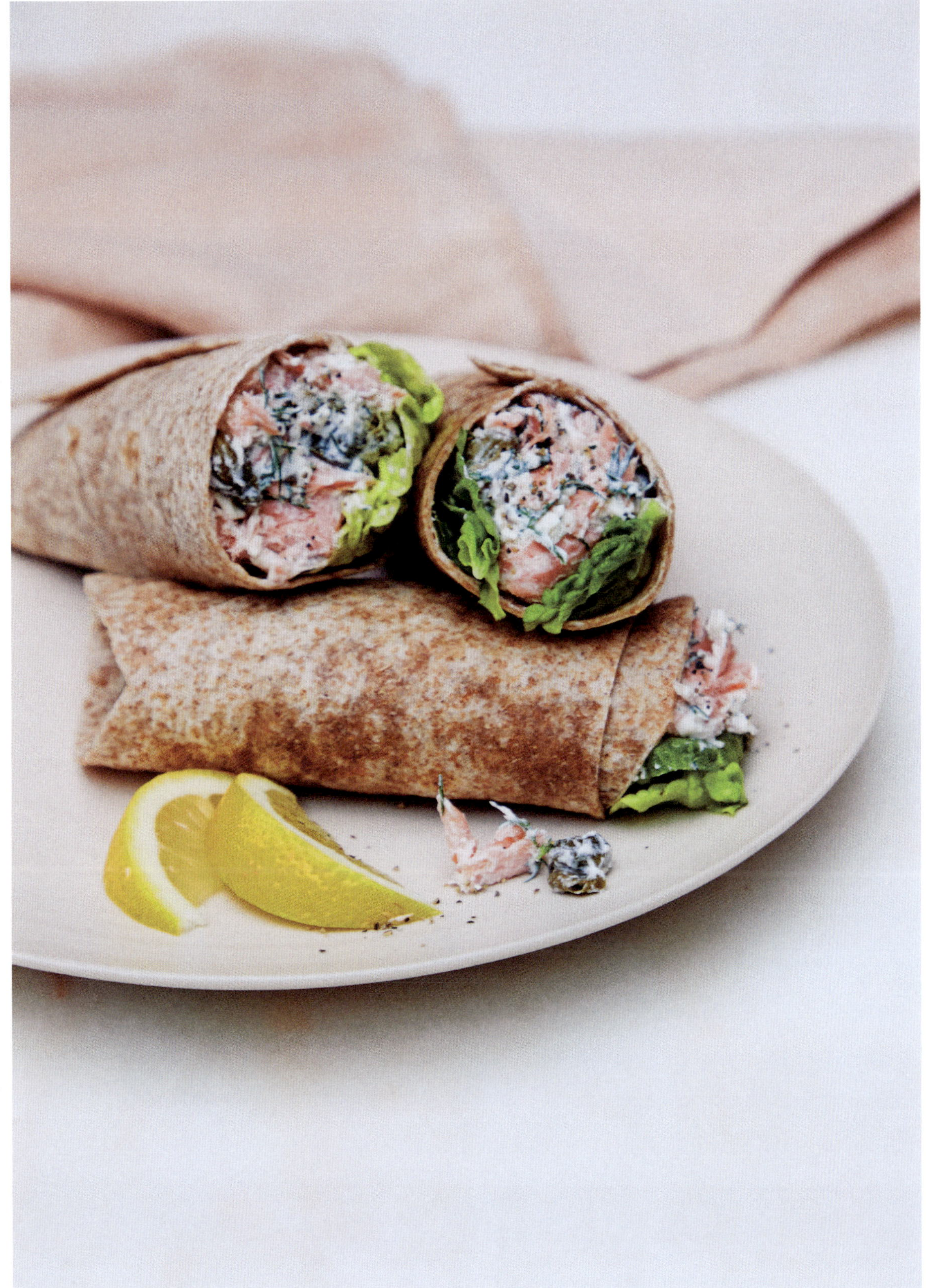

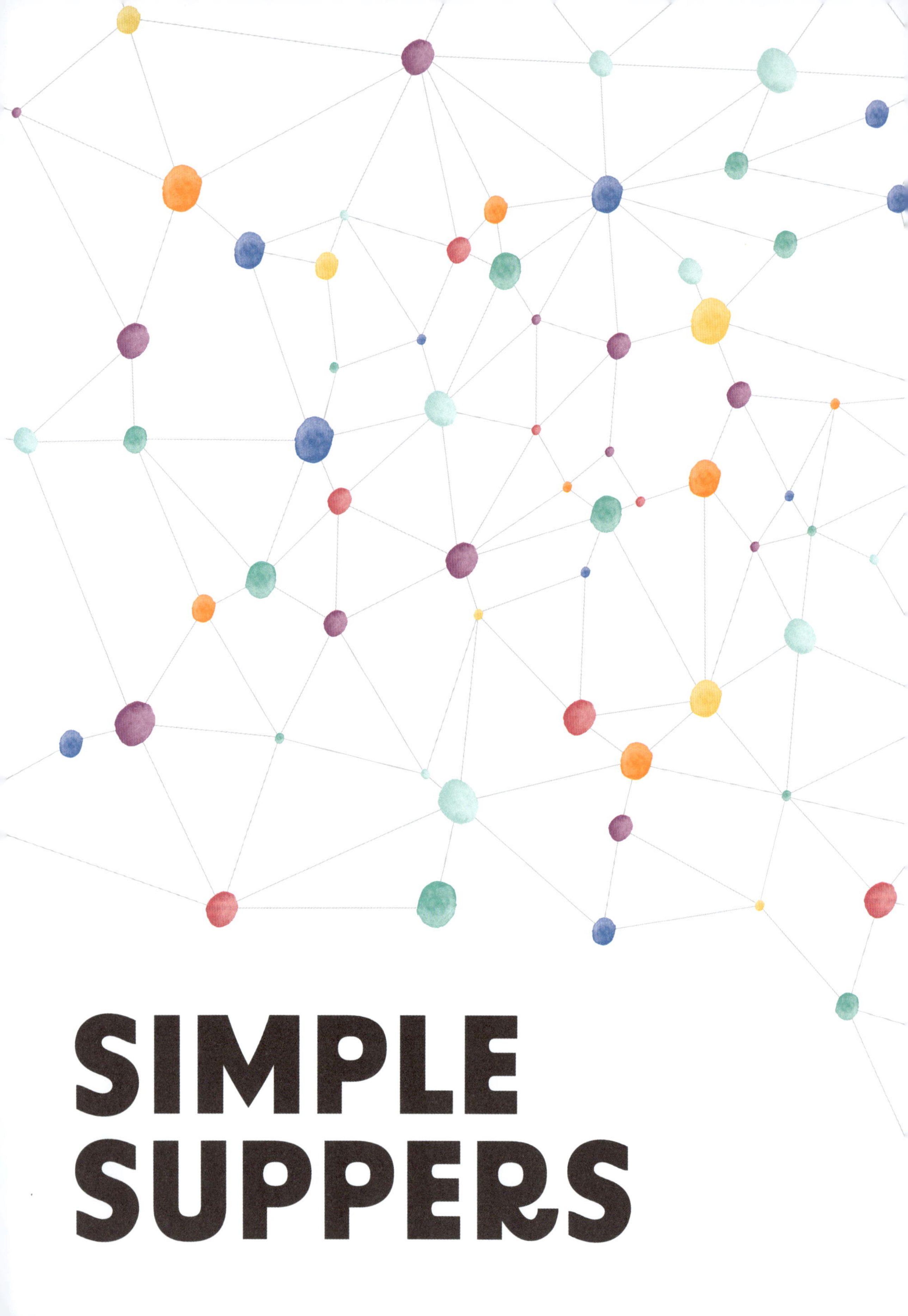
SIMPLE
SUPPERS

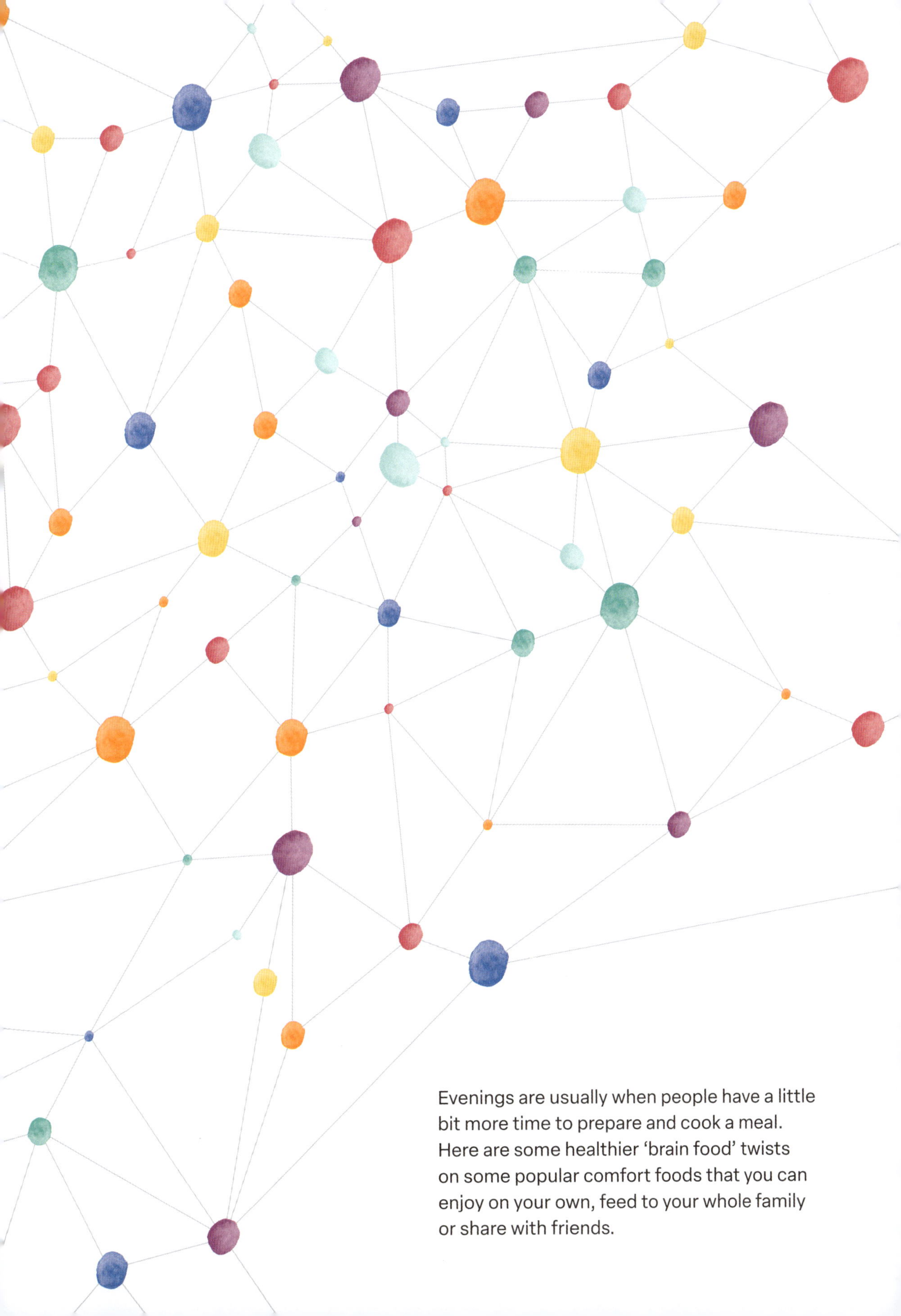

Evenings are usually when people have a little bit more time to prepare and cook a meal. Here are some healthier 'brain food' twists on some popular comfort foods that you can enjoy on your own, feed to your whole family or share with friends.

NATUREDOC CHICKEN NUGGETS

Serves 4

4 skinless, boneless chicken thighs, preferably organic or free-range
40g (¼ cup) red lentils
½ tsp ground paprika
40g (scant ½ cup) ground (powdered) almonds
½ tsp dried oregano
2 eggs, preferably free-range
2 Tbsp olive oil
salt and black pepper

Chicken nuggets the NatureDoc way! With a crunchy crust and soft moist chicken inside, you will be cooking these on repeat. They are a brilliant first step for selective eaters to try a twist on the shop-bought ultra-processed nuggets.

I use chicken thighs as they contain more iron and are less dry than the breast. The red lentils also contain iron and the almonds are rich in calcium. Serve with peas and home-made sweet potato fries.

Cut the chicken thighs into nugget-shaped pieces – I use kitchen scissors to do this.

Put the red lentils, paprika and some salt and pepper in a food processor fitted with a grinding blade and whizz for 1 minute to a fine powder.

Mix the ground (powdered) almonds with the oregano on a plate. Crack the eggs into a wide, shallow bowl and mix well with a fork. Spread the lentil powder on a third plate.

Dip each nugget of chicken first in the almonds, then the egg and finally the lentils. Ensure at each stage that each piece is covered evenly and well. Heat the olive oil in a large frying pan (skillet) over a medium heat. Without overcrowding the pan, add some of the coated nuggets, turning every couple of minutes so that they are crisp on all sides. Cook until the chicken is cooked all the way through (test one nugget by cutting it open to check it is no longer pink in the centre).

Repeat cooking in batches until all the chicken nuggets are cooked through.

Once cooked, these store in the refrigerator for 3 days or in the freezer for 3 months. To cook: spread out on a large baking tray and put in a preheated oven at 200°C/180°C fan/400°F/Gas mark 6, for 15–20 minutes from the refrigerator and 25–30 minutes if frozen.

Swap the ground almonds for gram (chickpea) flour, tapioca flour or rice flour.

dairy-free

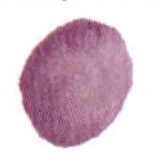

gluten-free

nut-free

sesame-free

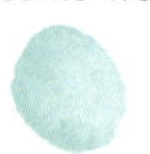

soy-free

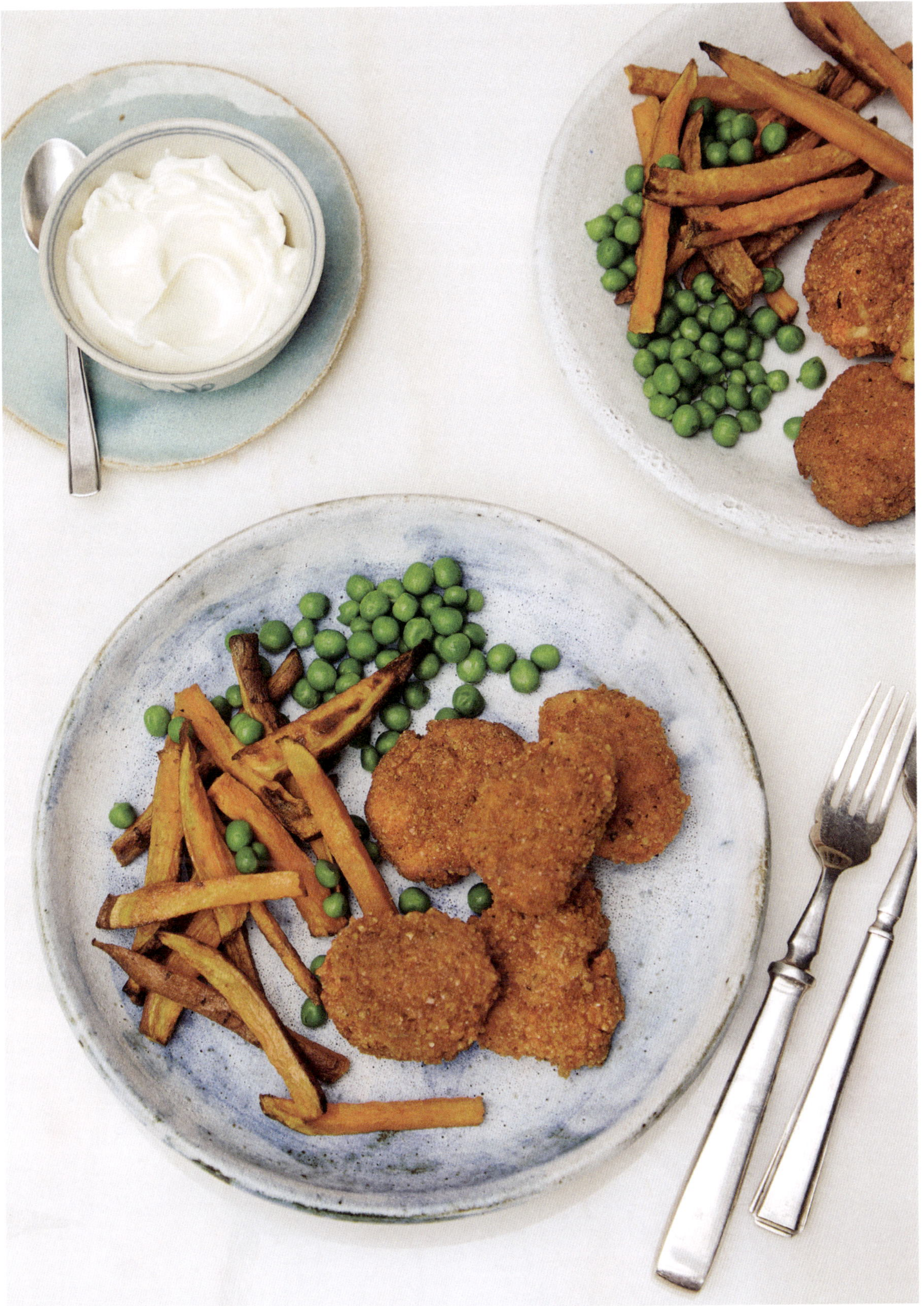

BUTTERNUT SQUASH & SAGE LASAGNE

Serves 4–6

Meat layer
2 Tbsp olive oil
1 onion, finely diced
1 garlic clove, crushed
400g (14oz) sausage meat or minced (ground) pork
2 chicken livers, trimmed and roughly chopped
1 red (bell) pepper, deseeded and finely diced
2 tsp fennel seeds
2 tsp fresh thyme leaves or 1 tsp dried
2 tsp smoked paprika
4 Tbsp tomato purée (paste)
125ml (½ cup) chicken stock or bone broth

Butternut squash layer
1 butternut squash, seeds removed, peeled and cut into chunks
2 Tbsp olive oil
2 tsp ground nutmeg
small handful of sage leaves, roughly chopped
1 Tbsp butter
150g (scant ¾ cup) ricotta or goat's cheese
salt and black pepper

Creamy layer
100g (½ cup minus 1 Tbsp) ricotta or goat's cheese or almond cheese
½ tsp ground nutmeg
handful of cavolo nero or kale, roughly chopped

6 oven-ready lasagne sheets, or 2 courgettes (zucchini) finely sliced or spiralized into ribbons
2 Tbsp grated Parmesan or pecorino
2 Tbsp pumpkin seeds
1 Tbsp chopped sage leaves, plus 5–6 whole leaves

A delicious and comforting lasagne with a brainy twist! Aromatic sage is helpful for mood and memory, the chicken liver contains plenty of iron and vitamin B12, while zinc-rich pumpkin seeds are a great topping. Make this with traditional lasagne sheets, or there's the option to use courgette ribbons to help reduce a blood glucose spike.

Lasagne is ideal to feed a crowd, but you can assemble this as individual servings and store these, uncooked, in the freezer.

First make the meat layer. Heat the olive oil in a large frying pan (skillet) or saucepan and sauté the onion for 3–5 minutes until soft and translucent. Add the garlic, sauté for a further minute, then add the sausage meat and livers and cook, stirring, until well browned.

Add the red pepper, fennel, thyme, paprika, tomato purée and finally the stock or broth. Bubble gently for at least 45 minutes, stirring from time to time. You want a nice thick meaty sauce.

Meanwhile, prepare the butternut squash layer. Lightly coat the squash in the oil, then sprinkle with the nutmeg and some salt and pepper. Roast in a preheated oven at 200°C/180°C fan/400°F/Gas mark 6 for 45 minutes. Add the sage for the last 5 minutes.

Blend the butternut squash with the butter and ricotta. Set aside.

The creamy layer is easy: simply blend the ricotta and nutmeg together and stir in the cavolo nero. Set aside.

Take an ovenproof dish measuring about 29 x 22cm (11.5 x 8.5in) and assemble as follows. Spoon a third of the meat sauce over the base of the dish. Cover with 3 lasagne sheets or half the courgette ribbons in a single layer. Cover with half the butternut squash mixture, spreading it evenly. Repeat those layers using half the remaining meat sauce, all the remaining lasagne sheets or courgette and all the butternut squash. Make a further layer using the rest of the meat sauce, then top with the creamy ricotta to make a final layer. Sprinkle with the Parmesan, pumpkin seeds and chopped sage.

Cook the lasagne in the preheated oven for 30 minutes. Rub a little extra oil over the 5 or 6 sage leaves. Remove the lasagne from the oven, top with the sage leaves, and return the dish to the oven for another 15–20 minutes until the cheese is golden and bubbling.

Store in the refrigerator for up to 3 days or in the freezer for up to 3 months. To reheat from chilled, cover the dish with foil and put in a preheated oven at 180°C/160°F fan/350°F/Gas mark 4 for 20–30 minutes until piping hot.

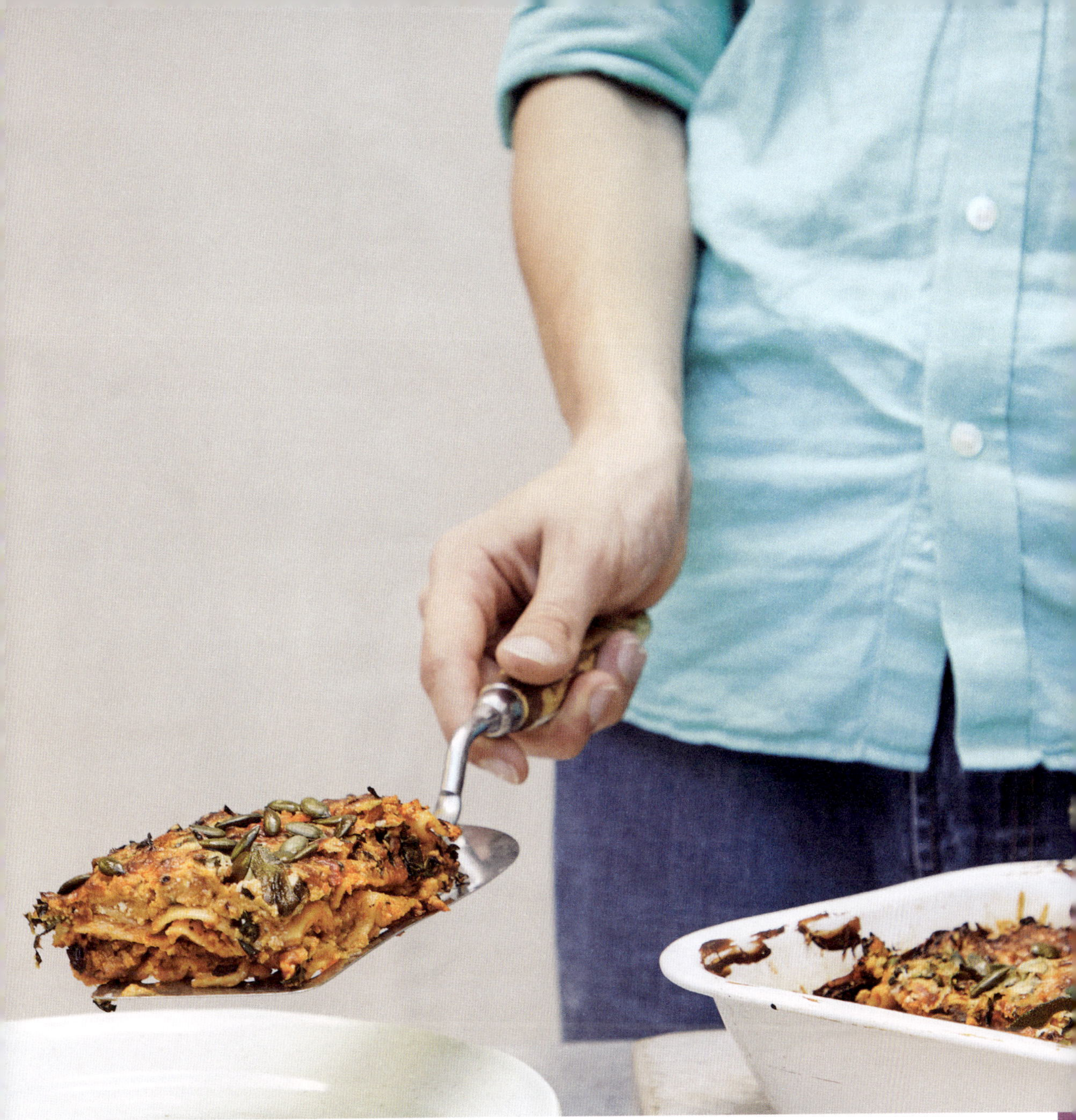

Use soft almond or cashew cheese and vegan spread.

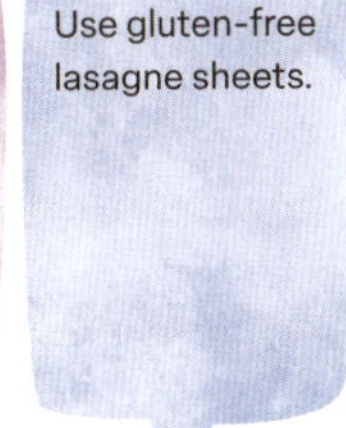

Use gluten-free lasagne sheets.

dairy-free

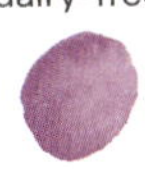

gluten-free

nut-free

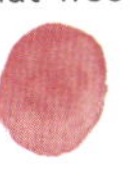

sesame-free

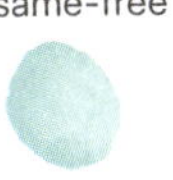

egg-free

soy-free

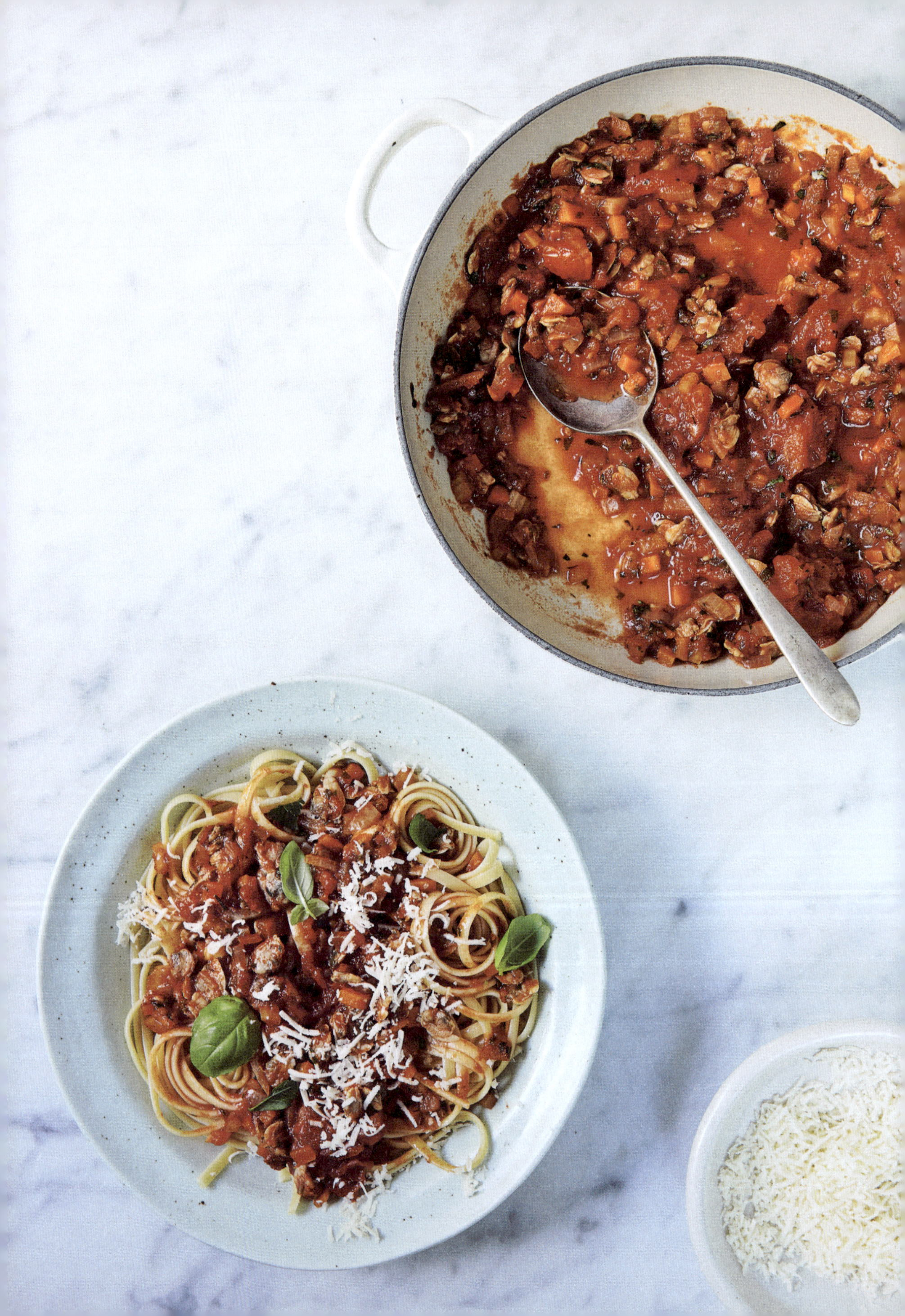

TOMATO & CLAM PASTA

Serves 4

2 Tbsp olive oil
1 small onion, finely chopped
2 garlic cloves, crushed
2 x 400g (14oz) cans plum tomatoes
1 carrot, peeled and diced
1 celery stick, diced
1 tsp apple cider vinegar
3 stems of fresh basil, leaves stripped and finely chopped, plus more to garnish, if liked
3 sprigs of fresh parsley, finely chopped
300g (10½oz) linguine or spaghetti
200g (7oz) jarred clams, drained
dried chilli flakes (optional)
Parmesan, grated (shredded), to serve (optional)
salt and black pepper

In my experience from talking to my clients, many neurodivergent people eat tomato pasta on repeat, and this can mean that, other than maybe a little grated Parmesan, their meal contains very little protein, so they may not feel full for that long.

Adding clams is a clever hack to help bolster the dish with protein as well as vitamin B12 without significantly changing the overall feel, smell or taste. Build up from a teaspoon of shelled clams in an entire bowl if you are cautious about introducing change.

Clams are small molluscs that have a soft texture and a very pleasant mild taste. They have the highest concentration of vitamin B12 of any food – which is important as B12 is a key nutrient for neurological health.

Heat the olive oil in a large saucepan over a medium heat. Add the onion and gently cook for 3–5 minutes until soft and translucent. Add the garlic and cook for a further minute.

Add the plum tomatoes and break up using a spatula, then add the carrot and celery. Stir in the apple cider vinegar, half the basil and half the parsley. Cook at a gentle simmer for 40 minutes, stirring from time to time.

About 10 minutes before the end of the cooking time, put the linguine or spaghetti in a large pan of boiling salted water and cook as per the packet instructions.

Add the rest of the basil and parsley and the clams to the tomato sauce and stir well. Test for seasoning and add salt, pepper and a few chilli flakes if you wish.

If you want the sauce to be very smooth and the clams not to be obvious, then cool down the sauce slightly and blend it using a stick blender directly in the pan. Serve with the pasta and topped with Parmesan cheese and some more basil, if liked.

Without the added clams the tomato sauce can be stored in the refrigerator for up to 3 days and the freezer for up to 3 months.

Use yeast flakes instead of Parmesan.
Use gluten-free pasta.

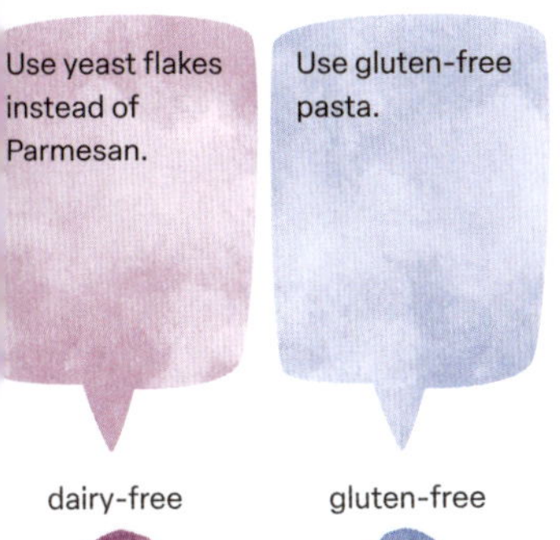

dairy-free · gluten-free · nut-free · sesame-free · egg-free · soy-free

LUCINDA'S SHEPHERD'S PIE

Serves 6–8

2 medium potatoes, peeled and quartered
1 whole cauliflower, leaves discarded and chopped into florets
1–2 Tbsp butter
glug of olive oil
1 onion, finely chopped
1 leek, finely chopped
400–500g (14oz–1lb 2oz) minced (ground) lamb
400g (14oz) can brown or green lentils, drained
2–3 carrots, peeled and cubed
2 sprigs of rosemary, needles finely chopped
1–2 Tbsp Worcestershire sauce
salt and black pepper

This is the dish I turn to when I need my brain to be fully focused. It is so comforting and delicious and is packed with nutrition and fibre. Making mash using cauliflower as well as potato reduces the starch content – use this combo whenever you make mash. My 'shepherd's pie' can easily be made plant-based by replacing the lamb with an extra can of lentils and using vegan Worcestershire sauce.

Cook the potatoes for 15 minutes in a large pan of boiling water and add the cauliflower florets halfway through. When both are soft, drain, mash well, then stir in the butter and a little salt and pepper to taste. Set aside.

While the potatoes and cauliflower are cooking, heat the olive oil in a large saucepan over a medium heat and fry the onion and leek until soft (about 5–7 minutes). Then add the lamb and brown on all sides over a slightly higher heat. Turn the heat down to medium and add the drained lentils, carrot, rosemary and Worcestershire sauce. Continue to cook until the carrots are soft. Season with salt and pepper and a little more Worcestershire sauce if you wish.

Preheat the grill (broiler) to high. Transfer the lamb mixture to an ovenproof dish measuring about 29 x 22cm (11.5 x 8.5in). Top with the mash and spread it evenly to cover. Grill (broil) until the topping is nice and crispy.

Store in the refrigerator for up to 3 days or in the freezer for 3 months. I recommend storing it once it is cooked through but not grilled. To reheat from chilled, cover the dish with foil and put in a preheated oven at 180°C/160°F fan/350°F/Gas mark 4 for 20–30 minutes until piping hot and then grill to crisp up the top.

Swap the butter for olive oil or a plant-based spread.

Replace the lamb with an extra can of lentils and use vegan Worcestershire sauce.

dairy-free
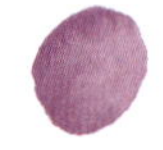
gluten-free

nut-free
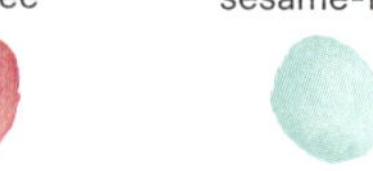
sesame-free
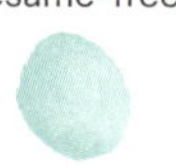
egg-free

soy-free

vegetarian
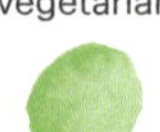

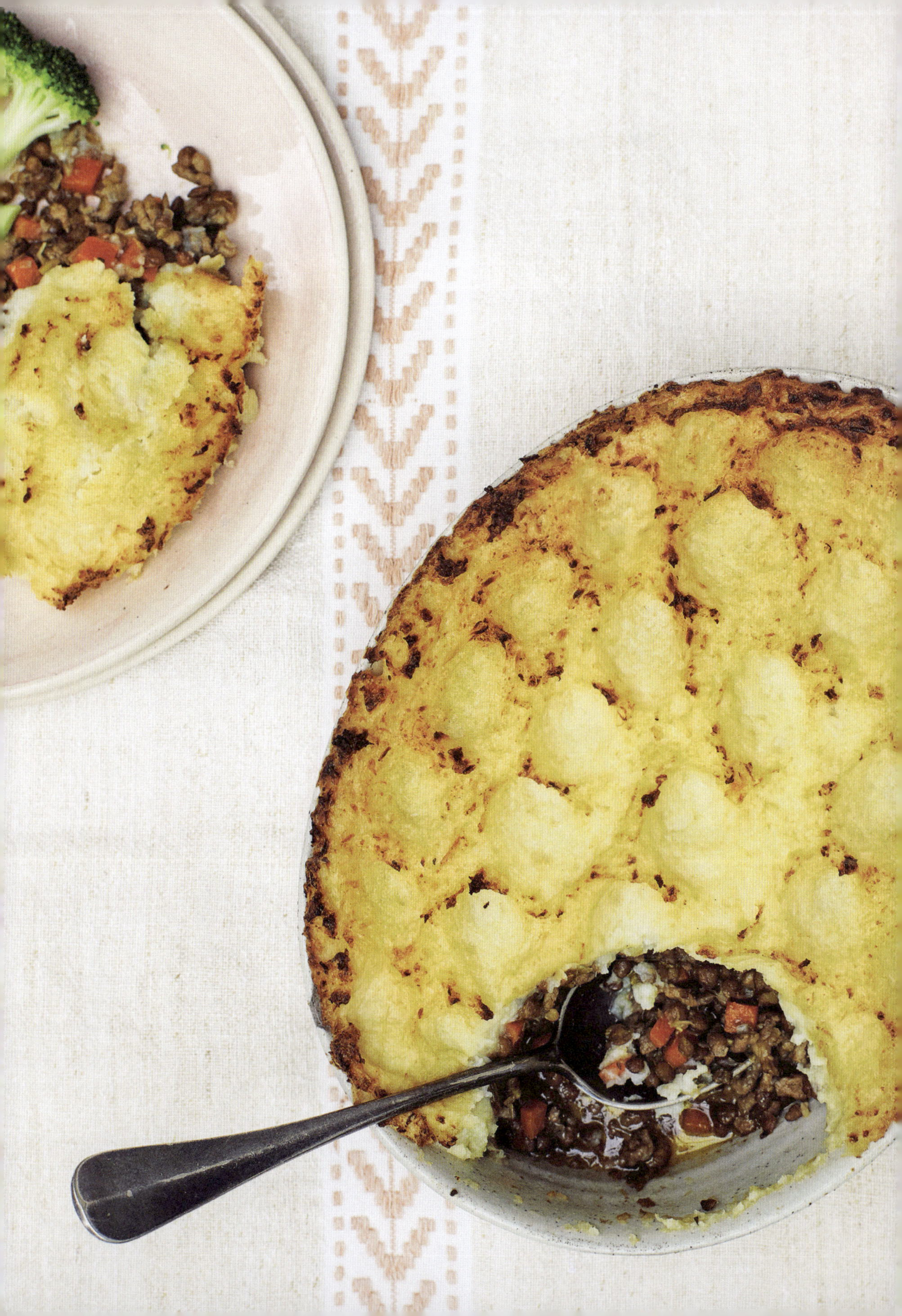

PRAWN EGG-FRIED RICE

Here's a one-pan meal that is easy to bring together: this egg-fried rice is tasty and packed with vegetables and omega-3-rich prawns. Five-spice and ginger are both soothing on the gut.

Serves 2

200g (1 cup) brown rice
2 Tbsp sesame oil
3 spring onions (scallions), finely chopped
1 red (bell) pepper, roughly chopped
3 tsp Chinese five-spice
large knob of ginger root, peeled and grated
2 eggs, preferably free-range
2 Tbsp tamari soy sauce
80g (scant ¾ cup) frozen peas
150g (generous 1 cup) cooked shelled prawns (shrimp)
15g (about 2 Tbsp) sunflower seeds
fresh coriander (cilantro) leaves and lime wedges to garnish (optional)

Rinse the rice and cook as per the packet instructions.

When the rice is almost cooked, gently heat the sesame oil in a large frying pan (skillet). Add the spring onions, red pepper, Chinese five-spice and ginger and stir-fry for 5 minutes.

Crack the eggs into a bowl and stir with a fork so the whites and yolks are well blended.

Add the cooked rice to the pan then add the tamari and the eggs and cook, stirring continuously, for a couple of minutes until the eggs start to scramble slightly. Stir in the frozen peas and prawns (shrimp). Cook for a further 2 minutes until they are heated through.

Sprinkle over the sunflower seeds and garnish with some coriander and lime wedges, if liked.

You can reheat this until piping hot once within 24 hours. Discard any remaining leftovers after 24 hours.

dairy-free

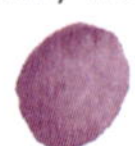

gluten-free

nut-free

sesame-free

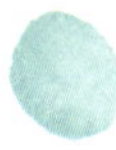

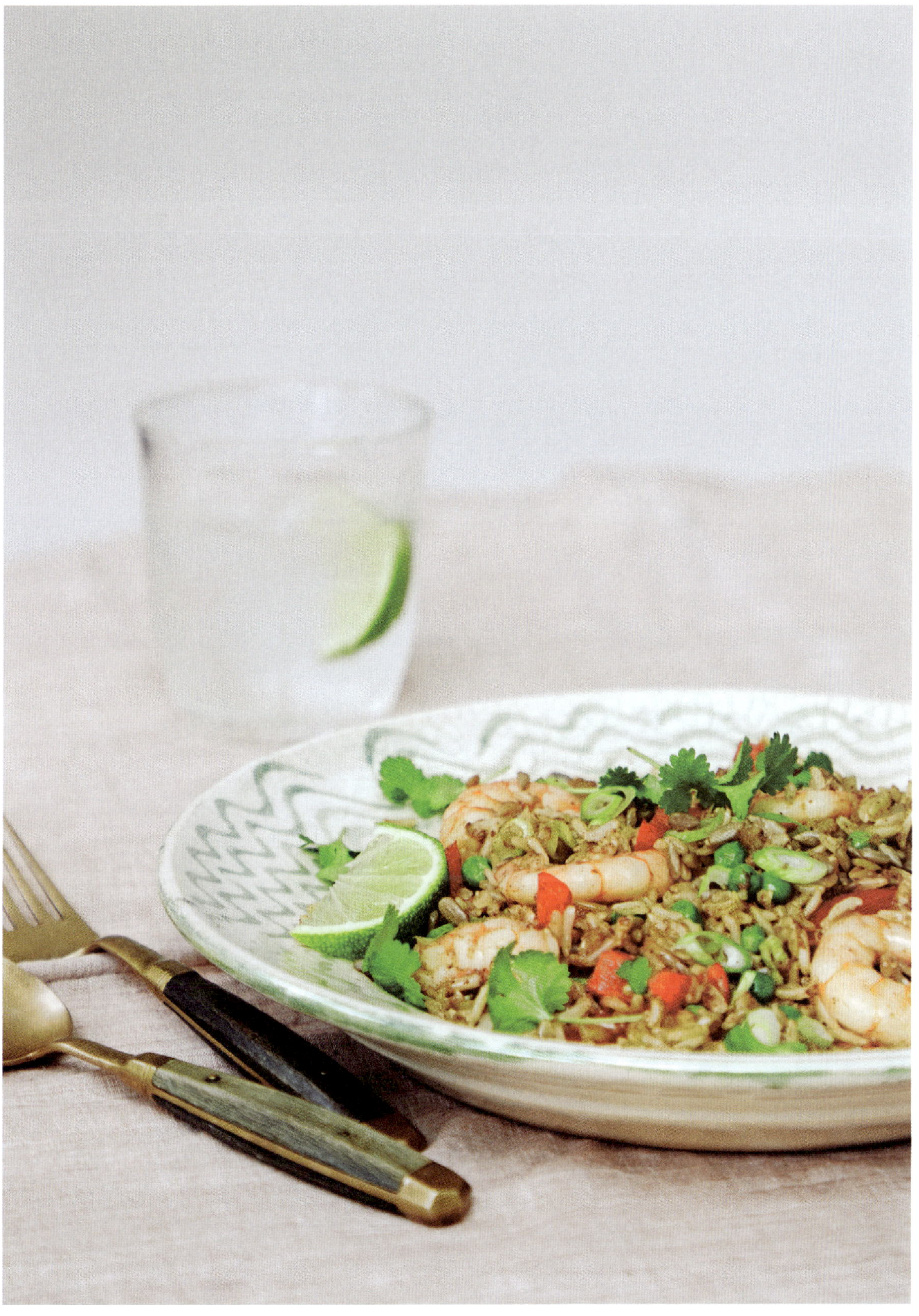

CRAB & PEA PESTO PASTA

Serves 2

150g (5½oz) fresh or dried pasta of choice
70g (scant ½ cup) frozen peas
170g (5¾oz) can white crab meat, drained weight 120g (4½oz) or 120g (4½oz) freshly cooked white crab meat

Pesto
60g (about 2 cups) fresh basil, leaves and stems
1 small garlic clove
30g (¼ cup) pine nuts, toasted
30g (1oz) Parmesan, grated
juice of ½ lemon
4 Tbsp olive oil

Most people love pesto pasta but find it isn't filling enough. To feel fuller for longer and to balance blood glucose levels better, you can include important protein by adding crab meat and frozen peas, both of which are protein-rich. Crab is also rich in zinc, iron, vitamin B12 and folate.

This combination makes a super-quick and filling supper, ticking all the nutrition and taste boxes. It's perfect for anyone who is not keen on eating fish or seafood, as the crab meat is soft and its flavour melds beautifully into the pesto.

You can buy fresh pesto and use canned crab meat to make this meal even easier. Fresh pasta containing egg is another way to get more protein into this meal and it's even quicker to cook.

Cook the pasta as per the packet instructions, adding the peas for the last 2 minutes, then drain.

Meanwhile, make the pesto by putting all the ingredients into a mini food processor and blitzing them until you have a bright green sauce. Add a little more olive oil if it seems too dry.

Add the pesto and the crab to the pasta and peas and stir gently to ensure everything is well coated in pesto.

Serve immediately. Any leftovers can be stored in the refrigerator for no more than 24 hours. Reheat thoroughly until piping hot.

TIP
For crab-free, use 120g (4½oz) drained bottled clams or 1 salmon steak (approx. 120g/4½oz).

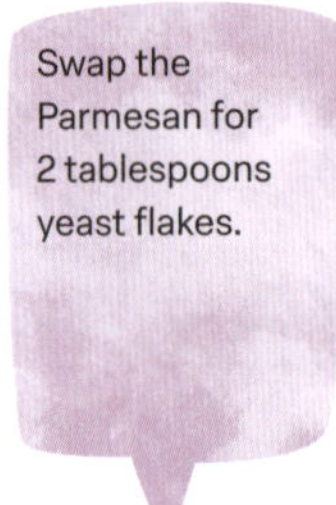

Choose a gluten-free pasta.

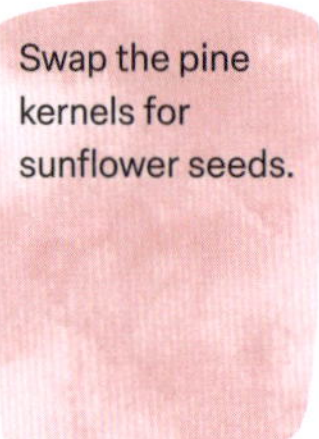

dairy-free

gluten-free

nut-free

sesame-free

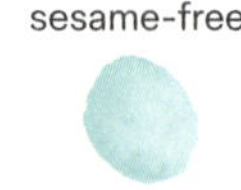

egg-free

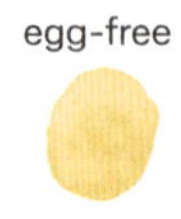

soy-free

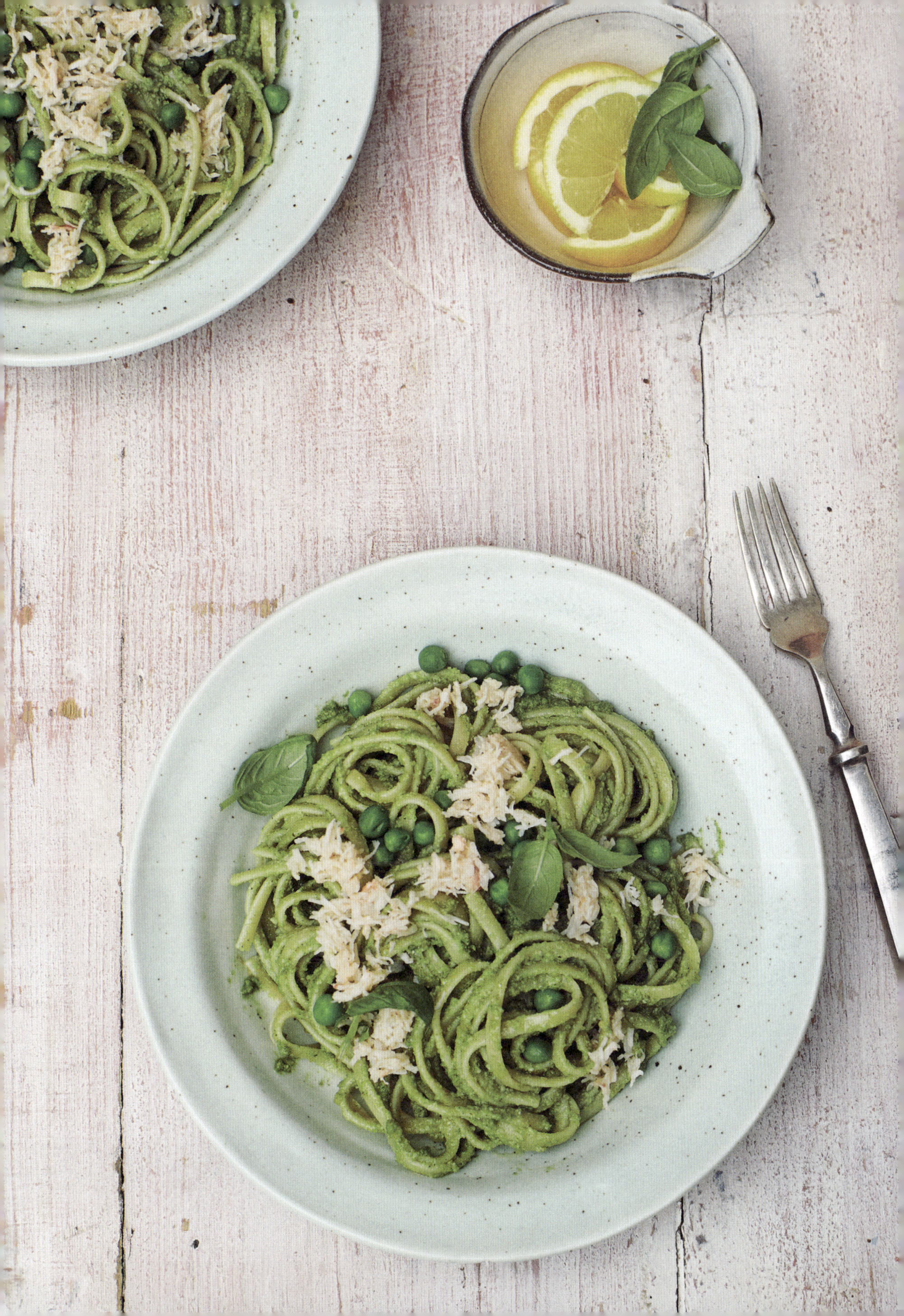

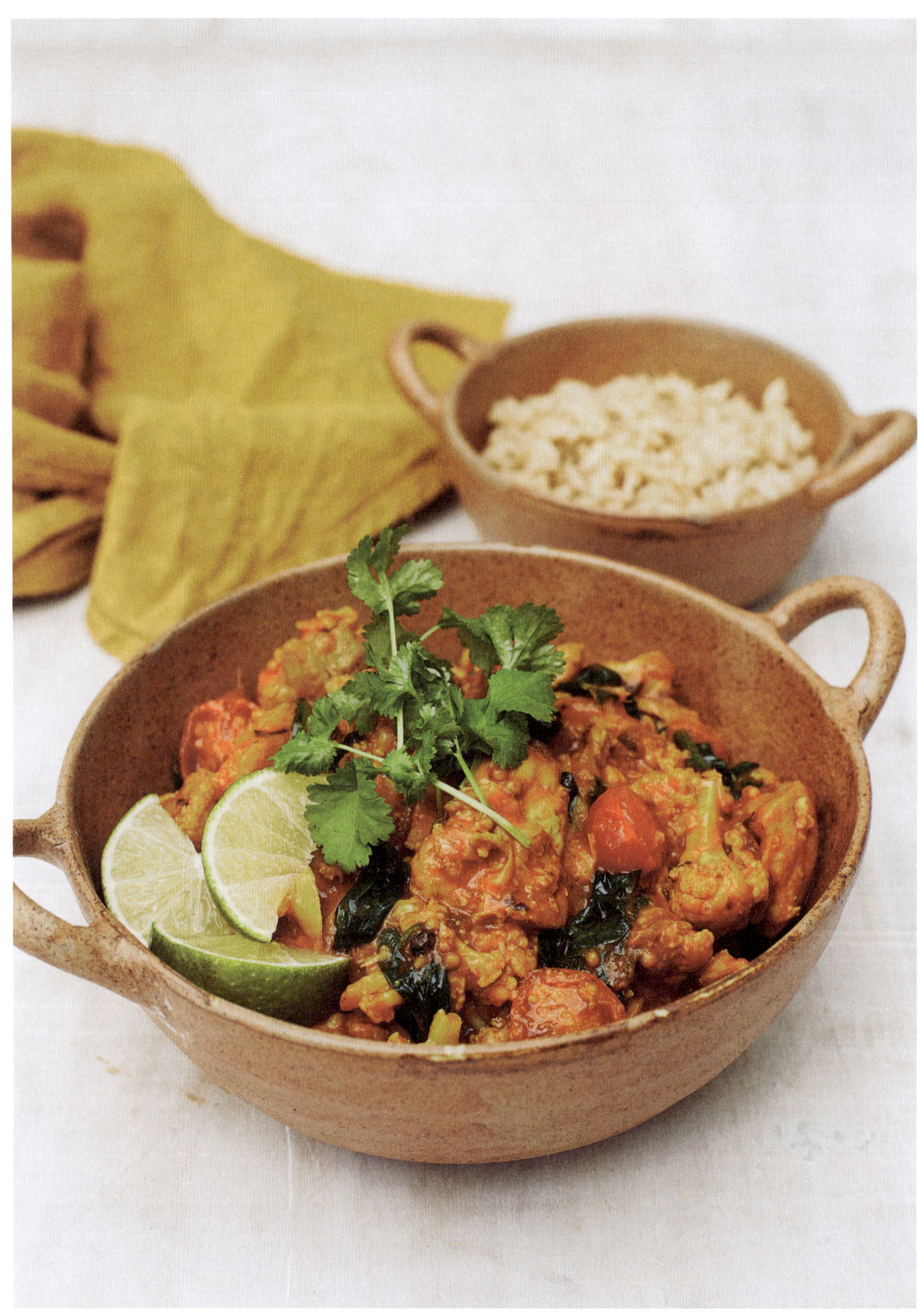

CHICKEN & CAULIFLOWER COCONUT CURRY

This is a light and fresh South Indian style curry with a creamy coconut sauce and delicious spices that are anti-inflammatory in nature. It is a real winner when you need some comfort food and something to recharge your brain. Swap the chicken for 50:50 diced firm tofu and green lentils if you want to make this plant-based. Chicken, tofu and lentils are all rich in protein and contain some iron to help nourish the blood.

Serves 4–6

Paste

2 garlic cloves
1 Tbsp mustard seeds
6 curry leaves
1 tsp tamarind paste
1 tsp ground turmeric
½ tsp peppercorns
100ml (scant ½ cup) coconut milk
1 fresh green chilli, deseeded

Curry

2 Tbsp coconut oil
1 onion, finely chopped
thumb of fresh ginger root, very finely chopped
6 skinless, boneless chicken thighs (about 600g/1lb 5oz), cut into bite-sized pieces
1 garlic clove, finely chopped
3 Tbsp tomato purée (paste)
300ml (1¼ cups) coconut milk
zest and juice of 1 lime
12 small cauliflower florets
8 cherry tomatoes, halved
handful of baby spinach
salt and black pepper
fresh coriander (cilantro) leaves, to garnish (optional)

First make the paste by putting all the ingredients into a mini food processor. Blend for 2 minutes to a fine paste.

Next make the curry. Heat the coconut oil in a large frying pan (skillet) over a medium heat and fry the onion and ginger for 3–5 minutes until the onion is translucent and soft. Next add the chicken and cook, turning the pieces until brown on all sides.

Add the garlic, tomato purée, coconut milk, lime zest and juice and the cauliflower florets. Bring to a simmer, then stir in the curry paste. Cover and simmer for 12–15 minutes, so that the chicken cooks through and the sauce reduces and thickens a little. Add salt and pepper to taste.

Stir in the tomatoes and spinach and, when the spinach starts to wilt, turn off the heat.

Serve with brown rice, sprinkled with fresh coriander.

You can prepare the paste in larger batches and store in the freezer. Any leftover curry sauce can be stored in the refrigerator for up to 3 days and frozen for up to 3 months.

Swap the chicken for 50:50 diced firm tofu (beancurd) and green lentils

dairy-free
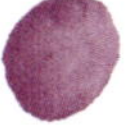
gluten-free

nut-free

sesame-free
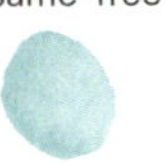
egg-free
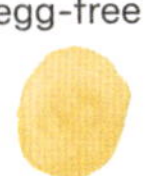
soy-free

vegetarian

ORANGE & GINGER STIR-FRY DUCK NOODLES

Orange, ginger and duck make a delicious combination, and this wholesome meal is rich in iron. The Chinese five-spice, garlic and ginger are great for digestion and help with immunity. Strips of duck breast are soft and easy to chew, making them easier for anyone who normally struggles to eat large chunks of meat.

Serves 4

350g (12oz) duck breast strips for stir-fry
200g (7oz) rice noodles
1 Tbsp sesame oil
250g (9oz) pak choi (bok choy), roughly chopped
1 tsp sesame seeds
fresh coriander (cilantro) leaves to garnish (optional)

Marinade
zest and juice of 1 unwaxed orange
3 Tbsp tamari soy sauce
1 tsp sesame oil
1½ Tbsp honey
1 tsp Chinese five-spice
1 garlic clove, finely chopped
1½ tsp grated or minced ginger root (fresh or frozen)

First make the marinade: put all the ingredients in a medium non-metallic bowl and gently whisk together. Add the duck strips, cover and leave for at least 10 minutes (or make ahead and leave it overnight in the refrigerator).

Cook the noodles as per the packet instructions, drain and set aside.

Meanwhile, heat the sesame oil in a large frying pan (skillet) then add the marinated duck strips. Stir-fry for 3–4 minutes, then add the remaining marinade. Cook for a further 3 minutes until the duck is cooked through. Remove the strips from the pan and set aside to rest.

Stir-fry the pak choi in the marinade left in the frying pan until it is soft, around 4–6 minutes, then add the cooked noodles and lastly the duck. Stir gently to coat everything lightly in the marinade. Sprinkle with the sesame seeds and garnish with coriander, if liked.

If not eating straight away, the stir-fried duck and pak choi can be cooled and stored in the refrigerator for up to 48 hours. Discard the cooked noodles within 24 hours of cooking.

Switch to olive oil or coconut oil and crunchy sunflower seeds.

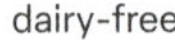

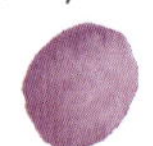

gluten-free

nut-free

sesame-free

egg-free

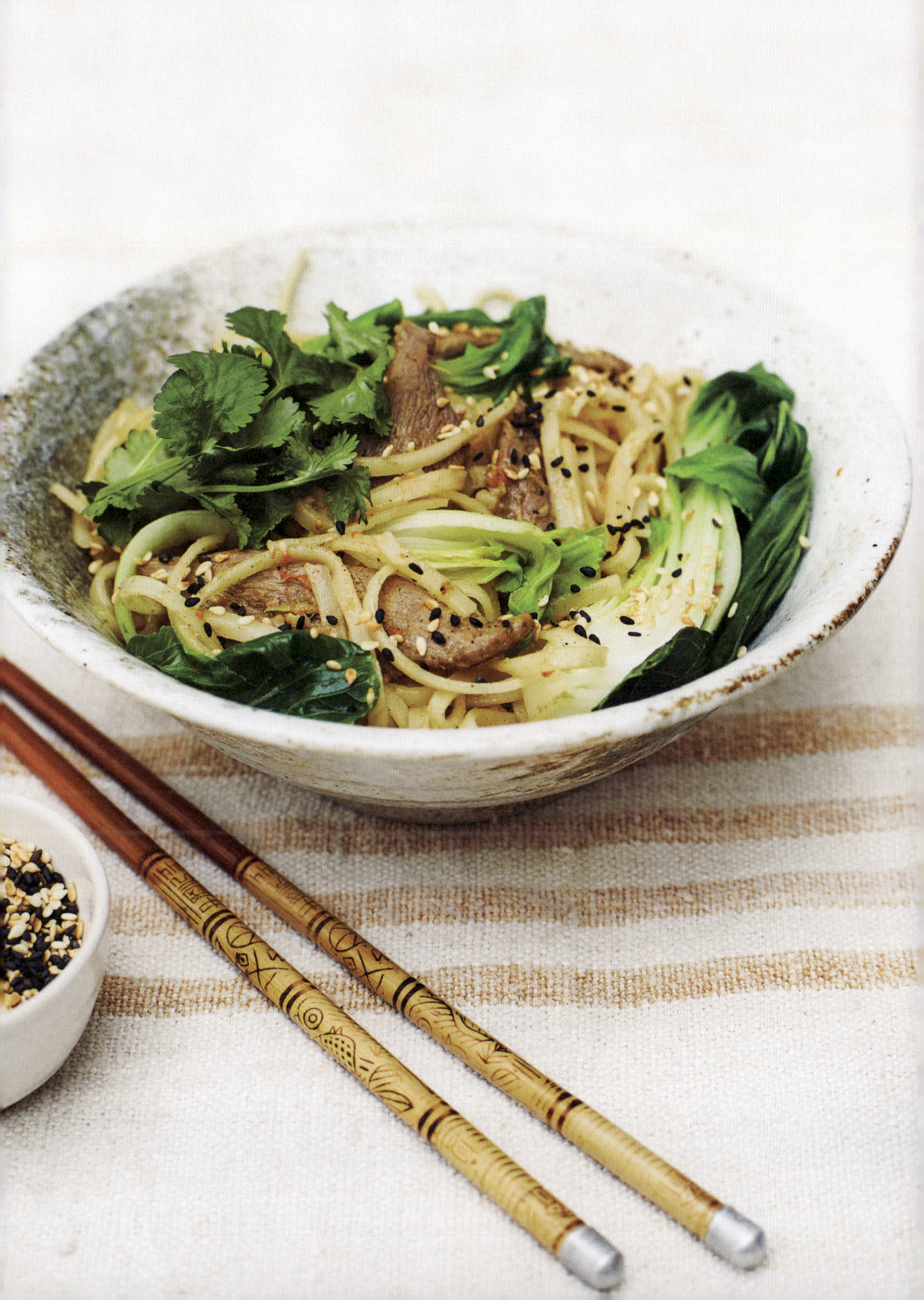

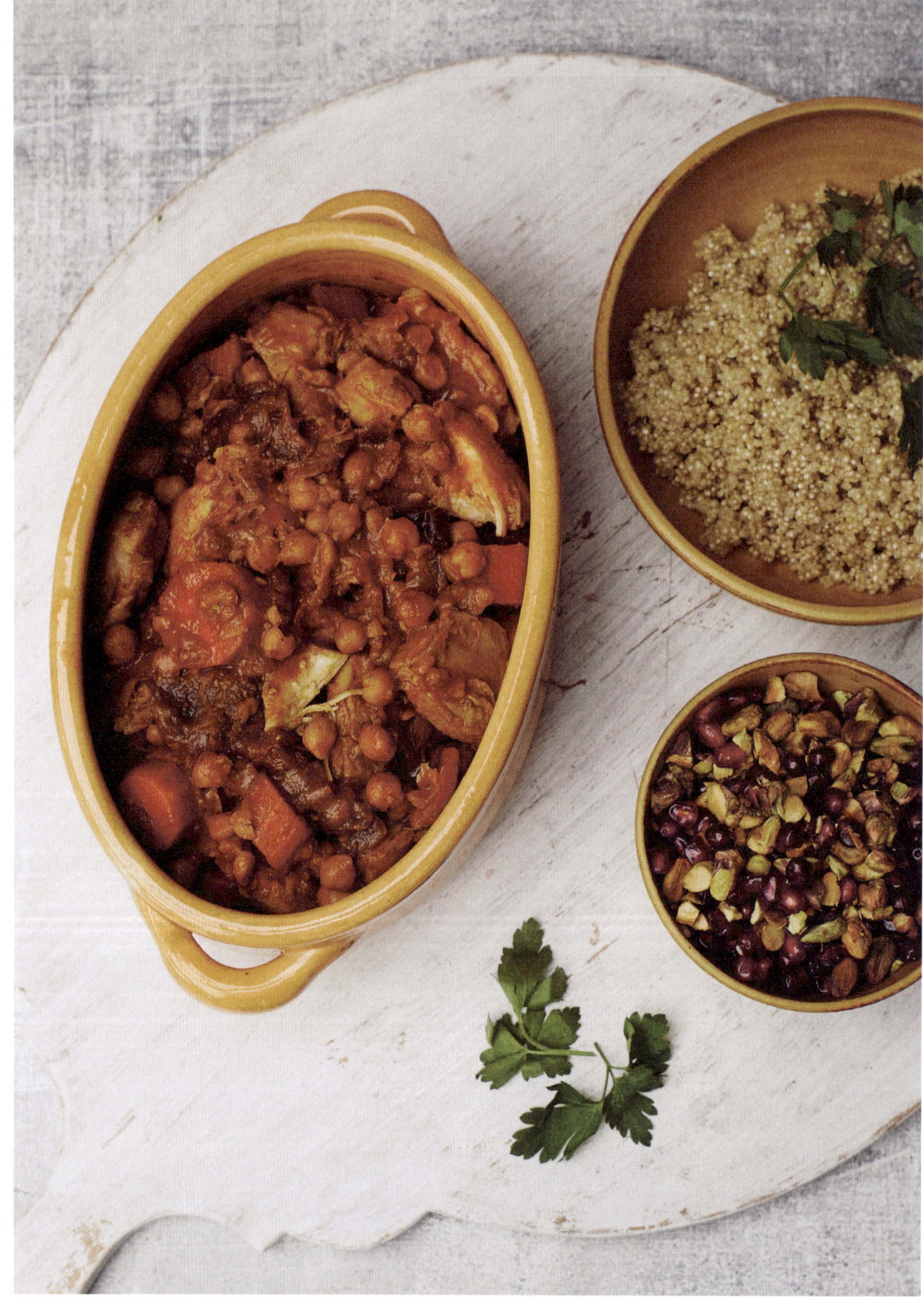

CHICKEN, APRICOT & SAFFRON TAGINE

Serves 4–6

1 pat of butter
2 Tbsp olive oil
6 skinless, boneless chicken thighs (about 600g/1lb 5oz), cut into bite-sized pieces
1 red onion, diced
240ml (1 cup) fresh chicken stock or bone broth
1 Tbsp tomato purée (paste)
2 carrots, peeled and cut into large chunks
12 stoned apricots (ideally natural brown and unsulphured), quartered
400g (14oz) can chickpeas (garbanzo beans), drained
1 Tbsp peeled and crushed fresh ginger root
2 cinnamon sticks
1 tsp ground turmeric
3 saffron strands
salt and black pepper

Optional
1 Tbsp shelled pistachios, roughly chopped
1 Tbsp chopped fresh parsley
1 Tbsp pomegranate seeds

Tagine is a Moroccan dish that uses gentle warming spices, all of which are anti-inflammatory and support the diversity of the gut microbiome. This version has a wonderful combination of sweet apricot and a kick of ginger. Saffron is soothing on the mood and can help with focus.

Chicken, apricots and chickpeas contain good amounts of iron, making this a good recipe if you are feeling tired, run-down or washed out. Typically, tagine is served with couscous, but rice or quinoa are options as well as flatbreads or pitta bread.

Heat the butter and oil in a large saucepan over a medium heat and brown the chicken pieces on all sides. Transfer the chicken to a plate, keeping as much of the butter and oil in the pan.

Fry the onion in the butter and oil for 3 minutes, then add all the remaining ingredients. Cover and cook for a further 10 minutes.

Return the chicken to the pan and give it a good stir. You can either continue to cook this, covered, over a gentle heat for 20 minutes or transfer it to an ovenproof dish and cook in a preheated oven at 180°C/160°C fan/325°F/Gas mark 3 for 20 minutes. For a real depth of flavour, leave it to cook for up to an hour over a very low heat.

Serve garnished with pistachios, parsley and pomegranate seeds, if you like.

The tagine can be cooled and stored in the refrigerator for up to 3 days, and for 3 months in the freezer.

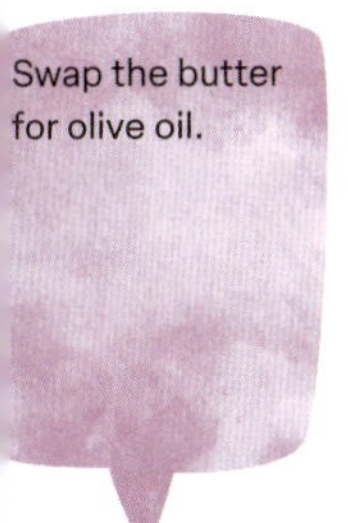

dairy-free
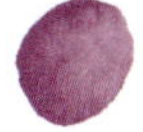

gluten-free
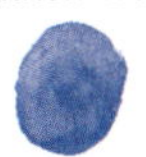

nut-free

sesame-free
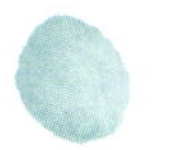

egg-free
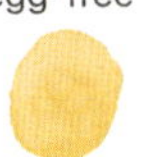

soy-free

BLACK BEAN & SWEET POTATO CHILLI

Black beans and sweet potato make the most delicious and nourishing pairing that works well in a Mexican chilli. The warming mellow spices – paprika, cumin and coriander and a touch of chilli – are a winning combination for gut health. This recipe contains five veggies as well as garlic and beans, so it is a great way of getting your five a day. To speed up the prep, you can use a food processor to finely grate the veg.

Serves 4–6

2 Tbsp olive oil
1 small onion, finely diced
2 garlic cloves, crushed
1 sweet potato, peeled and finely grated (shredded)
1 carrot, peeled and finely grated (shredded)
½ courgette (zucchini), finely grated (shredded)
1 red (bell) pepper, finely diced
2 x 400g (14oz) cans black beans, drained
3 Tbsp tomato purée (paste)
250ml (1 cup plus 1 Tbsp) vegetable stock
1 Tbsp smoked paprika
1 Tbsp ground cumin
1 Tbsp ground coriander
½ tsp chilli powder or 1 fresh red chilli, deseeded and finely sliced, or to taste
salt and black pepper

To serve
2 Tbsp chopped fresh coriander (cilantro)
lime wedges
full-fat plain yoghurt
cooked rice or quinoa

Heat the olive oil in a large saucepan over a medium heat and add the onion. Cook for 3–5 minutes until soft, then add the garlic and cook for a further minute.

Add the sweet potato, carrot and courgette, then add in the red pepper, black beans, tomato purée, stock and spices. Cover and cook over a medium heat for 40 minutes, stirring from time to time. Add some extra stock if the mixture is looking a bit dry. Season with salt and pepper, and chilli powder or fresh chilli if you like, adding it cautiously.

Sprinkle with chopped coriander and serve with lime wedges, yoghurt and rice or quinoa.

Store leftovers in the refrigerator for 3 days or in the freezer for 3 months.

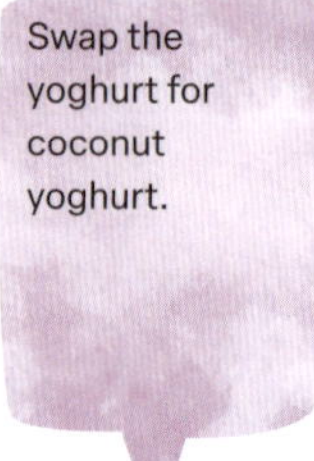

dairy-free
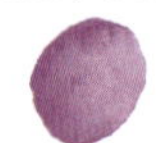
gluten-free

nut-free

sesame-free

egg-free

soy-free
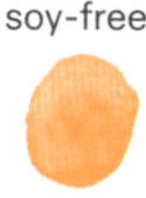
vegetarian
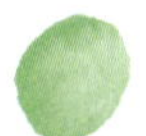

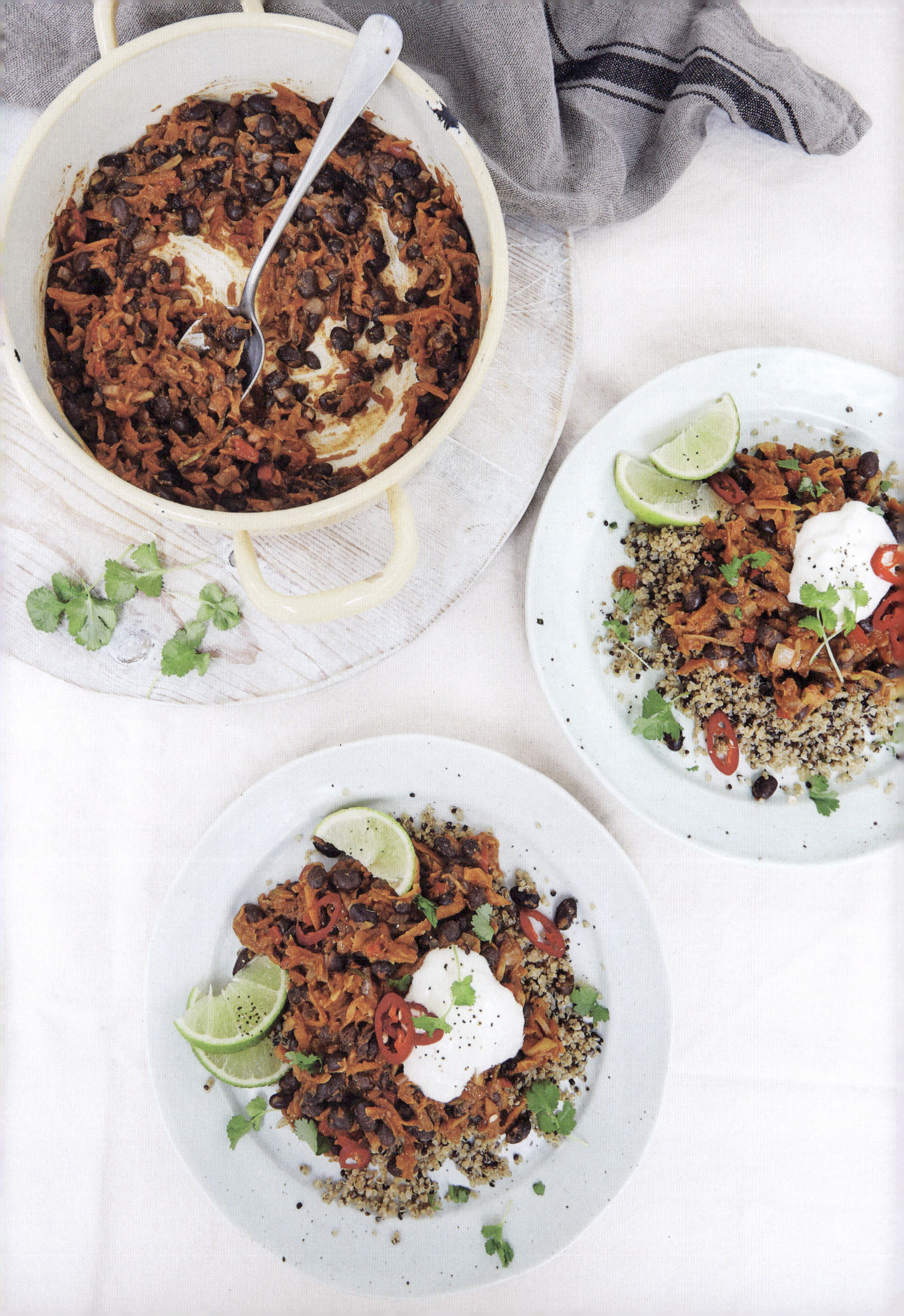

TOFU PAD THAI NOODLES

Here's how to make a comforting and nourishing supper of noodles packed with iron-rich tofu (beancurd) and six vegetables in a delicious Pad Thai sauce. Sheer happiness in a bowl!

Serves 2

200g (7oz) wide rice noodles (uncooked weight)
2 Tbsp sesame oil
15g (½oz) tamarind paste
280g (10oz) firm tofu (beancurd), cubed
½ small onion, sliced
120g (4¼oz) French (green) beans, topped, tailed and halved
¼ spring (white) cabbage, sliced
2 eggs, preferably free-range
300g (10½oz) beansprouts, fresh or canned and drained
1 carrot, peeled and ribboned
2 Tbsp roughly chopped spring onions (scallions)

Pad Thai sauce
85g (3oz) tamarind paste
2 Tbsp coconut sugar (or soft brown sugar)
2 pinches of salt

To serve
2 Tbsp unsalted roasted peanuts, crushed
fresh coriander (cilantro) leaves
2 lime wedges

Cook the noodles as per the packet instructions.

Make the Pad Thai sauce by stirring together the tamarind paste and coconut sugar with the salt.

Heat the sesame oil in a large frying pan (skillet) or wok and stir in the tamarind paste. Add the tofu and stir-fry until it is gently browned on all sides.

Add the onion and stir-fry for 3 minutes, then add the green beans and cabbage and cook for a further 3 minutes – you may need a little more sesame oil. Next, add the cooked rice noodles and Pad Thai sauce. Stir gently to coat the noodles, tofu and veg.

Crack in the eggs and gently stir through, so that they break up a little and cook for 2–3 minutes. Finally, stir in the beansprouts, carrot ribbons and spring onions to warm through.

Pop the Pad Thai on plates, sprinkle on the peanuts and coriander leaves and serve with lime wedges.

Store any leftovers in the refrigerator and eat within 24 hours of cooking. Reheat thoroughly to ensure the noodles are piping hot.

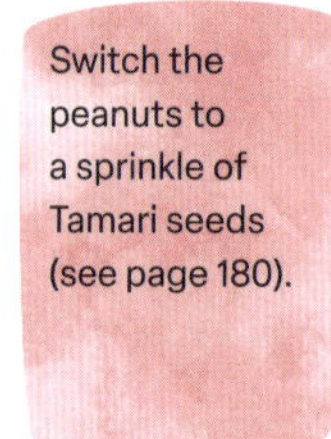

Switch to olive or coconut oil.

Combine 30g gram flour with 40ml water and use instead.

dairy-free
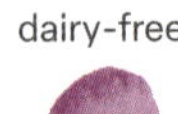

gluten-free

nut-free

sesame-free

egg-free

vegetarian
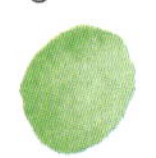

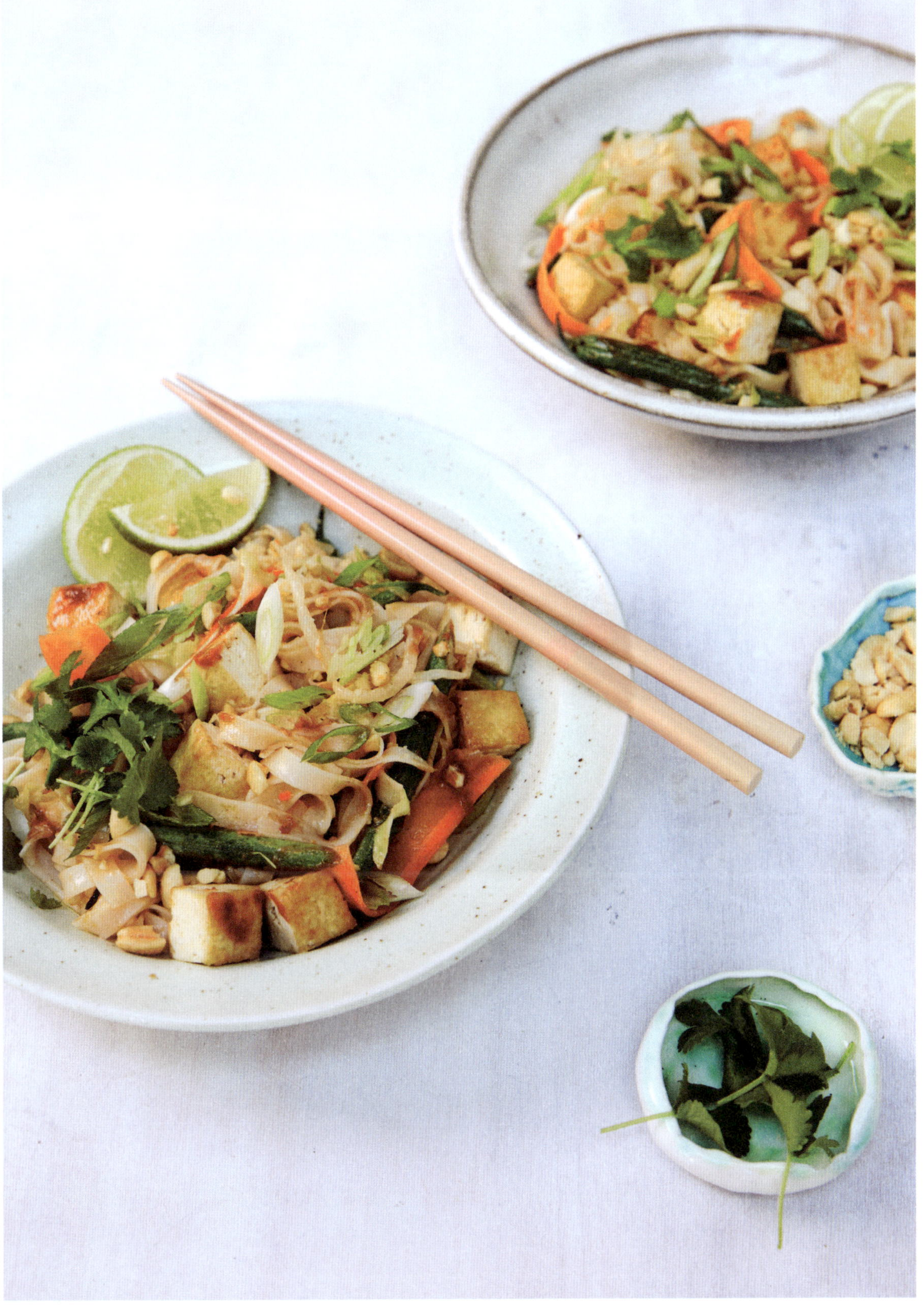

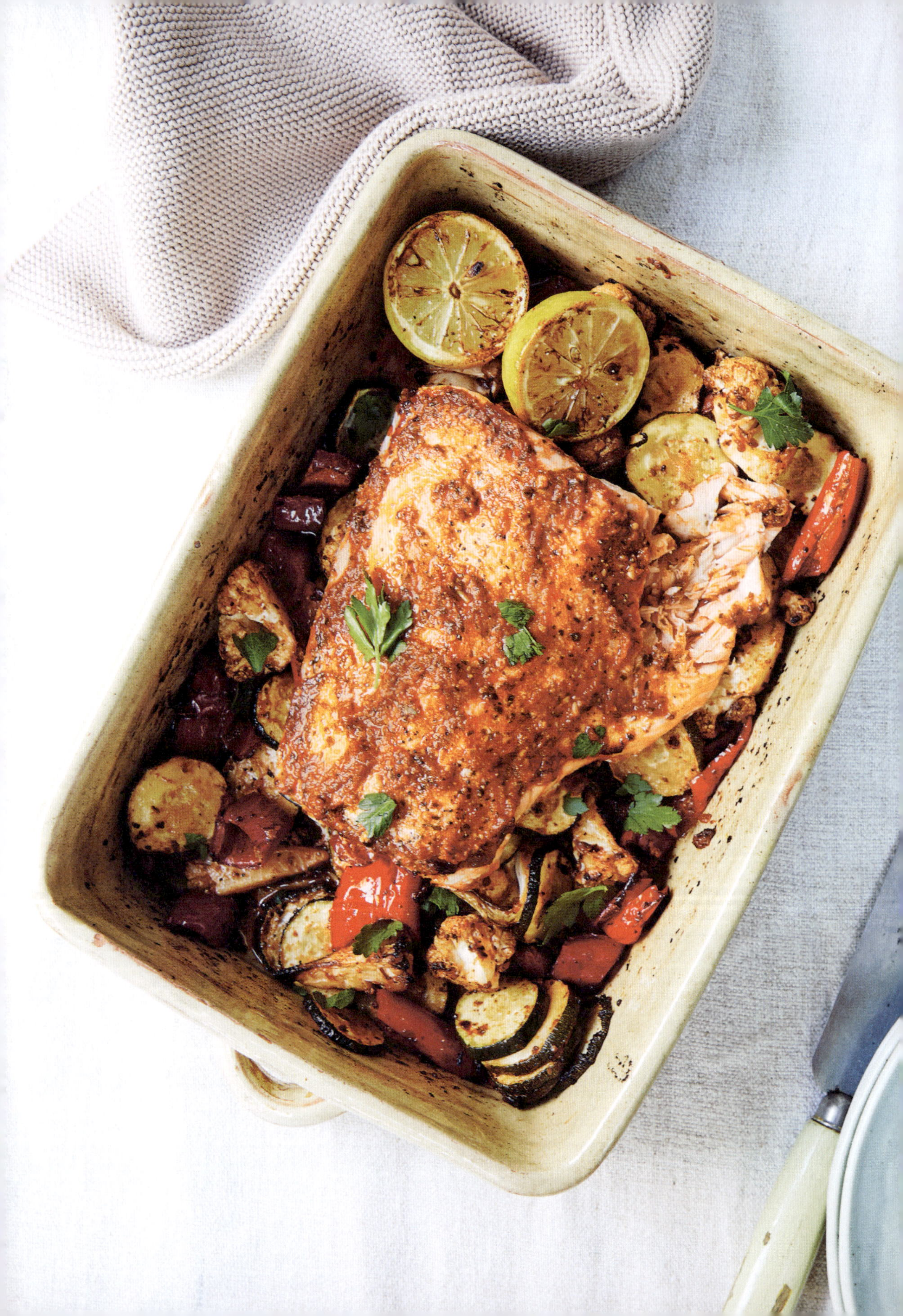

RED PESTO SALMON TRAYBAKE WITH MEDITERRANEAN ROAST VEGETABLES

This is a great way to eat the Mediterranean way and top up with your omega-3 fatty acids. Serve with quinoa, brown rice, gnocchi or egg pasta for a filling, nutritious and delicious meal. Any leftovers make a great lunchbox filler, as this one can be enjoyed cold as well as hot.

Serves 4

3 Tbsp red pesto paste
3 Tbsp olive oil
1 cauliflower, chopped into small florets
400g (14oz) salmon fillet, skin on
2 courgettes (zucchini), sliced into rounds
2 red (bell) peppers (ideally Romano), deseeded and chopped into 2cm (¾in) pieces
1 lemon, halved
flat-leaf parsley, chopped, to garnish

Preheat the oven to 200°C/180°C fan/400°F/Gas mark 6.

Mix the red pesto and olive oil in a small bowl to make a dressing.

Scatter the cauliflower florets into a large roasting tray and drizzle over 2 heaped tablespoons of the red pesto dressing. Pop into the oven for 15 minutes.

Rub 1 tablespoon of pesto dressing over the salmon. Set aside.

After the cauliflower has roasted for 15 minutes, add the courgette, red pepper and lemon to the roasting tray, coat with the remaining pesto dressing and toss everything together. Return the tray to the oven for 20 minutes.

Add the salmon, skin-side up, and roast for a final 15 minutes or until the flesh is almost completely opaque and flakes easily; the time will depend on the thickness of the fillet. Remove the skin from the salmon before serving. Garnish with chopped parsley.

Store any leftovers in the refrigerator for up to 48 hours.

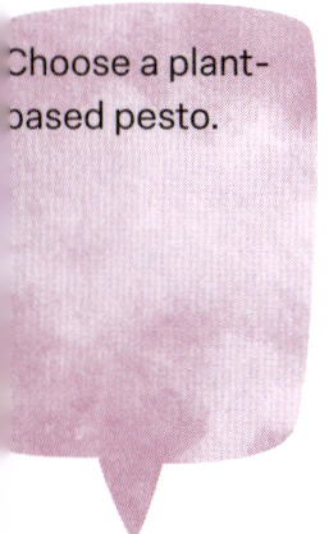

Choose a nut-free pesto.

dairy-free

gluten-free

nut-free

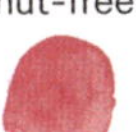

sesame-free

egg-free

soy-free

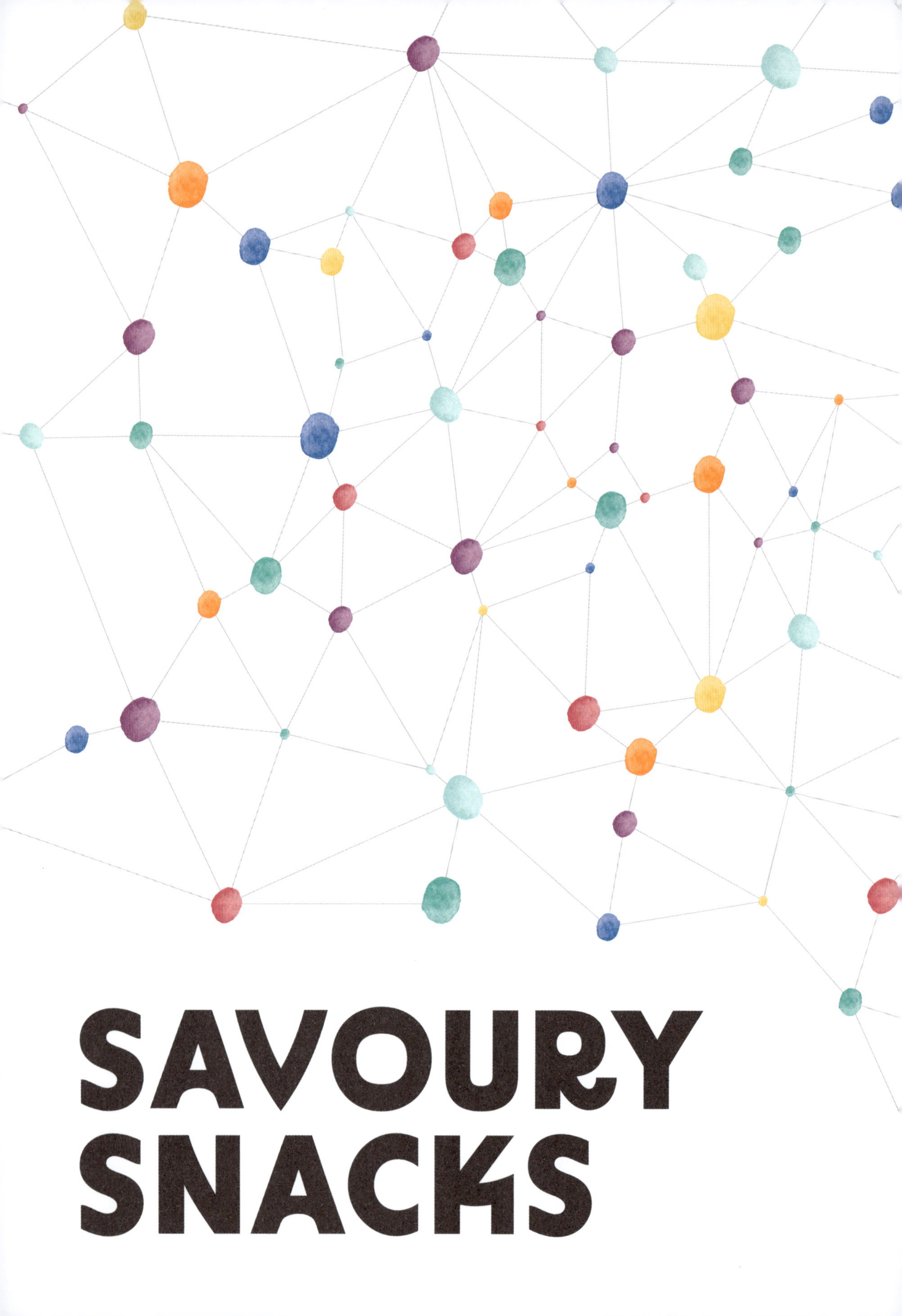

SAVOURY SNACKS

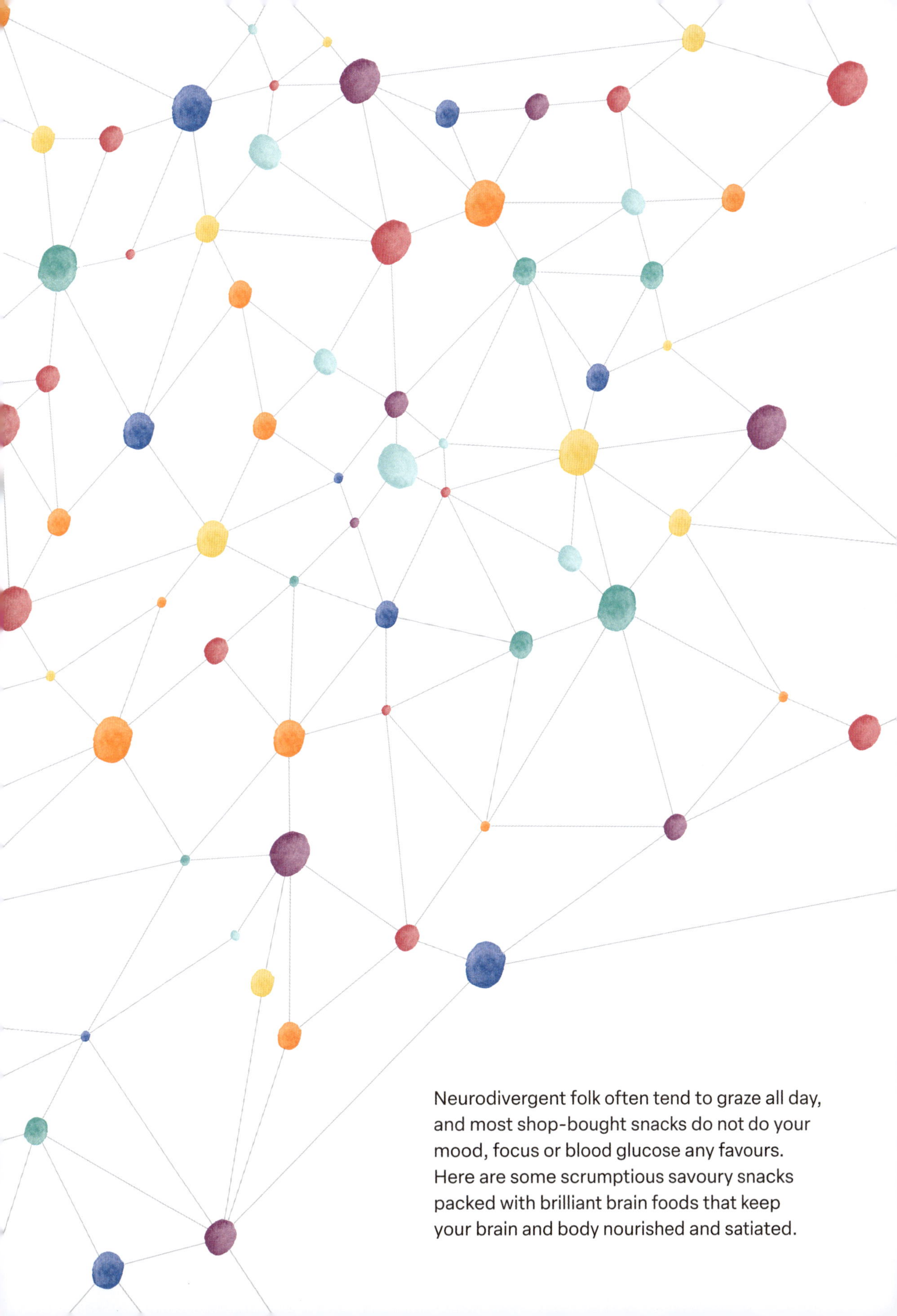

Neurodivergent folk often tend to graze all day, and most shop-bought snacks do not do your mood, focus or blood glucose any favours. Here are some scrumptious savoury snacks packed with brilliant brain foods that keep your brain and body nourished and satiated.

MARGHERITA PIZZA WAFFLES

A crunchy pizza-style snack that is so much more nutritious than pizza! It is made with nutrient-rich spelt flour, eggs and milk as well as two types of cheese. Waffles are always a winner with all ages and even better when they taste like a margherita pizza!

Makes 6

320g (2½ cups minus 1 Tbsp) spelt flour
1 tsp baking powder
150g (scant 1½ cups) grated (shredded) Cheddar or firm mozzarella
100g (1½ cups) grated (shredded) Parmesan
3 tsp Italian seasoning
2 eggs, preferably free-range
250ml (1 cup plus 1 Tbsp) milk of choice
4 Tbsp sundried tomato purée (paste)
1½ Tbsp melted butter
salt and black pepper
olive oil, for greasing

Set your waffle-maker to heat up while you make the batter.

Put the flour, baking powder, both cheeses, Italian seasoning and some salt and pepper in a large bowl. Mix well.

In a second bowl, combine the eggs, milk, tomato purée and melted butter. Add the wet mixture to the dry ingredients and stir lightly until just combined.

When the waffle-maker is hot, grease the waffle irons with a little oil if not non-stick and spoon in enough batter just to fill each waffle iron (you can usually cook two waffles at a time); try not to overfill them or the batter will spill and make a mess. Cook the waffles for 5 minutes, checking them after around 4 minutes and turn them over for the final minute. They should be ready once the steam has stopped coming out of the waffle-maker.

Place on a wire rack to cool slightly while you make the rest.

Serve the waffles warm, or cool and add to lunchboxes. You can also freeze them in a single layer on a tray and then store them in the freezer for up to 3 months. Pop them into the toaster to defrost and reheat.

Use a vegan mozzarella.
Use a gluten-free flour blend or sorghum flour.
dairy-free
gluten-free

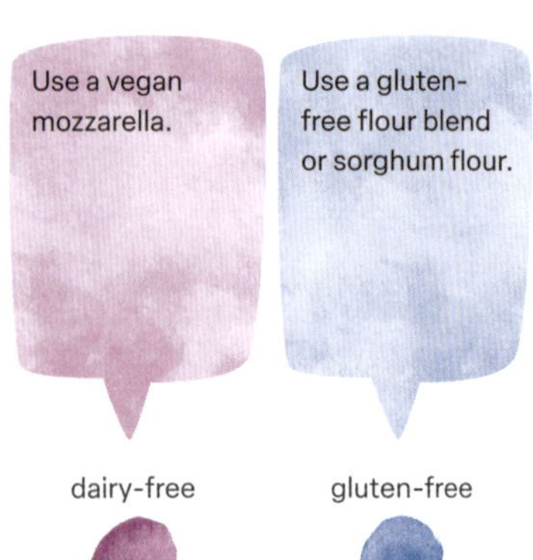

Omit the eggs and use a mix of 50:50 spelt:gram (chickpea) flour.

nut-free

sesame-free

egg-free

soy-free

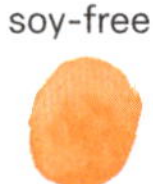

vegetarian

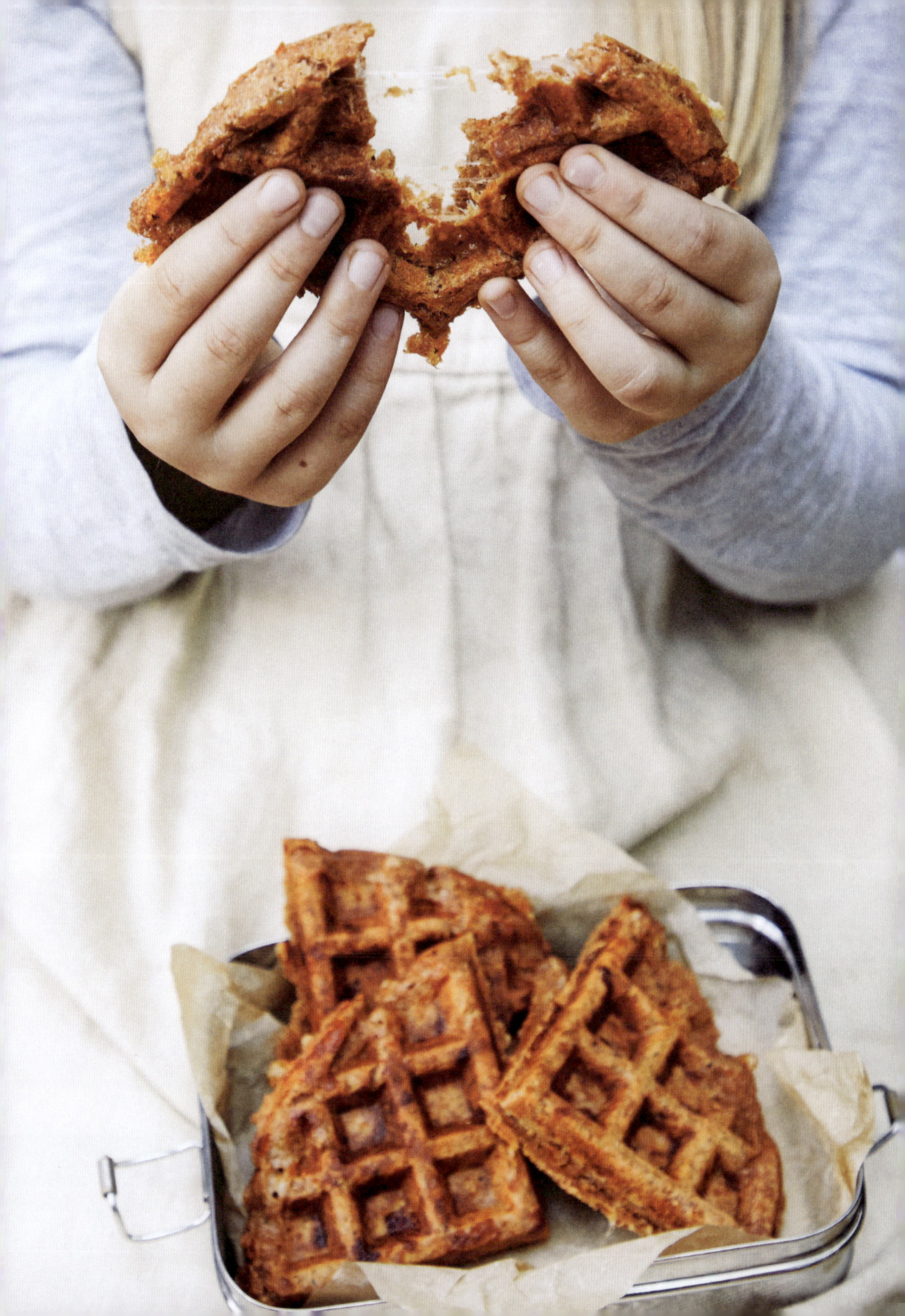

ROSEMARY & GARLIC CHICKPEA FOCACCIA

Rosemary is one of the best culinary herbs to lift the mood and help with focus. This gluten-free and grain-free focaccia-style bread is packed with protein and fibre, rich in iron and choline, and tastes just incredible. It is a great recipe for those neurodivergent folk who tend to like eating only beige food and need more nourishment.

Psyllium husk helps to bind all the ingredients together to make a bread that does not crumble. This natural fibre is gentle on the gut if you have a tendency to get bunged up!

Serves 4

2 tsp active dry yeast
80ml (⅓ cup) lukewarm water
2 tsp maple syrup or honey
150g (generous 1½ cups) gram (chickpea) flour
10g (¼oz) psyllium husk powder
1½ tsp baking powder
½ tsp sea salt flakes (kosher salt)
1 egg plus 2 egg whites, preferably free-range
3 generous Tbsp extra virgin olive oil, plus extra for greasing
2 tsp apple cider vinegar

Topping
1 Tbsp finely chopped fresh rosemary or ½ Tbsp dried
1 finely sliced garlic clove
1½–2 Tbsp extra virgin olive oil
1 tsp sea salt flakes (kosher salt)

Activate the yeast by putting it in a medium bowl with the warm water and maple syrup. Stir and leave for 7 minutes – it should start fermenting and bubble a little.

Meanwhile put the gram flour, psyllium husk, baking powder and salt into a large bowl and stir well to combine.

Add the egg, egg whites, olive oil and apple cider vinegar to the yeast mixture and whisk with a fork for a couple of minutes to make the mixture light and frothy.

Fold the wet ingredients into the dry ingredients and combine to form a thick dough.

Line a baking tin with baking paper or use a silicone baking sheet. Grease with a little olive oil so the dough does not stick. Tip the dough onto the baking sheet and use a spatula to spread it evenly, so it is around 1cm (½in) thick. Cover with a clean tea towel and leave to rise in a warm dry place for 40–50 minutes.

After about 40 minutes, preheat the oven to 200°C/180°C fan/400°C/Gas mark 6.

continued overleaf

Omit the eggs and use 4 tablespoons of whipped aquafaba (chickpea water).

dairy-free
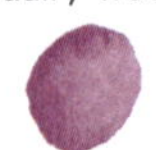
gluten-free

nut-free

sesame-free

egg-free

soy-free
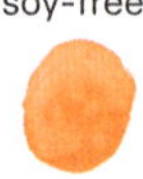
vegetarian
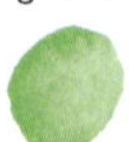

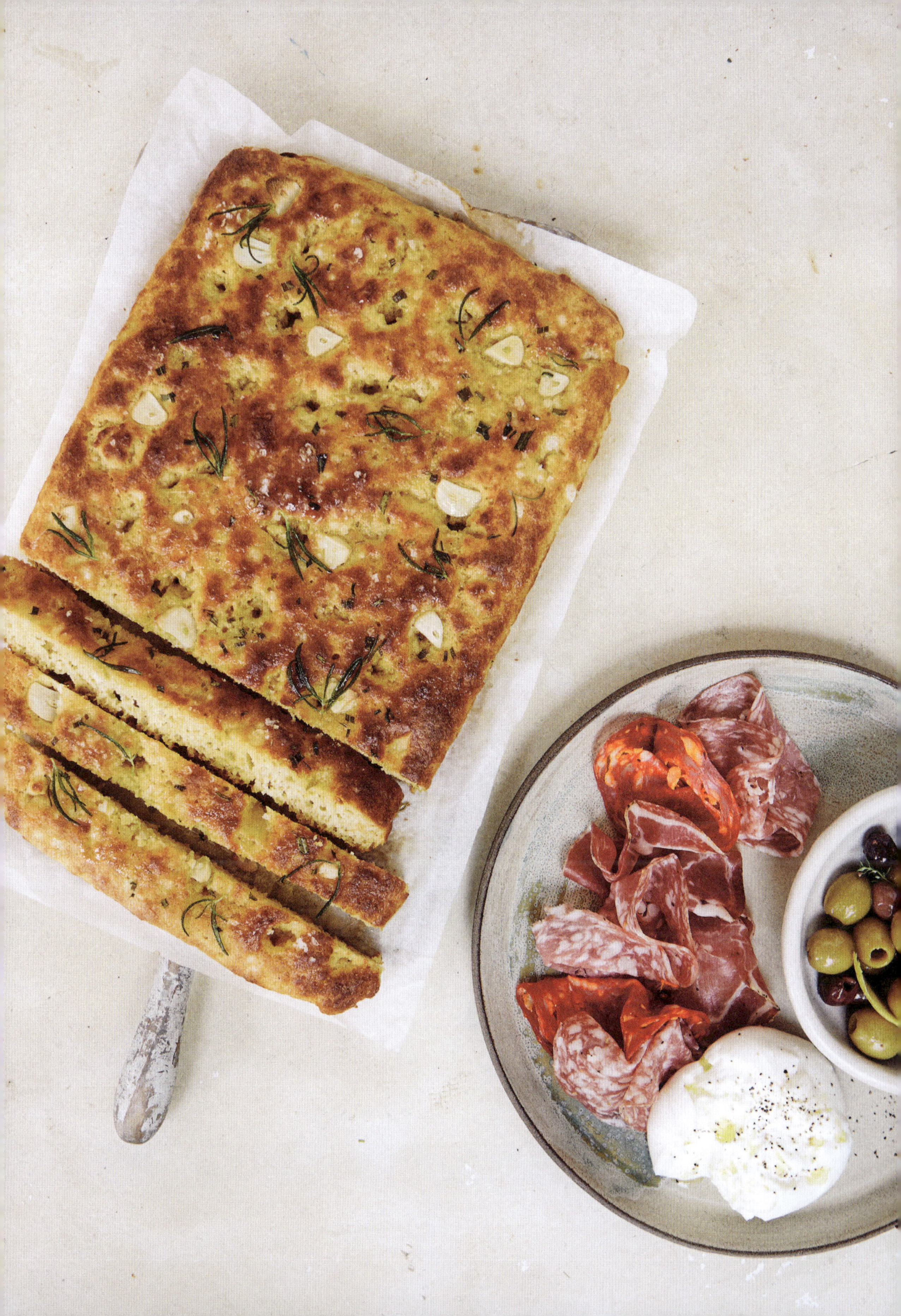

ROSEMARY & GARLIC CHICKPEA FOCACCIA CONTINUED

Once the dough has risen, use wet fingers to create indentations in the focaccia, then sprinkle it with chopped rosemary, garlic slivers, extra virgin olive oil and sea salt flakes. Bake the focaccia in the middle of the oven for 18 minutes, covering the top with baking paper after about 10 minutes to stop it burning. Check it after 15 minutes (some ovens run hotter than others).

Take out of the oven and cool the focaccia completely on a wire rack before serving – the texture is much nicer that way.

Slice and dip into balsamic vinegar and olive oil and serve with olives, cheese or ham.

Store in an airtight tin or sealed container for up to 3 days or, wrapped, in the freezer for 3 months.

ANTS ON LOGS

Serves 2

2 celery sticks
6 tsp almond butter
18 dried cranberries

This is a fun and yummy way to eat a nutritious snack. Celery is a great source of luteolin that can support speech and communication (see page 86), almond butter is packed with protein and healthy fats, while sweet dried cranberries are rich in antioxidants. If you keep all three ingredients to hand, you can put these little logs together very quickly

In place of almond butter you can also use cream cheese, ricotta, cottage cheese, cashew/almond nut cheese, hummus or chicken liver pâté.

Clean and trim the celery sticks and cut into 3 or 4 even pieces.

Carefully fill the celery with almond butter using a teaspoon and top with dried cranberries.

Store in the refrigerator in a sealed container for up to 3 days.

Use a soft cheese, hummus or pâté instead of the almond butter.

dairy-free
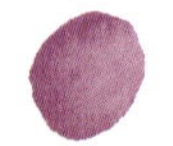

gluten-free

nut-free

sesame-free

egg-free

soy-free
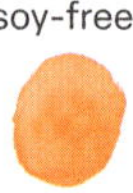

vegetarian
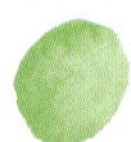

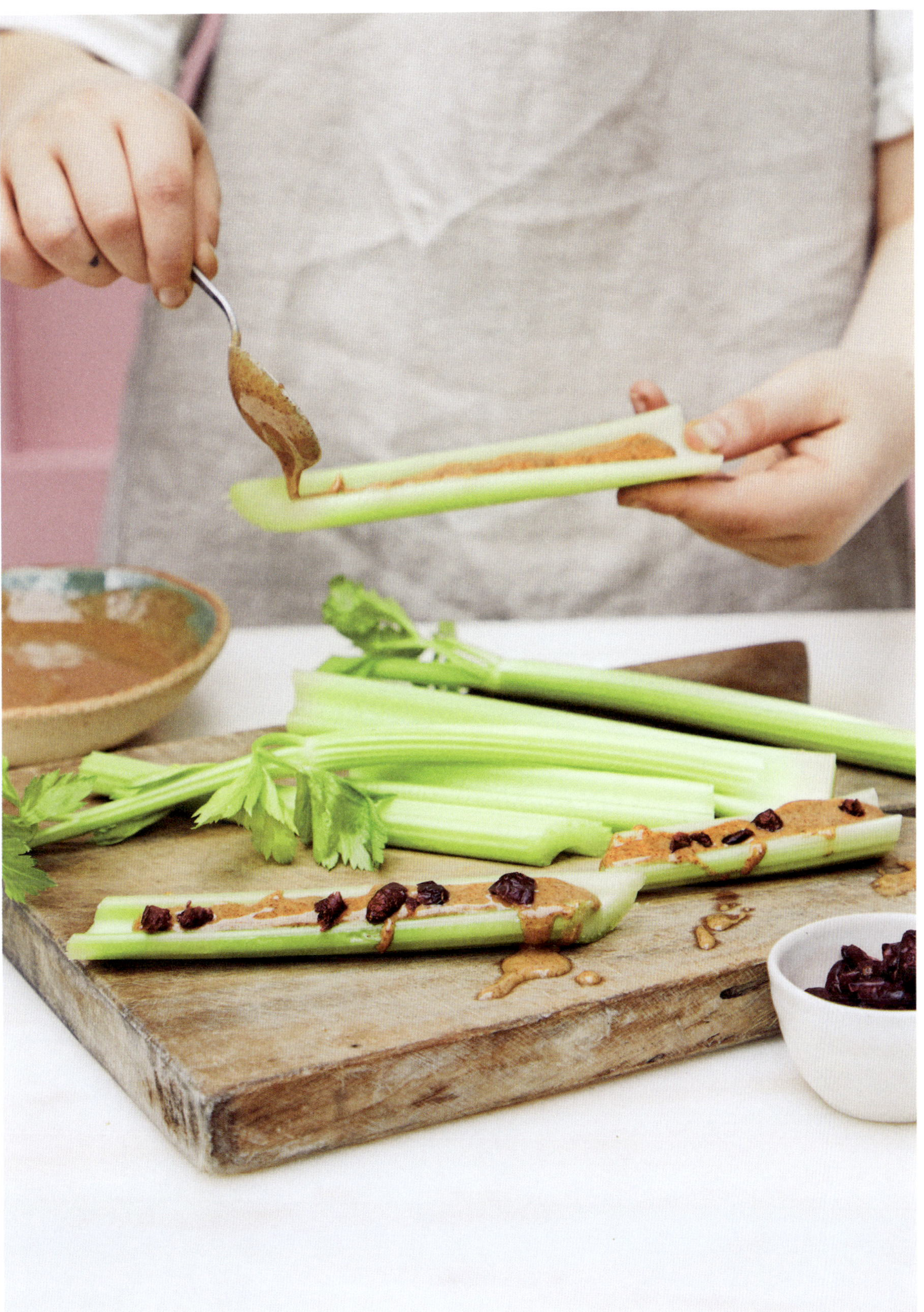

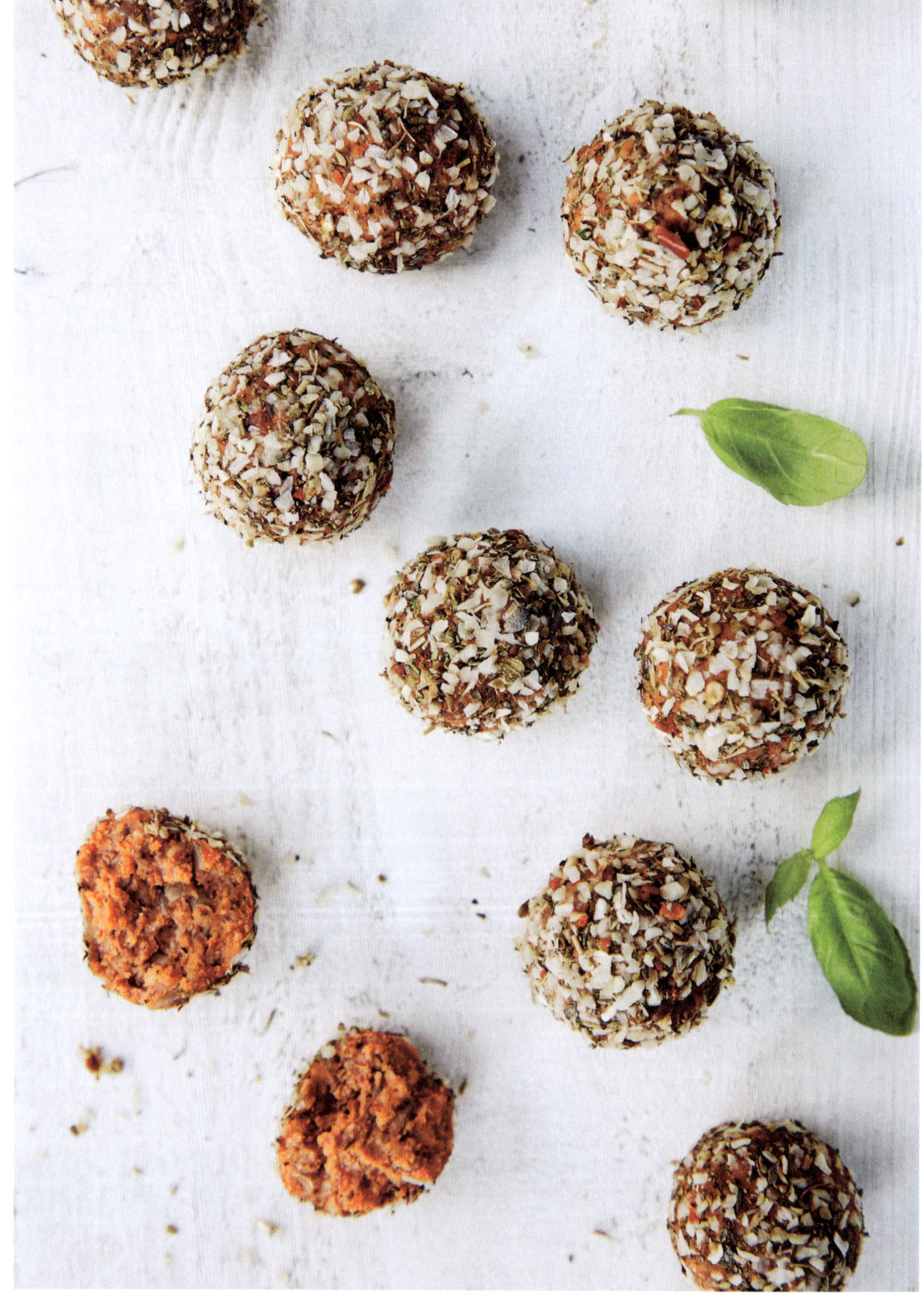

PIZZA ENERGY BALLS

These delicious savoury energy balls taste like pizza with their Italian-style flavours but are packed with protein and nutrient-dense ingredients. They are a perfect snack when you're out and about. They are also nut-free so you can add to your children's lunchboxes.

Makes 12 balls

130g (4½oz) canned cannellini beans (drained weight)
35g (about ⅓ cup) rolled oats
35g (about 4 Tbsp) sunflower seeds
6 sundried tomatoes
2 Tbsp grated (shredded) firm mozzarella
3 tsp Italian seasoning (or used dried mixed herbs, oregano or basil)
salt and black pepper
1 Tbsp onion granules

Rinse and drain the cannellini beans and put into a blender along with the oats, sunflower seeds, sundried tomatoes, mozzarella, 2 teaspoons of the Italian seasoning and some salt and pepper. Blend for 2–3 minutes to make a thick, smooth mixture. You will need to stop the machine and use a spatula to push the mixture down between bursts of blending.

Scoop out tablespoonfuls of the mixture and roll into balls. Scatter the onion granules and the remaining teaspoon of Italian seasoning on a plate and roll the balls to coat.

Pop in the refrigerator to firm up. Keep refrigerated and use within 3 days. You can also freeze them for up to 3 months.

TIP

Use the leftover cannellini beans from the can to make a dip, or add to stews or salads.

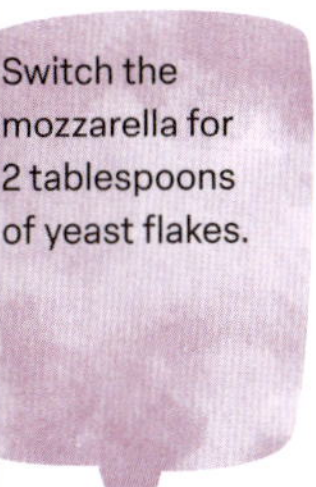

Use gluten-free oats.

dairy-free

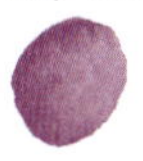

gluten-free

nut-free

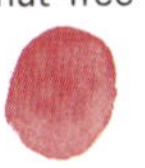

sesame-free

egg-free

soy-free

vegetarian

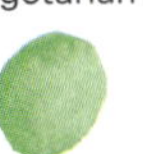

EAT YOUR GREENS MUFFINS

The idea of eating green veg can be very off-putting for some neurodivergent folk, and sometimes you have to think out of the box to find a great solution to help them get enough folate into their diet.

These savoury muffins are packed with greens and have a lovely cheesy flavour. Serve on their own as a snack or part of a packed lunch, alongside soup or spread with pâté or cream cheese.

Makes 12

handful of kale or cavolo nero (stalks removed)
4 Tbsp olive oil, plus extra for cooking
1 small shallot, finely diced
160g (1 cup plus 2 Tbsp) spelt or wholemeal (whole wheat) flour
100g (1 cup) ground (powdered) almonds
1 tsp baking powder
¼ tsp bicarbonate of soda (baking soda)
250g (generous 1 cup) full-fat plain yoghurt
2 eggs, preferably free-range
90g (3¼oz) feta cheese, crumbled, plus extra to sprinkle
1 courgette (zucchini), finely grated (shredded)
1 tsp fresh thyme leaves or ½ tsp dried
salt and black pepper

Topping
1 Tbsp sunflower seeds
1 Tbsp pumpkin seeds

Preheat the oven to 180°C/160°C fan/350°F/Gas mark 4 and line a 12-hole muffin tray with paper cases.

Prepare the kale by removing the hard stems and finely slicing the leaves. Warm a little olive oil in a frying pan (skillet), then sauté the kale and shallot for about 4–5 minutes until soft. Set aside to cool.

Meanwhile, combine the spelt flour, ground almonds, baking powder, bicarbonate of soda and some salt and pepper in a large mixing bowl. Set aside.

In a second large bowl, mix the yoghurt, eggs and 4 tablespoons of olive oil. Stir in the crumbled feta, courgette and thyme, along with the cooled kale and shallots.

Tip the wet ingredients into the dry ingredients and stir until just combined to make the muffin dough – don't overmix.

Use an ice-cream scoop to fill the muffin cases with dough. Sprinkle each muffin with a little extra feta and a few sunflower seeds and pumpkin seeds. Bake in the preheated oven for 15–18 minutes, until risen, golden and cooked through (test with a skewer). Every oven is different so watch the muffins closely from 14 minutes.

Cool for 30 minutes on a wire rack then serve.

These muffins stay fresh in an airtight tin for up to 4 days. They also freeze well for up to 3 months.

Use mild-tasting coconut yoghurt or soft nut cheese and replace the feta with 2 tablespoons of yeast flakes, plus a little extra to sprinkle on top of the muffins.

Use a gluten-free flour or a baking blend. Sorghum flour works well.

Replace the almonds with 100g gram (chickpea) flour.

Swap the eggs for 2 tablespoons of ground flaxseed, mixed into 3 tablespoons of water and soaked for at least 10 minutes.

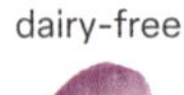

dairy-free

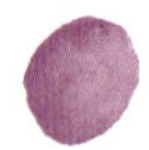

gluten-free

nut-free

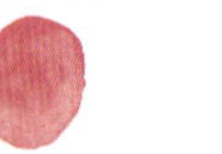

sesame-free

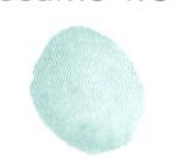

egg-free

soy-free

vegetarian

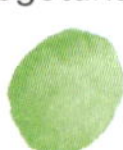

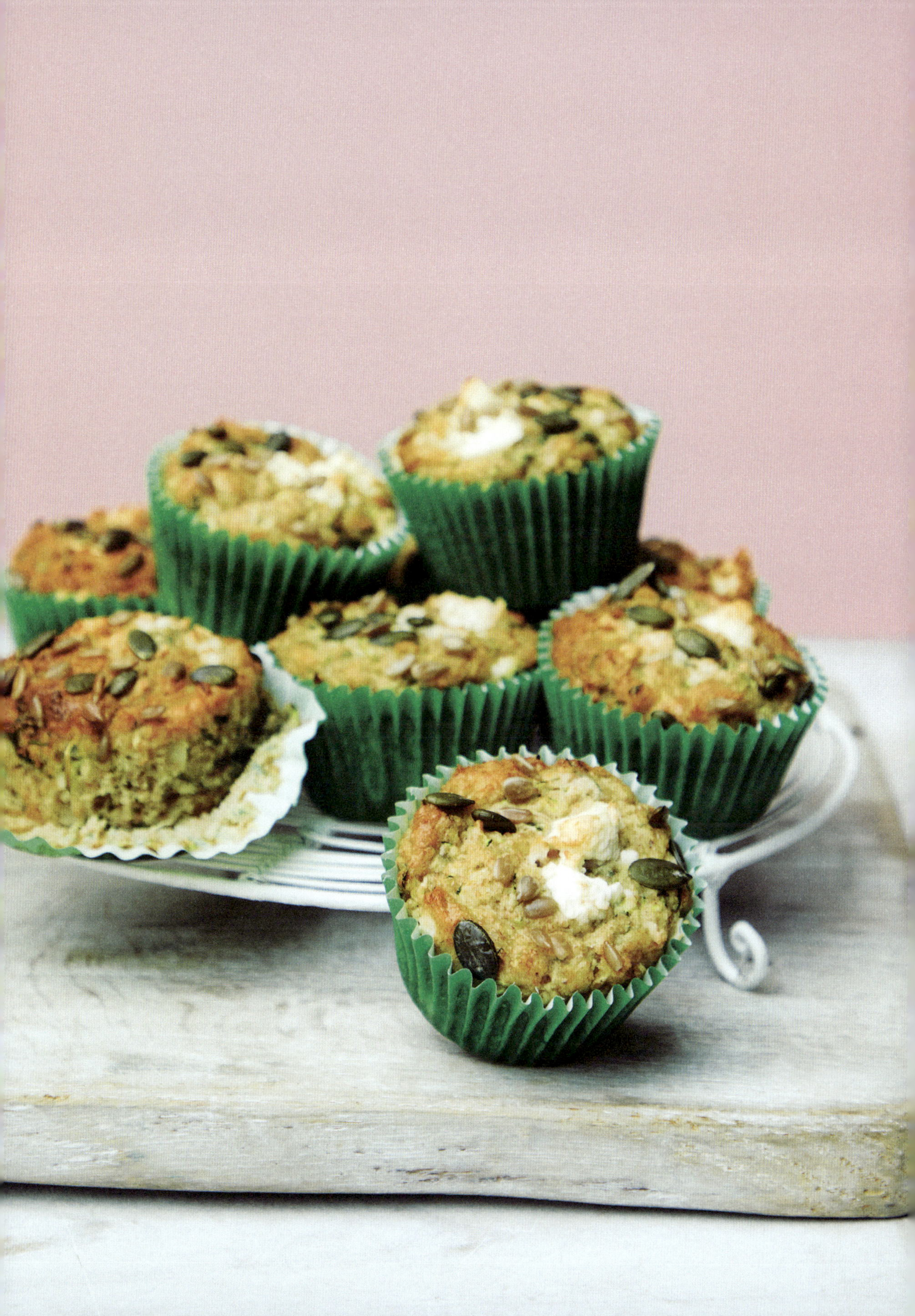

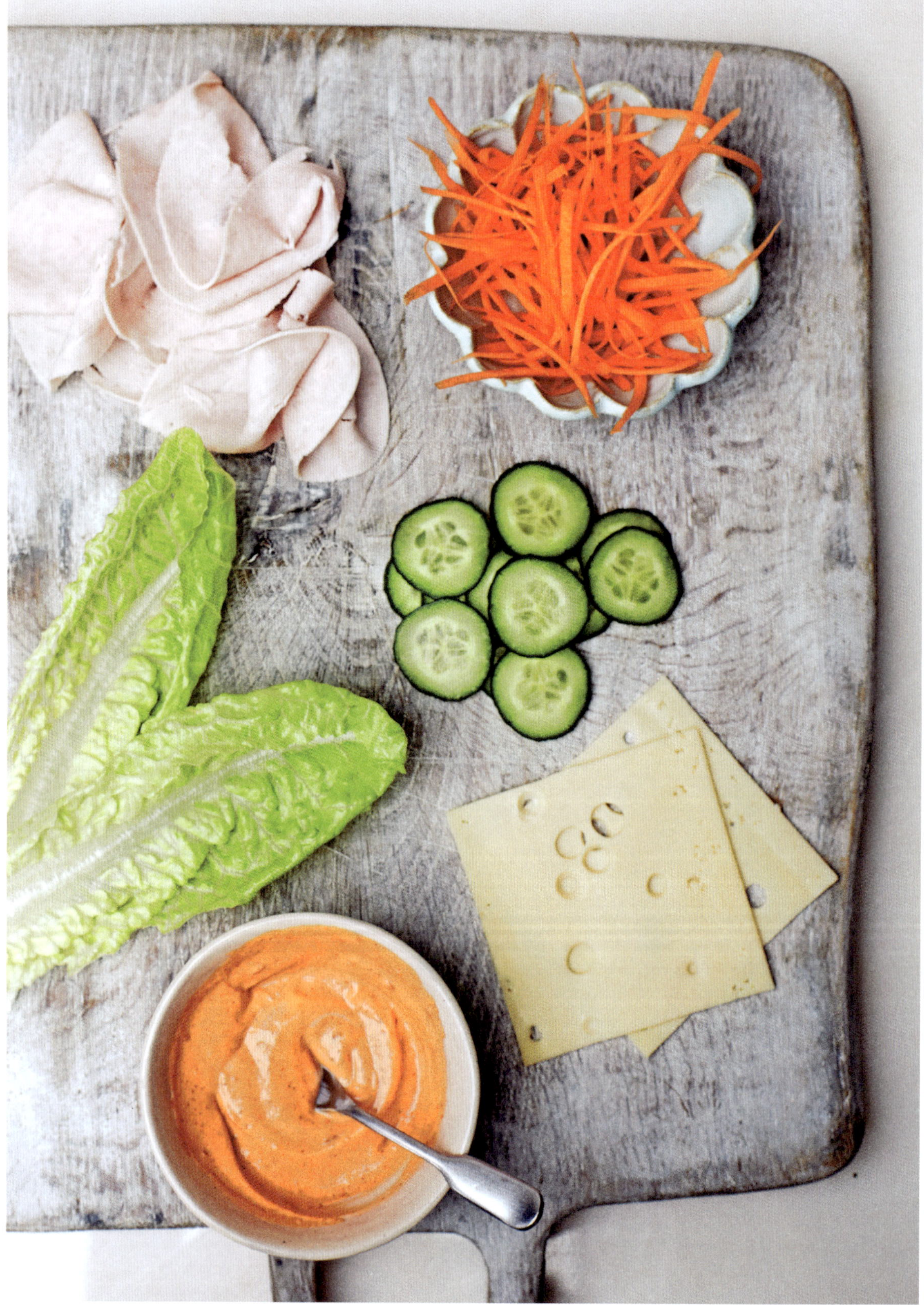

LETTUCE, TURKEY & CHEESE ROLL UPS

Makes 2

2 Romaine lettuce leaves (Little Gem/ Boston lettuce or young spring green leaves are fine)
2 tsp mayonnaise
1 dash of harissa paste
4 slices of cooked turkey
2 slices of Emmental or Cheddar cheese
1 small carrot, grated (shredded)
6 thin slices of cucumber

A wrap without the bread! Use lettuce or young spring green leaves instead of a wheat-based wrap and roll these around a delicious filling of turkey, cheese and crunchy salad veg with a harissa mayonnaise.

Turkey is an important source of tryptophan, which helps to create our happy neurotransmitter serotonin. You can swap the turkey slices for Parma ham, cooked chicken slices, smoked mackerel or smashed chickpeas if you prefer. You can source harissa mayonnaise to make this recipe even simpler.

Lay the lettuce leaves flat, one slightly overlapping the other.

Mix the mayonnaise with the harissa paste and spread on top of the lettuce leaves.

Layer on the turkey slices, then the cheese slices, followed by the carrot and cucumber. Roll up tightly to hold the ingredients together then cut in two.

Serve immediately or store in the refrigerator for up to 24 hours.

Use dairy-free mayonnaise and replace the cheese with smashed chickpeas (garbanzo beans) mixed with an extra 2 teaspoons of dairy-free mayonnaise.

Swap the turkey slices for smashed chickpeas.

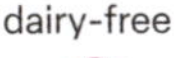

dairy-free

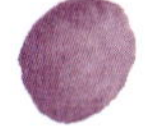

gluten-free

nut-free

sesame-free

egg-free

soy-free

vegetarian

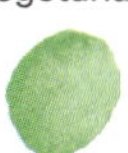

TURMERIC HUMMUS

Serves 4

3 dried apricots (ideally natural brown and unsulphured), pitted
400g (14oz) can chickpeas (garbanzo beans), drained
1 Tbsp tahini (sesame paste)
juice of 1 lemon
3 Tbsp olive oil
1 garlic clove, crushed
1 tsp ground turmeric
1 tsp ground ginger
1 tsp dried mint
1 tsp ground cumin
salt and black pepper

Sweet and tangy, this yummy hummus is packed with gut-health goodies that all help dial down inflammation. It's a brilliant way to enjoy the benefits of turmeric, and when I was testing this recipe my teenage son ate a whole bowlful within 5 minutes!

Simply serve with crunchy sliced crudités or spread on a wrap or crackers. You can also eat this hummus alongside a salad or use it as a filling for a baked sweet potato. The chickpeas can be swapped for other white beans, such as cannellini or flageolets.

Soak the dried apricots in water for at least 10 minutes to rehydrate and soften them, then discard the water.

Rinse and drain the chickpeas and tip into a blender. Add the rehydrated apricots along with the tahini, lemon juice, olive oil, garlic, turmeric, ginger, mint, cumin and some salt and pepper. Blitz for 2–3 minutes until smooth, or stop sooner if you like the texture to be a bit chunkier. Every minute or so stop and scrape down the sides so everything is blended properly. Add in a little extra olive oil or a tablespoon of water if the mixture is too thick for your liking.

Store in the refrigerator for up to 3 days.

Swap the tahini for cashew butter, sunflower seed butter or sunflower seeds. (You can also omit the tahini entirely if there are multiple allergies.)

dairy-free
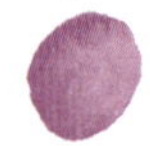
gluten-free

nut-free

sesame-free

egg-free

soy-free

vegetarian
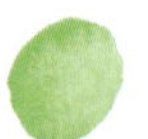

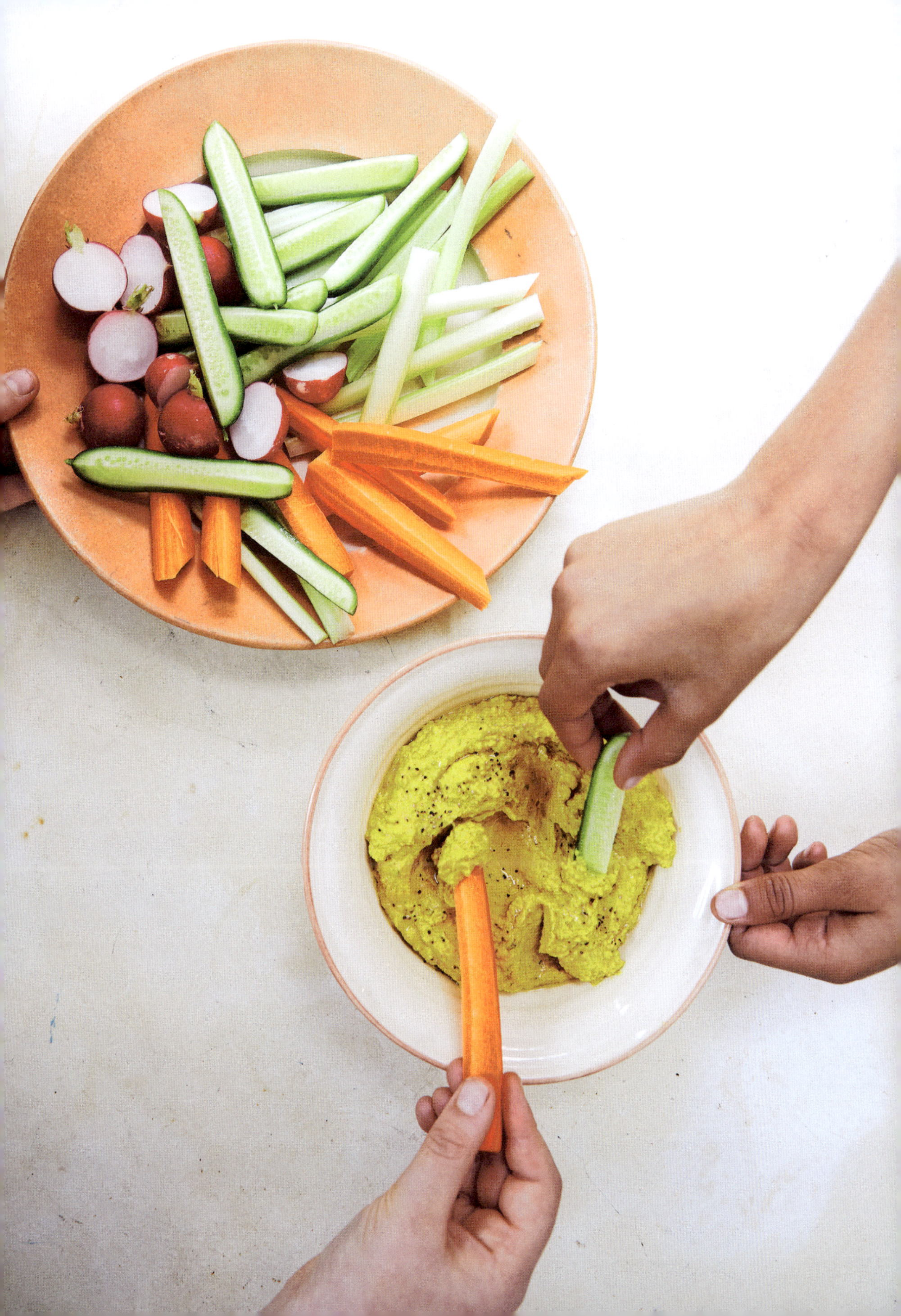

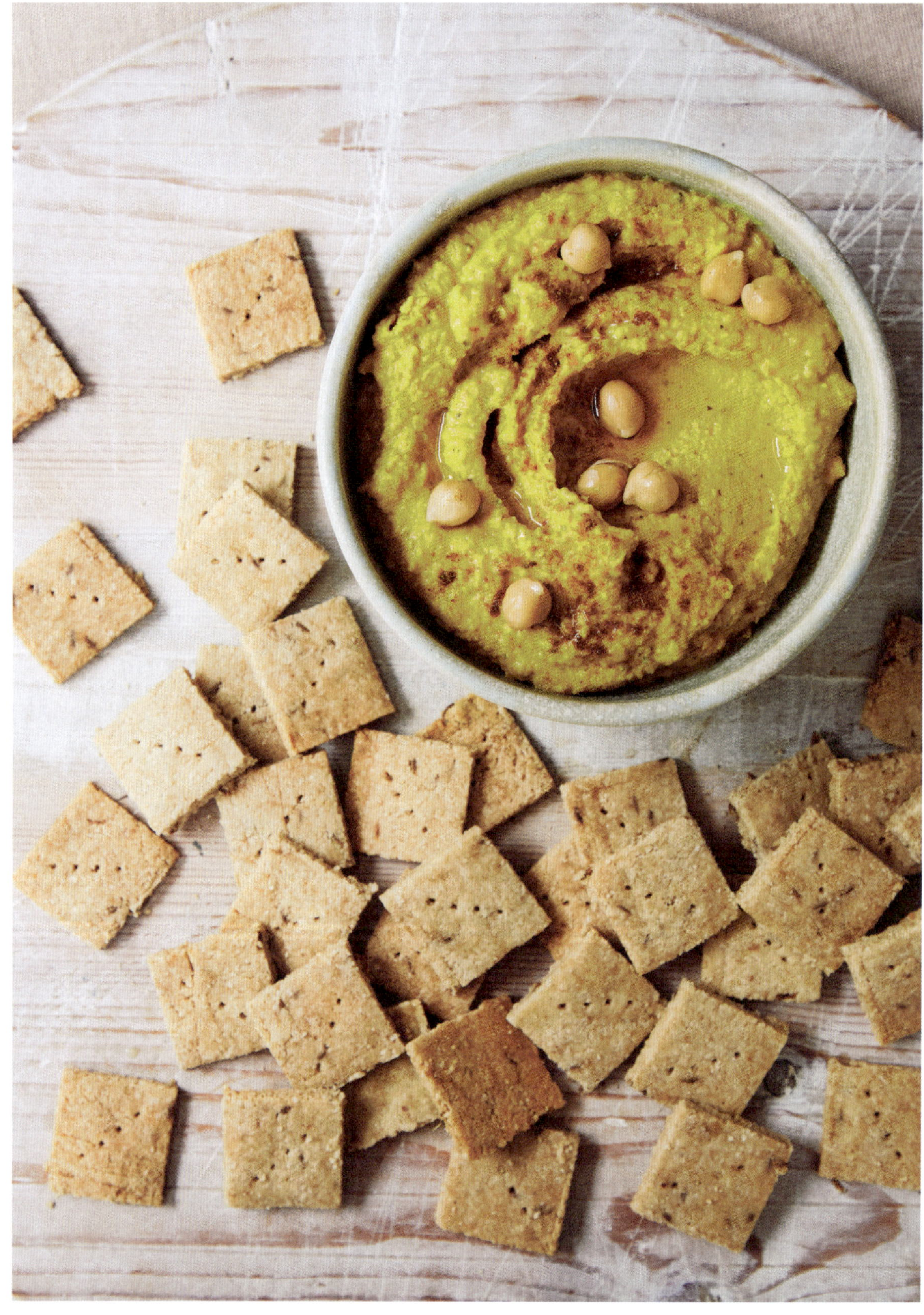

CUMIN & CORIANDER ALMOND CRACKERS

These crunchy crackers have a lovely mellow cumin and coriander flavour. There is no flour; instead, they are made with ground almonds, which are packed with calcium and protein. Serve with olives or my Turmeric Hummus (page 176).

Makes 12–16

- 160g (1½ cups) ground (powdered) almonds
- 2 tsp whole cumin seeds
- 1 Tbsp ground coriander
- ½ tsp sea salt flakes (kosher salt)
- 1 Tbsp olive oil
- 1 large egg, preferably free-range

Preheat the oven to 170°C/150°C fan/340°F/Gas Mark 3½. Combine the ground almonds, cumin, ground coriander and salt in a bowl.

Whisk together the olive oil and egg in a small bowl.

Pour the wet ingredients into the dry ingredients and mix with a spoon or your hands until well combined. Roll the dough into a ball. Then press the dough between two large sheets of baking paper and roll with a rolling pin into a flat oval or square shape that is around 3mm (⅛in) thick.

Remove the top sheet of paper and transfer the bottom sheet with rolled-out dough onto a baking tray. Score or cut the dough into 3cm (1¼in) square shapes with a pizza cutter or knife and prick them with a fork. Bake in the preheated oven for 12–15 minutes, until the crackers are light golden brown and a bit crispy. The squares on the edges will be better cooked than those in the middle, so you may need to remove the outermost squares and then pop the rest back in the oven for a further 2 minutes to crisp up.

Let the crackers cool on the baking sheet for 30 minutes and then devour!

These store in a sealed container for 3 days or in the freezer for 3 months. If you need to crisp them up, pop them in a preheated oven at 170°C/150°C fan/340°F/Gas Mark 3½ for 2–3 minutes.

Omit the egg and add 1 tablespoon of ground flaxseed mixed with 2 tablespoons of water.

dairy-free

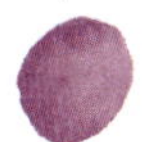

gluten-free

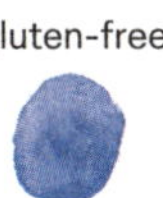

sesame-free

egg-free

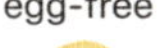

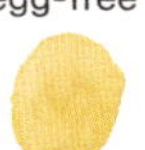

soy-free

vegetarian

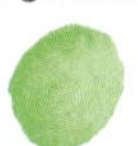

FENNEL & PAPRIKA ROASTED CHICKPEAS

Makes 1 x 350g (12oz) jar

400g/14oz canned chickpeas (garbanzo beans)
1 Tbsp olive oil
2 tsp smoked paprika
2 tsp dried mixed herbs
2 tsp fennel seeds
1 tsp salt

With warming spices, crispy chickpeas (garbanzo beans) make a perfect snack to nibble, or they can be sprinkled onto salads to given them a protein and fibre boost.

Preheat the oven to 200°C/180°C fan/390°F/Gas mark 6.

Drain and rinse the chickpeas in a sieve and shake off any excess liquid. Spread the chickpeas on paper towels and gently pat dry.

Mix the olive oil, paprika, herbs, fennel seeds and salt in a bowl, then add the chickpeas. Stir to coat them well with the mixture. Spread the chickpeas on a baking tray and roast for 30–40 minutes, or until brown and crunchy. Check frequently towards the end of the cooking time to avoid burning. Eat warm or at room temperature.

Store in a glass jar in the refrigerator for up to 3 days.

dairy-free
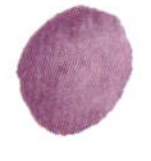
gluten-free

nut-free

sesame-free
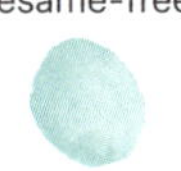
egg-free

soy-free

vegetarian
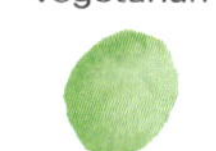

TAMARI TOASTED SEEDS

Makes 1 jar

100g (about ¾ cup) pumpkin seeds
100g (about ¾ cup) sunflower seeds
2 tsp tamari soy sauce

This is one of the tastiest and easiest snacks to have to hand. Make a batch and store them in a jar for when you need to nibble on a quick snack that also enriches you with healthy fats, iron, choline and Vitamin E. They also make delicious sprinkles for salads and dips as well as a crunchy savoury toast topper.

Japanese tamari soy sauce is naturally gluten-free and has a more mellow umami flavour than Chinese soy sauce.

Heat a dry frying pan (skillet) over a high heat and add the seeds to the pan, stirring constantly. Toast the seeds until they just start turning brown and then turn off the heat entirely.

Add the tamari soy sauce and keep on stirring. The sauce will become sticky quite quickly, so it is important that it coats all the seeds evenly.

Remove from the pan, spread out on a plate and allow to cool completely, then store in a jar for up to 3 months.

dairy-free
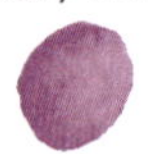
gluten-free

nut-free

sesame-free
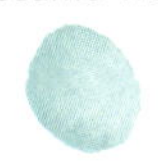
egg-free

vegetarian

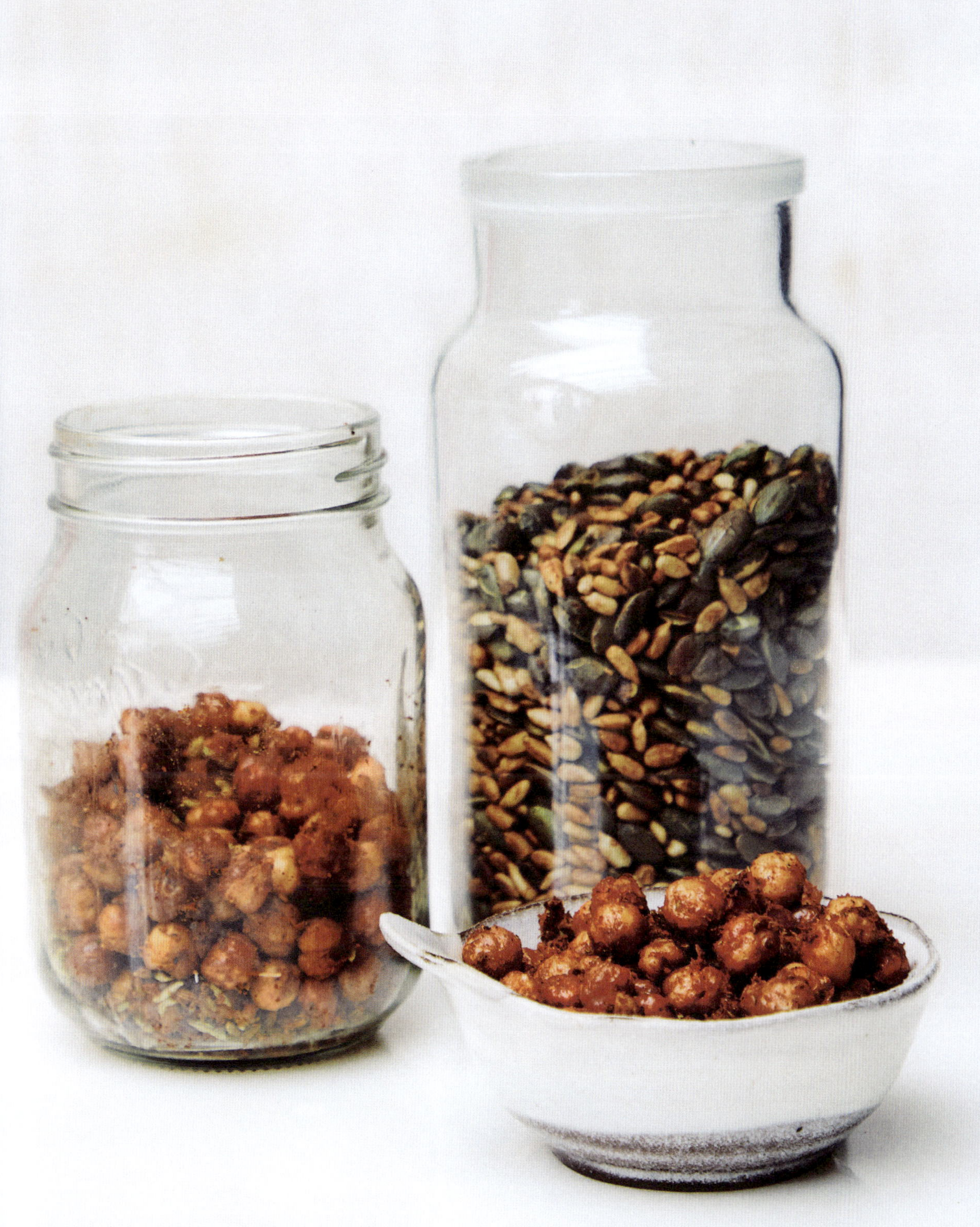

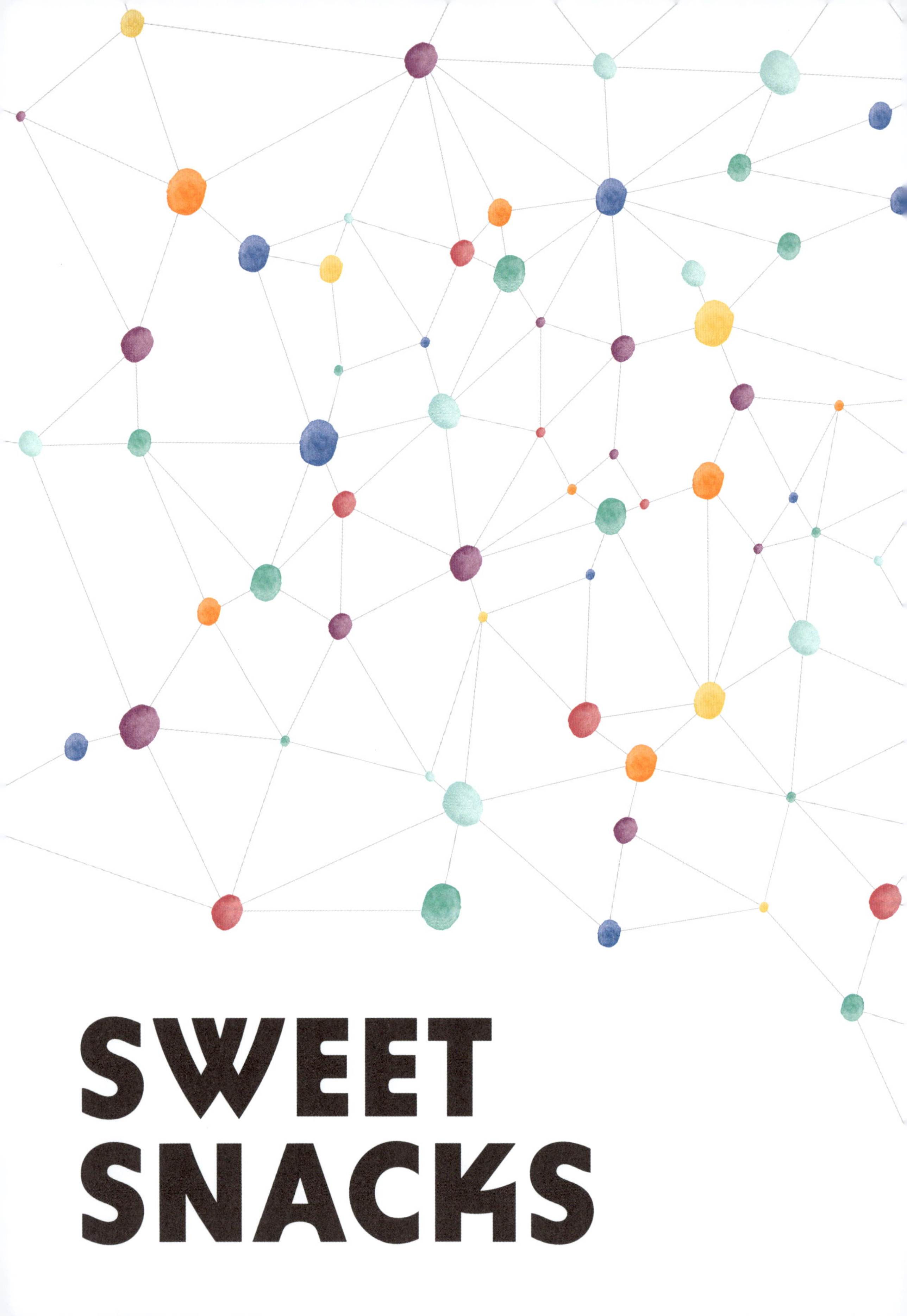
SWEET
SNACKS

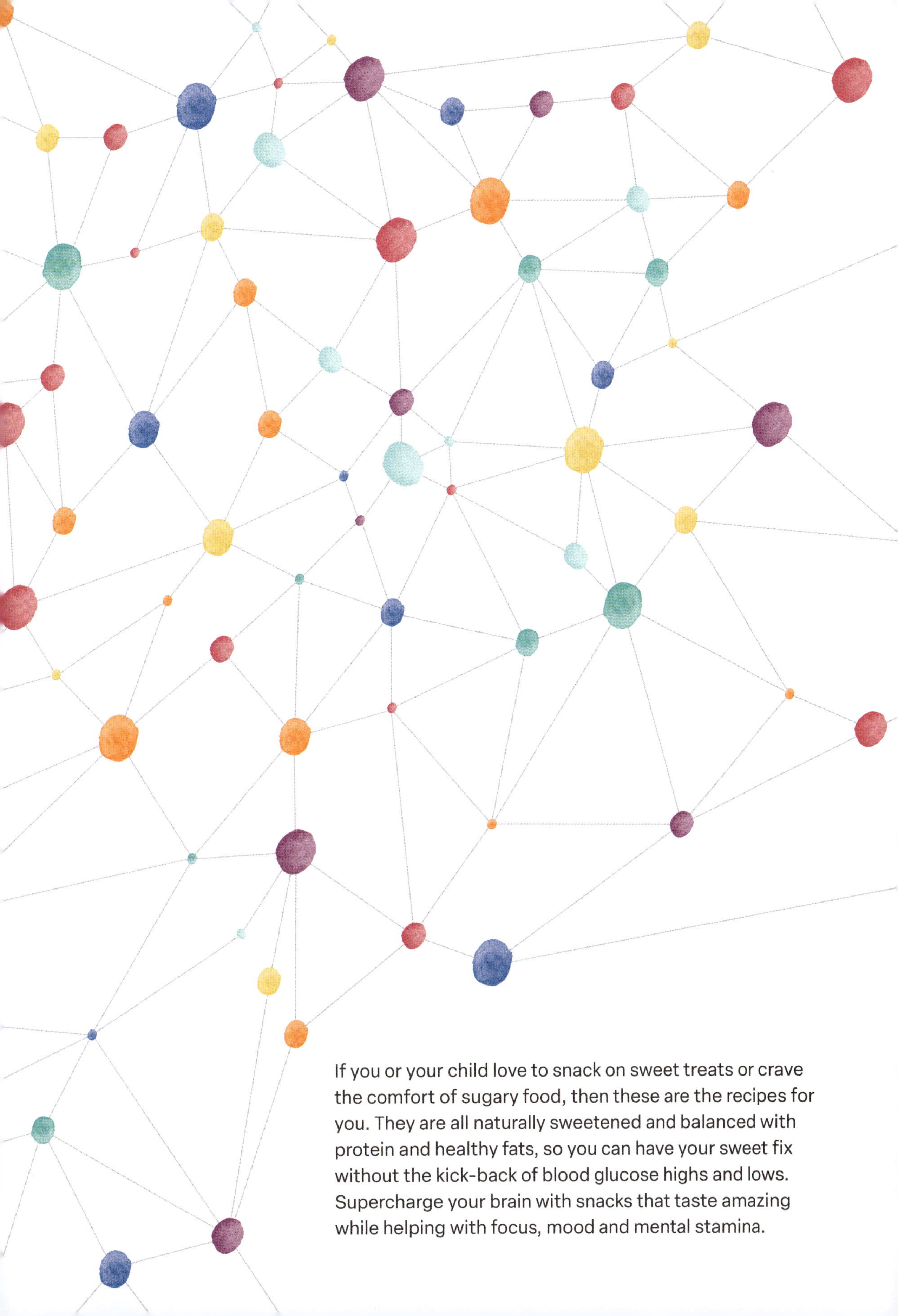

If you or your child love to snack on sweet treats or crave the comfort of sugary food, then these are the recipes for you. They are all naturally sweetened and balanced with protein and healthy fats, so you can have your sweet fix without the kick-back of blood glucose highs and lows. Supercharge your brain with snacks that taste amazing while helping with focus, mood and mental stamina.

APPLE & CINNAMON CLOUD COOKIES

Makes 16

120g (½ cup) butter
110g (¼ cup plus 2 Tbsp) maple syrup
1 egg plus 1 egg yolk, preferably free-range
160g (1 ⅓ cups) gram (chickpea) flour
½ tsp baking powder
1 apple, peeled, cored and finely diced
2 tsp ground cinnamon
½ tsp sea salt flakes (kosher salt)

The classic combination of apple and cinnamon gives these light, fluffy cookies their delicious taste and aroma. They are beautifully soft and melt in the mouth, making them suitable for anyone who struggles to chew their food. They are also gluten- and grain-free and packed with protein, fibre, iron and choline. Gram (chickpea) flour (you can also use besan flour) is easily available – you can also blitz dried chickpeas in a food processor with a grinding blade (or a Nutribullet) for 2 minutes to make a fine flour.

For a dairy- and egg-free alternative, replace the flour, eggs and butter with 400g (14oz) canned drained chickpeas and ½ cup almond/peanut butter or tahini. This results in cookies with a slightly different consistency – more dense, chewy and less fluffy.

Preheat the oven to 180°C/160°C fan/350°F/Gas mark 4. Prepare and line 3 baking trays with baking paper (or, if you don't have multiple trays/oven shelves, work in batches).

Melt the butter in a small saucepan over a low heat, then set aside to cool slightly.

Put the maple syrup, egg and egg yolk into a mixing bowl and whisk with a fork. Pour in the slightly cooled butter and whisk everything together until frothy and creamy.

In a separate bowl, mix the flour, baking powder, diced apple, cinnamon and salt.

Tip the dry ingredients into the wet ingredients and mix to form a loose dough. Scoop tablespoonfuls of the dough onto the baking tray(s), spaced well apart – the cookies will spread as they cook. Bake for 12–15 minutes until lightly browned all over and firm at the edges. Let them cool slightly on the baking tray and then transfer to a wire rack to cool further and firm up. However, they are delicious eaten warm!

Store for up to 2 days in an airtight container. The cookies can also be frozen, preferably on the day they are baked, for up to 3 months.

Swap the butter for coconut oil or a dairy-free spread.

See the recipe introduction.

See the recipe introduction.

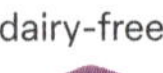

dairy-free

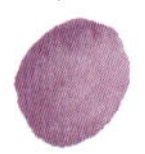

gluten-free

nut-free

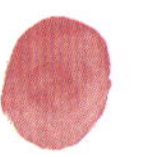

sesame-free

egg-free

soy-free

vegetarian

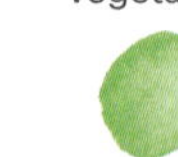

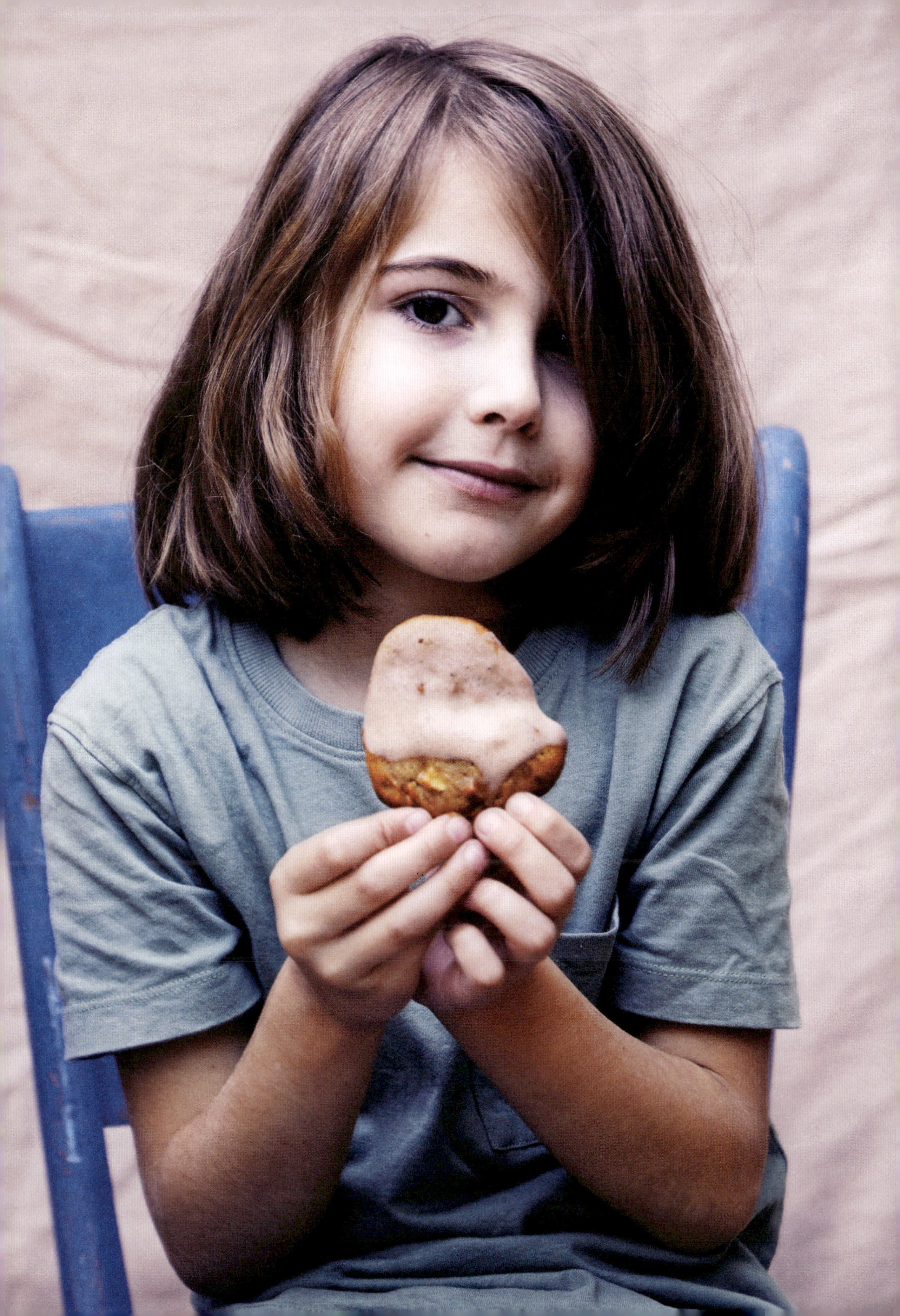

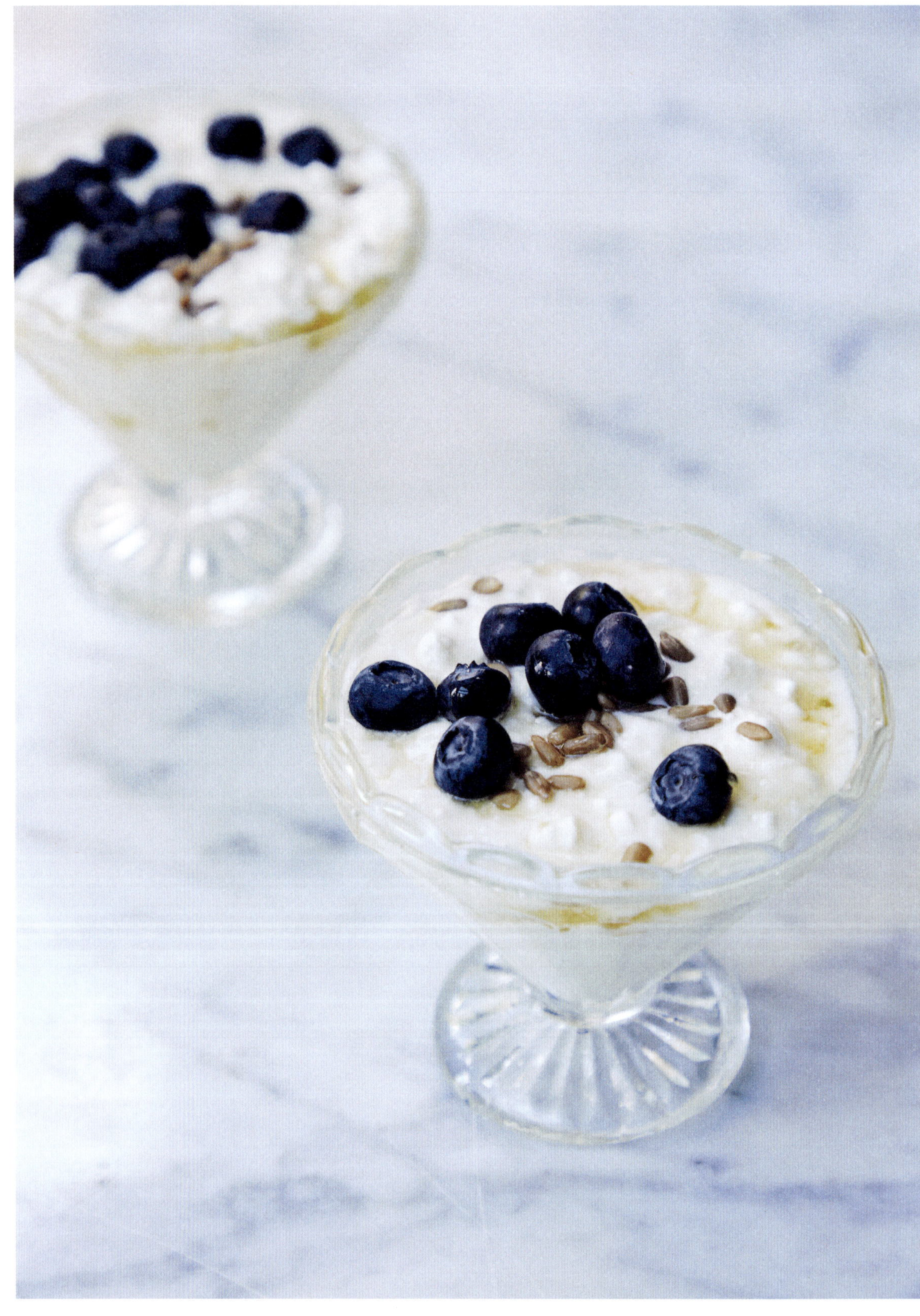

BLUEBERRY & VANILLA COTTAGE CHEESE POTS

Serves 2

300g (scant 1½ cups) full-fat cottage cheese
1 tsp vanilla extract
1 tsp honey or maple syrup
2 tsp sunflower seeds
handful of blueberries

These little treats give a blast of creamy protein that is brilliant for a speedy breakfast or quick snack. Blueberries contain flavonoids, which are thought to improve memory, learning and general cognitive function. Sunflower seeds add a nice crunch as well as a hit of choline and Vitamin E.

If you or your child prefer a smoother texture, blitz the cottage cheese, vanilla and honey in a blender for 1 minute. The blueberries and sunflower seeds can also be stirred into the blitzed-up cottage cheese and the mixture then frozen into ice lollies or ice cream.

Enjoy these with other fresh seasonal or frozen fruit, such as raspberries, strawberries, mango, nectarines, peaches, plums or cherries.

Stir together the cottage cheese, vanilla and honey or maple syrup until well combined.

Transfer to small bowls and serve sprinkled with the sunflower seeds and blueberries.

Swap the cottage cheese for 300g (10½oz) of silken tofu (beancurd) or 300g (generous 2 cups) of cashew nuts, soaked for 2 hours then drained and blended.

dairy-free
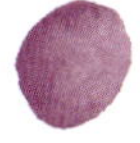
gluten-free

nut-free
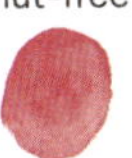
sesame-free
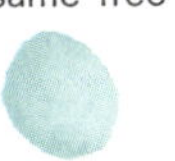
egg-free

soy-free

vegetarian
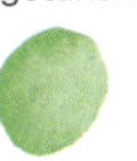

BLISS BALLS

Makes 12

For Choccy Miso Bliss Balls
12 pitted dates
100g (1 cup) rolled oats
70g (generous ½ cup) cacao or cocoa powder
4 tsp miso paste
3 Tbsp tahini (sesame paste)
1 Tbsp maple syrup

Salty miso combined with creamy tahini and sweet dates is a moreish taste sensation. These bliss balls are a quick and easy no-cook treat that is packed with nutritious calcium and iron as well as fermented miso, which feeds the gut microbiome. My family and I tend to eat them straight from the freezer!

If the dates are dry or hard, soak them in warm water for 10 minutes, then drain.

Put all the ingredients in a food processor and pulse for 2–3 minutes until a ball of dough starts to form.

Take 2 teaspoons of the mixture and roll between your palms to form a ball. (It helps if you dampen your hands first to stop the dough sticking to your fingers; you also get a lovely smooth finish.)

Repeat until you have used up all the mixture – this should make around 12 bliss balls.

Transfer to a tray or sealed container and put in the refrigerator for at least 30 minutes to firm up.

Store in the refrigerator for 3 days or 3 months in the freezer.

For Raspberry & Peanut Butter Bliss Balls
12 pitted dates
100g (1 cup) rolled oats
4 tsp peanut butter
3 Tbsp hulled hemp seeds
1 Tbsp maple syrup
12 raspberries, fresh or frozen

These raspberry and peanut butter bliss balls are packed with omega-3 and choline to help with focus and learning, plus a whole raspberry hidden in the centre.

If the dates are dry or hard, soak them in warm water for 10 minutes, then drain.

Put all the ingredients except the raspberries in a food processor and pulse for 2–3 minutes until a ball of dough starts to form.

Take 2 teaspoons of the mixture, flatten slightly and pop a raspberry in the middle. Fold the sides around carefully to enclose the fruit then roll between your palms to form a ball. (It helps if you dampen your hands first to stop the dough sticking to your fingers; you also get a lovely smooth finish.)

Repeat until you have used up all the mixture – this should make around 12 bliss balls.

Transfer to a tray or sealed container and put in the refrigerator for at least 30 minutes to firm up.

Store in the refrigerator for 3 days or 3 months in the freezer.

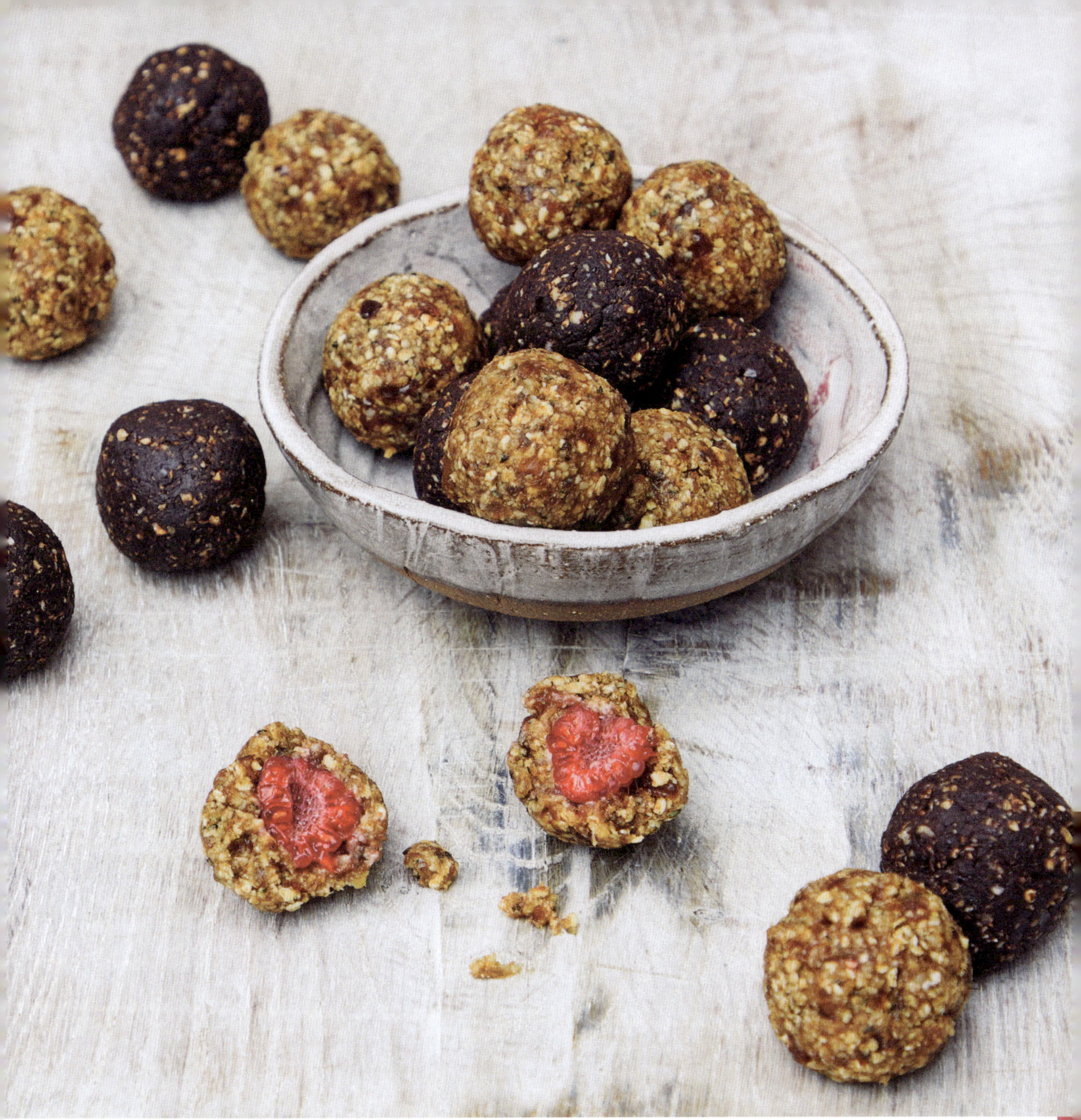

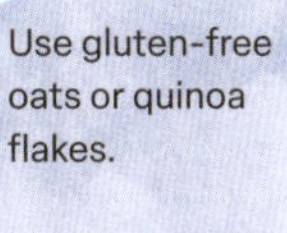
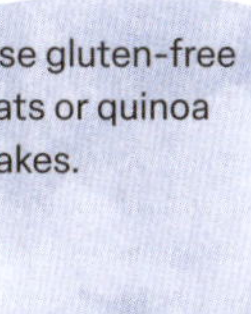

Use gluten-free oats or quinoa flakes.

Swap the peanut butter for sunflower seed butter or sunflower seeds.

Swap the tahini for almond butter or sunflower seed butter.

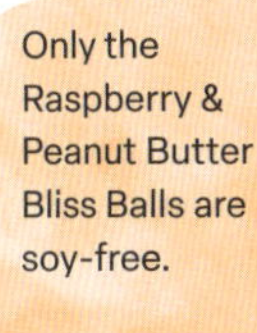

Only the Raspberry & Peanut Butter Bliss Balls are soy-free.

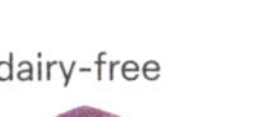

dairy-free

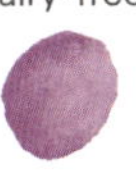

gluten-free

nut-free

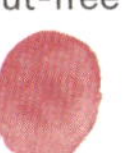

sesame-free

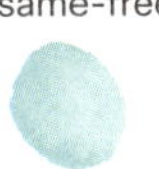

egg-free

soy-free

vegetarian

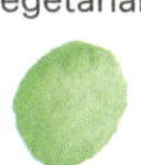

BRAIN BRILLIANCE ROCKY ROAD

Makes 10 slices or 20 small squares

225g (8oz) dark (plain) chocolate (70% cocoa), broken into pieces
2½ Tbsp coconut oil
1½ Tbsp maple syrup
150g (about 1 cup) drained chickpeas (garbanzo beans), jarred or canned
1½ Tbsp pre-roasted, chopped hazelnuts or roughly chopped hazelnuts
75g (½ cup) raisins
40g (3 generous Tbsp) pumpkin seeds
pinch of sea salt flakes (kosher salt), optional

A healthy version of Rocky Road that will become your go-to snack when you need more brain food. This has the perfect balance of crunchy and sweet in the form of hazelnuts, pumpkin seeds and raisins. Chickpeas are a brilliant way to add extra iron, protein and fibre. This combination makes a wholesome snack that helps to regulate blood glucose.

Line a small baking tray with baking paper.

Put the chocolate, coconut oil and maple syrup into a mixing bowl. Set over a pan of simmering water for a few minutes to gently melt the chocolate. Stir occasionally to speed this up.

Meanwhile, rinse and dry any excess water from the chickpeas.

Once the chocolate mixture has melted, stir in the chickpeas, hazelnuts, raisins and pumpkin seeds. Add a pinch of salt if using unsalted canned chickpeas rather than jarred ones. Press the mixture into the lined tray, and pop into the refrigerator to set for about 1 hour.

To serve, cut into 10 slices or 20 bite-sized squares. Store in the refrigerator for up to 3 days or in the freezer for up to 3 months.

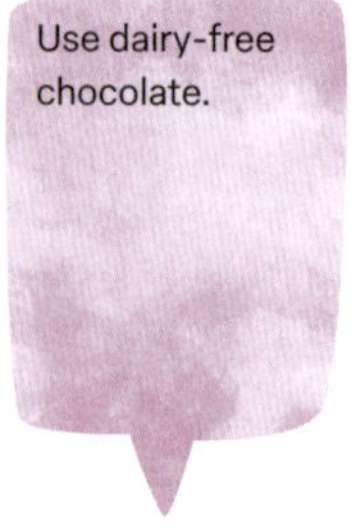

Swap the hazelnuts for sunflower seeds or chia seeds.

dairy-free
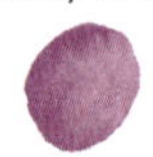
gluten-free

nut-free

sesame-free

egg-free

soy-free

vegetarian
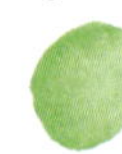

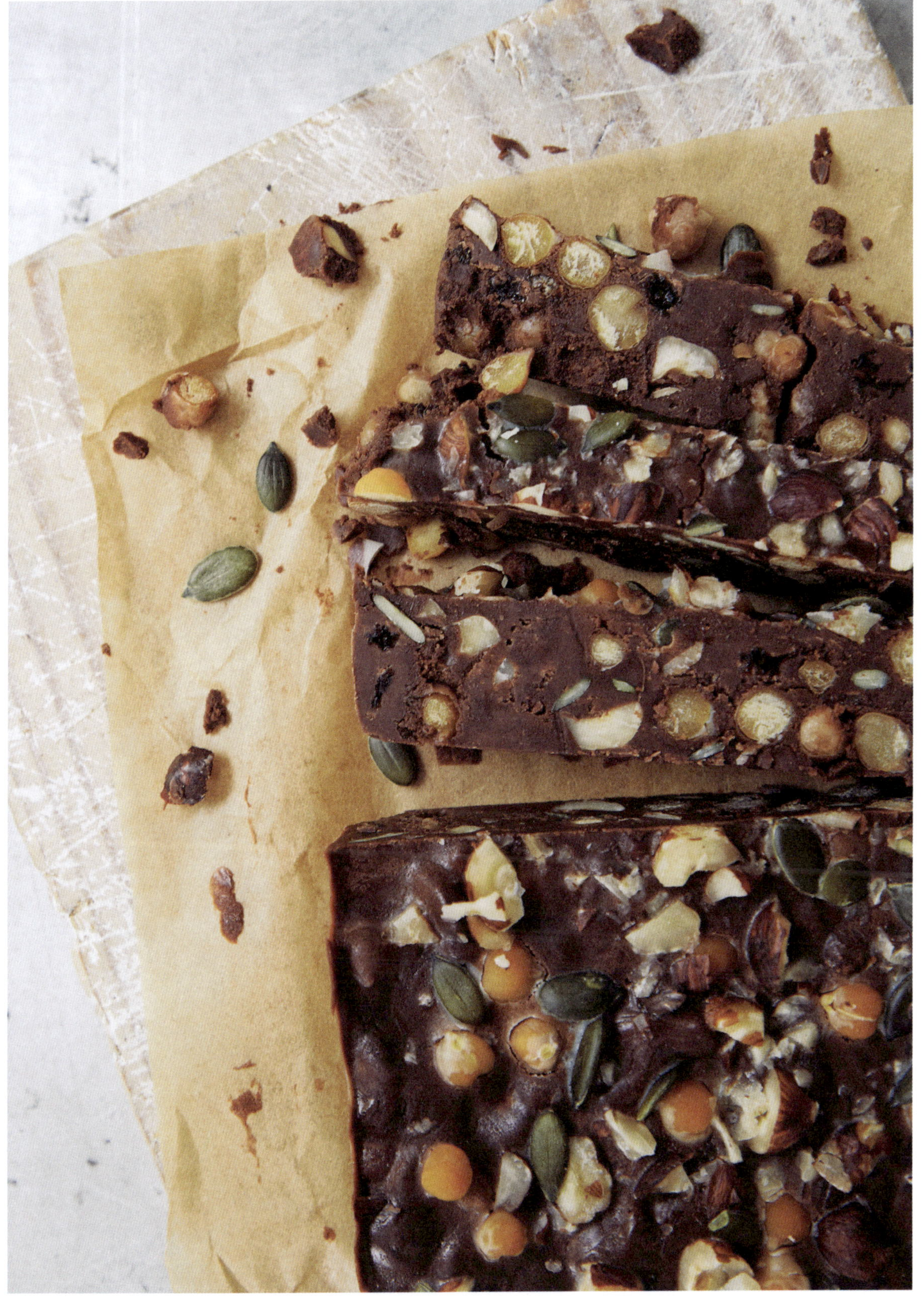

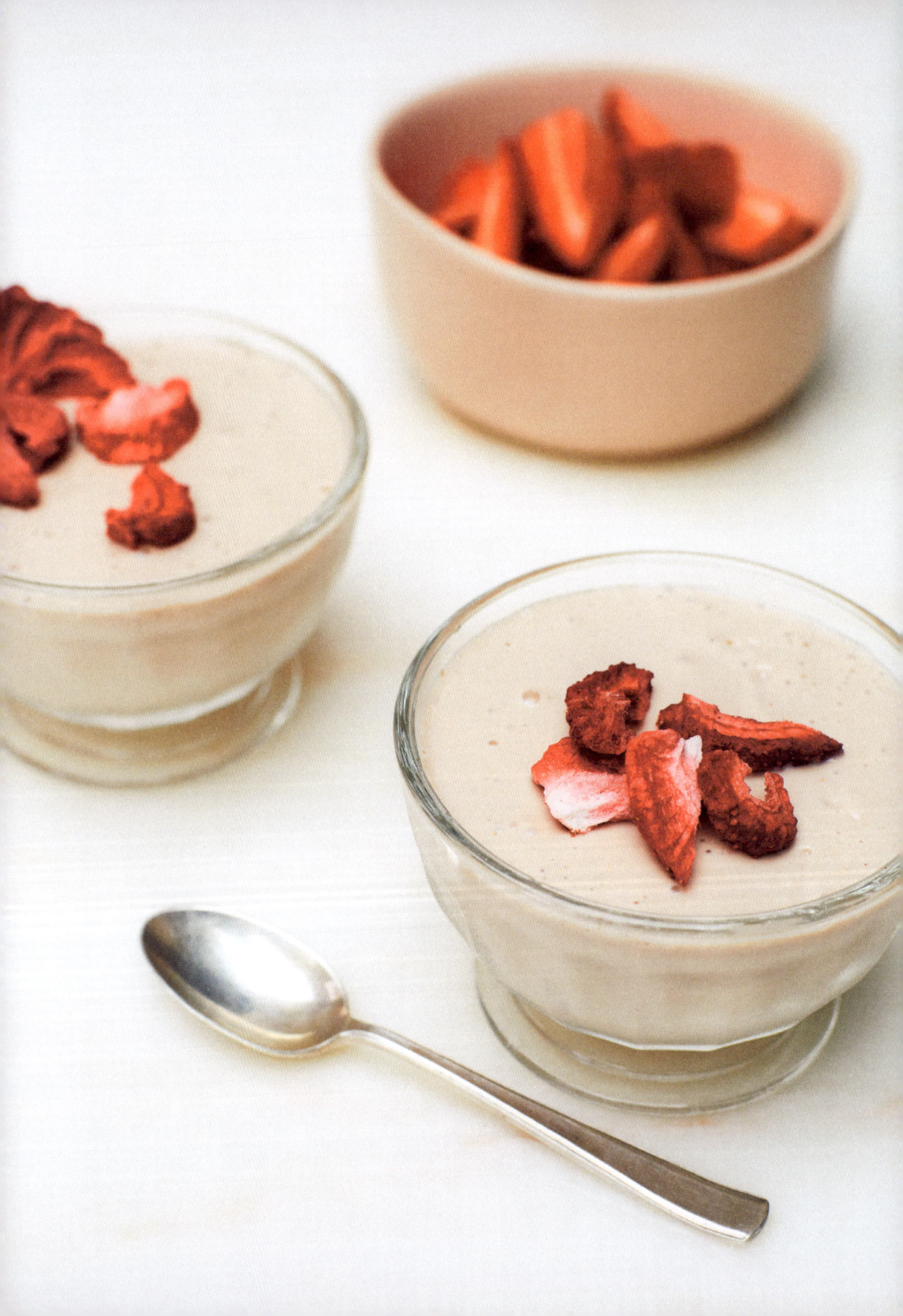

STRAWBERRY MOUSSE

This recipe makes a light and delicate mousse, packed with protein and perfect for breakfast, a quick snack or dessert. Ricotta is an excellent source of GABA – the neurotransmitter that keeps us cool, calm and relaxed. Eggs are full of choline, an essential nutrient that helps with memory, processing and emotional regulation. The strawberries bring their sweetness as well as Vitamin C.

Serves 4

1½ tsp butter
3 eggs, preferably free-range
125g (½ cup plus 1 Tbsp) ricotta cheese
200g (about 2 cups) strawberries, fresh or frozen
1 tsp vanilla extract
1½ Tbsp honey
Freeze-dried strawberry sprinkles or frozen strawberry pieces (optional)

Melt the butter in a frying pan (skillet) over a gentle heat. Crack in the eggs and mix with a spatula. Cook, stirring, to make sloppy scrambled eggs: they don't want to be runny or dry. Remove from the heat and leave to cool slightly.

Put the eggs, ricotta, strawberries, vanilla and honey in a blender and blitz for about a minute or until the mixture is smooth. Transfer into glasses or ramekins.

Top with freeze-dried strawberry sprinkles or frozen strawberry pieces and serve slightly warm, or pop in the refrigerator for 30–60 minutes to eat cold.

Store in the refrigerator for up to 3 days.

Swap the ricotta for 125g (4½oz) of silken tofu (beancurd) and use olive oil instead of butter.

dairy-free

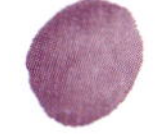

gluten-free

nut-free

sesame-free

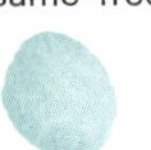

soy-free

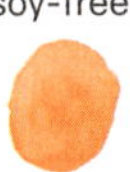

vegetarian

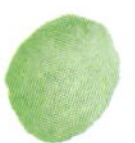

SALTED CARAMEL DOUGHNUTS

Makes 8 large or 16 mini doughnuts

1 tsp coconut oil, melted, plus extra for greasing
220g (generous 2 cups) ground (powdered) almonds
1 tsp mixed spice
½ tsp baking powder
¼ tsp bicarbonate of soda (baking soda)
4 Tbsp maple syrup
4 Tbsp milk of choice
3 eggs, preferably free-range
1 tsp vanilla extract
1 tsp apple cider vinegar

Topping
135g (5oz) or about 7 soft Medjool dates, pitted
6 Tbsp hot water
3 Tbsp cashew butter (for home-made, see the intro on page 203)
½ tsp sea salt flakes (kosher salt)

Doughnuts can be packed with lots of nutritious goodies if you want! These salted caramel doughnuts taste sublime and are easy to make, being baked not deep-fried. Using almonds not flour means they are grain- and gluten-free and high in protein, calcium and choline.

Preheat the oven to 200°C/180°C fan/400°F/Gas mark 6 and grease a doughnut pan with a little coconut oil.

Stir together the almonds, mixed spice, baking powder and bicarbonate of soda in a large bowl.

Whisk together the melted coconut oil, maple syrup, milk, eggs and vanilla extract in a small bowl.

Fold the wet ingredients into the dry ingredients. Finally add the apple cider vinegar and mix well to combine everything.

Spoon the mixture into the greased pan, filling each doughnut hole about two-thirds full. Cook for 12–15 minutes for mini doughnuts and 20–25 minutes for larger ones, or until the dough springs back when pressed. Allow the doughnuts to cool in the pan, then transfer to a wire rack to cool completely.

Meanwhile make the topping. Do ensure your dates are very soft. If they seem at all dry or hard, soak them in warm water for at least 10 minutes and then drain.

Blend the dates, hot water, cashew butter and salt in a high-speed blender until completely smooth, scraping down the sides with a spatula as needed. This will take a few minutes until you have a lovely smooth glaze.

When the doughnuts are fully cool, top each one with some of the glaze. Any leftover glaze can be used as a dip for fruit.

Store in an airtight tin for up to 3 days or in the freezer for up to 3 months.

Swap the ground almonds for coconut flour and replace the cashew butter with tahini (sesame paste).

dairy-free

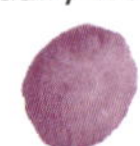

gluten-free

nut-free

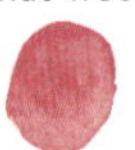

sesame-free

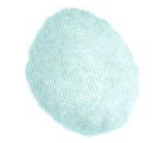

soy-free

vegetarian

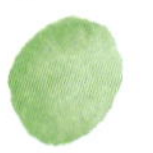

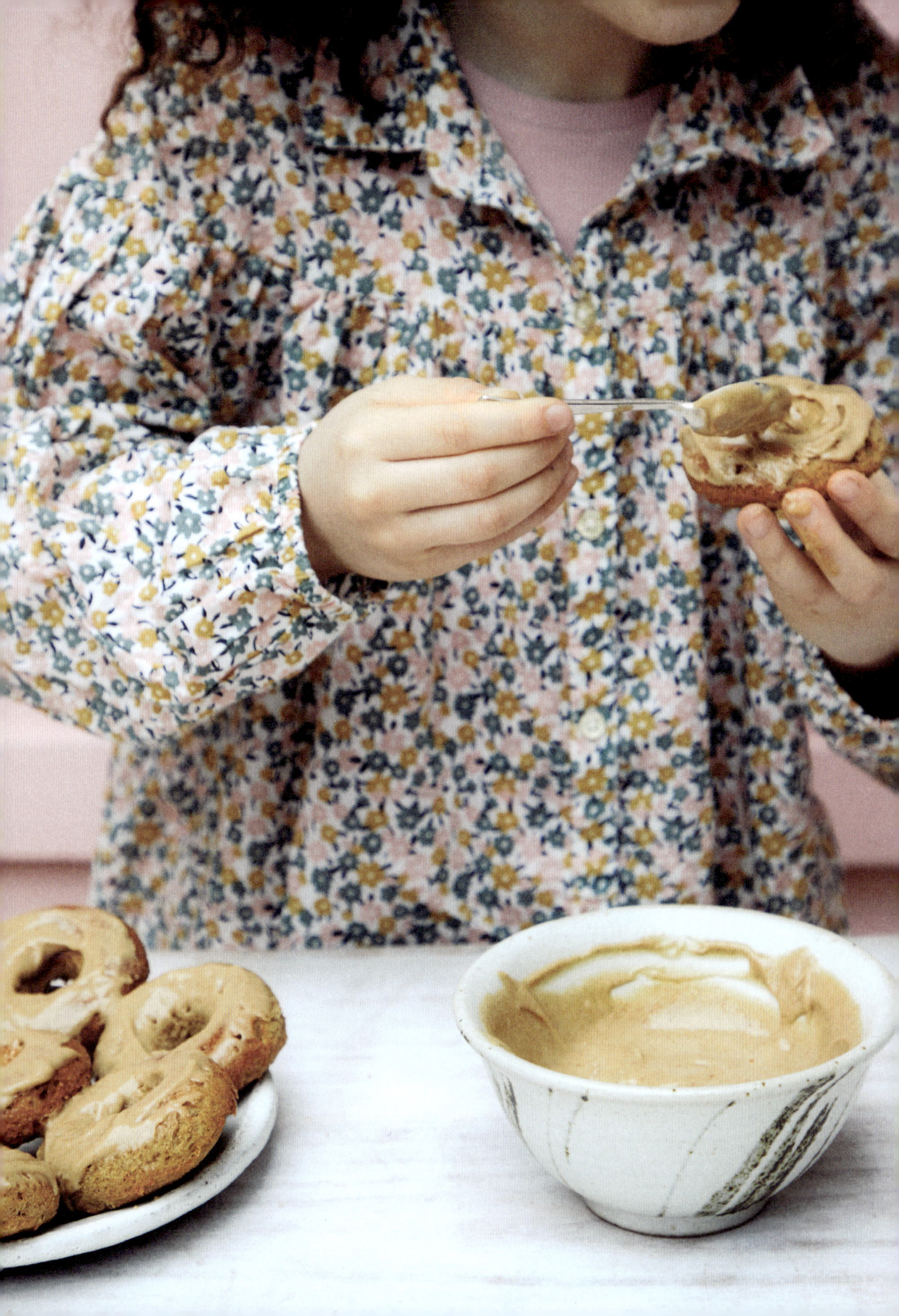

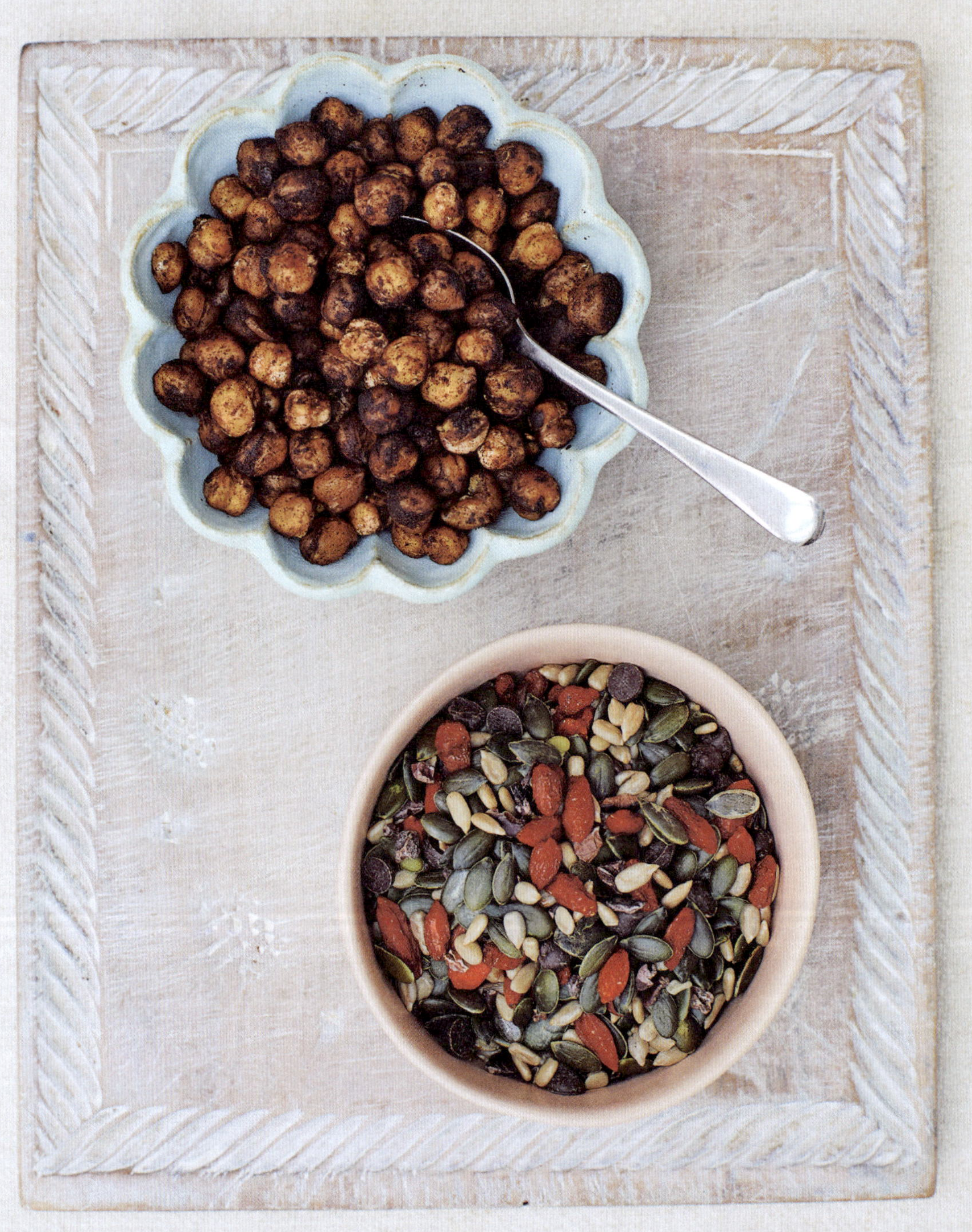

CINNAMON & VANILLA ROASTED CHICKPEAS

Makes 1 x 350g (12oz) jar

400g/14oz can chickpeas (garbanzo beans)
1 Tbsp olive oil
1 tsp vanilla extract
2 tsp ground cinnamon
2 tsp coconut sugar or light muscovado sugar
1 tsp sea salt flakes (kosher salt)

Sweet without the sugar rush, these roasted chickpeas (garbanzo beans) make a lovely snack rich in protein and fibre as well as iron. If you prefer your chickpeas savoury, then try my recipe for Fennel & Paprika Roasted Chickpeas (see page 180).

Preheat the oven to 200°C/180°C fan/390°F/Gas mark 6.

Drain the chickpeas in a sieve (strainer) and rinse well. Shake off any excess liquid and spread the chickpeas on paper towels, then gently pat dry.

Mix the olive oil, vanilla, cinnamon, coconut sugar and salt together in a small bowl, then stir in the chickpeas. Ensure they are coated well with the mixture. Spread out the chickpeas on a baking tray and roast for 30–40 minutes, or until brown and crunchy. Check frequently towards the end of the cooking time to avoid burning. Eat warm or at room temperature.

Store in a glass container in the refrigerator for up to 3 days.

GOJI TRAIL MIX

Makes 1 x 350g (12oz) jar

100g (about ¾ cup) pumpkin seeds
100g (about ¾ cup) sunflower seeds
50g (about ¼ cup) goji berries
50g (about ¼ cup) raw cacao nibs
30g (about ⅓ cup) dark or milk chocolate drops (optional)

This mix has been the go-to snack and breakfast topper for yoghurt and granola for me and my husband for the last ten years: we never tire of it. We always have a big jar in the kitchen, ready to grab when we need a bit of brain fuel and strength. The goji berries and the cacao nibs pair beautifully.

Goji berries are a good source of iron and vitamin C, and raw cacao nibs are rich in magnesium and zinc as well as iron. The other seeds are packed with vitamin E as well as zinc and magnesium. You should find all the ingredients in a large supermarket, or your local health food shop.

Tip all the ingredients into a jar and stir well. Store, sealed, for up to 3 months.

dairy-free

gluten-free

nut-free

sesame-free

egg-free

soy-free
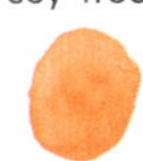
vegetarian

MELLOW MOOD ICE LOLLIES

Makes 4 ice lollies (popsicles)

240ml (1 cup) cloudy apple or pear juice
2 tsp dried chamomile, lemon balm and passionflower (leaves and flowers) – or a teabag containing one or a combination of all three
juice of ½ lemon
¼ cucumber, peeled, seeds removed

Many neurodivergent folk are in a state of fight or flight much of the time, and sometimes an ice lolly is all the food they can face. Sucking on a cooling lolly can be soothing in itself. This recipe contains a mixture of calming herbs that you can grow yourself or pick up in your local health food shop. Chamomile, lemon balm and passionflower all contain the neurotransmitter GABA, which helps us to keep cool, calm and relaxed and also helps us to sleep when we are stressed.

Heat the apple juice in a saucepan until it is simmering gently. Add the dried herbs or tea bag, cover the pan and continue to simmer for 5 minutes. Turn off the heat and let the herbs steep in the juice for a further 10 minutes at least while the juice cools down a little.

Once the infused juice has cooled down, remove the herbs using a small strainer or fish out the tea bag. Press the herbs or give the tea bag a quick squeeze to ensure you get all the lovely benefits from the herbs in the juice.

Transfer the liquid to a blender, add the lemon juice and cucumber and blend for 10–20 seconds until smooth.

Pour into ice-lolly moulds and pop on the tops. Place the moulds on a small tray or flat surface in the freezer for about 4 hours until fully frozen, then transfer to a bag and store the lollies in the freezer for up to 3 months.

dairy-free

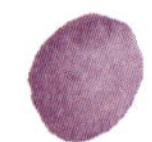

gluten-free

nut-free

sesame-free

egg-free

soy-free

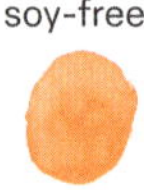

vegetarian

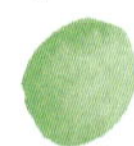

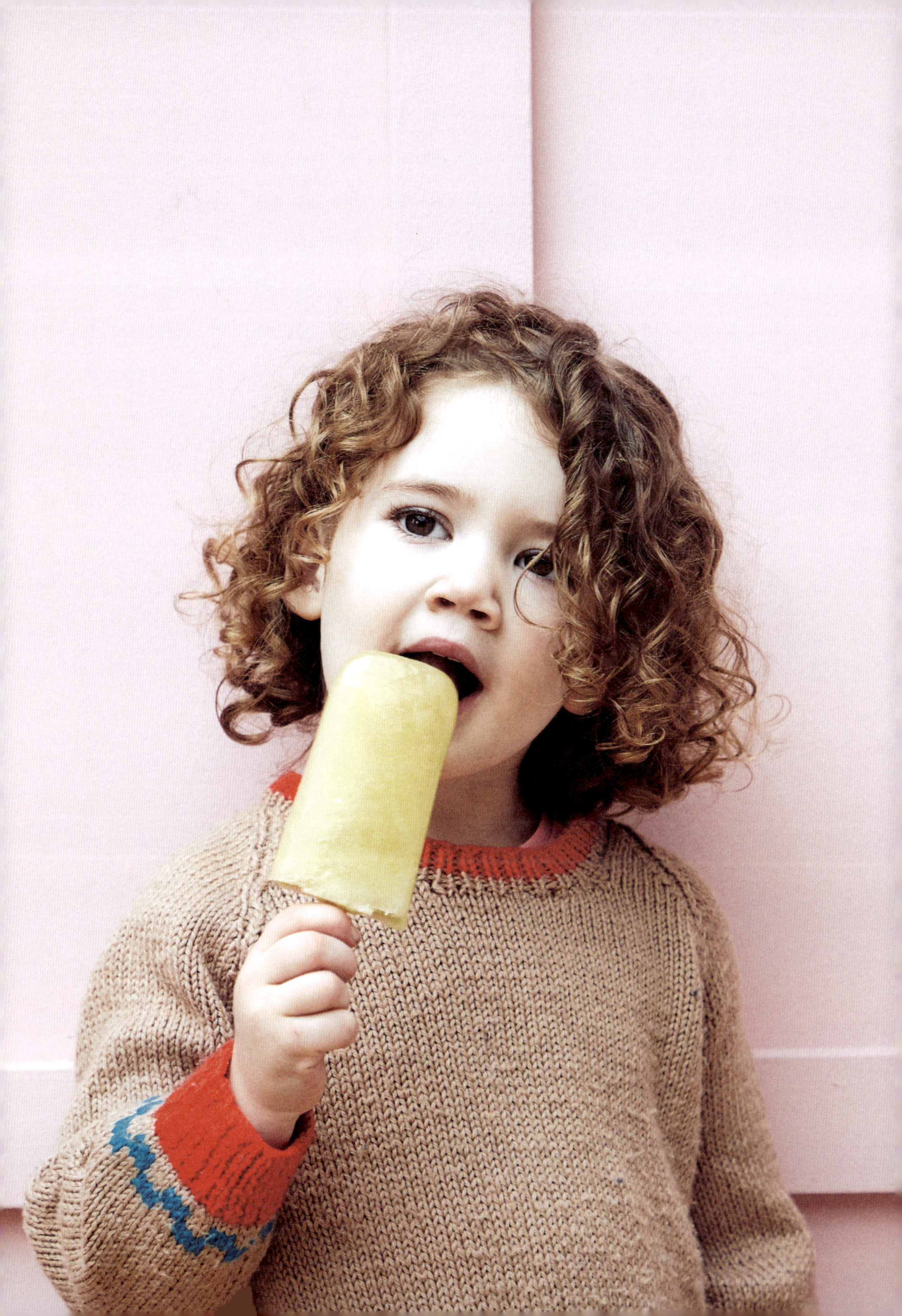

ZESTY TANGERINE SQUARES

Makes 25

100g (1 cup) rolled oats
250g (1⅔ cups) pitted dried apricots (ideally natural brown and unsulphured)
1 tsp allspice
25g desiccated (shredded) coconut
60g (scant ½ cup) pumpkin seeds
60g (scant ½ cup) pecan nuts
1 tsp vanilla extract
5 Tbsp cashew butter (for home-made, see the intro on page 203)
3 tsp coconut oil
zest and segments of 2 tangerines

Squidgy and citrusy, these filling squares of goodness are packed with zinc and magnesium. Sweetened only with iron-rich apricots and mellow allspice they are entirely plant-based and dairy-free – and you can easily make them gluten-free too. A treat to have in your freezer when you or your kids need a nutritious snack... NOW!

Pop all the dry ingredients into a food processor and blitz for about 30 seconds until the apricots are finely chopped.

Add the vanilla extract, cashew butter and coconut oil and blitz for a further 30 seconds.

With the machine running, slowly add the tangerine zest and flesh until the mixture forms a sticky ball.

Line a 20cm (8in) square cake tin with a sheet of baking paper and then use your hands to pack the oat mixture into the tin until it is evenly spread and pressed into the corners. Pop in the refrigerator for 45 minutes or the freezer for 20 minutes to firm up.

Slice into 16 squares. Store in the refrigerator for 3 days or in the freezer for up to 3 months.

Use gluten-free oats or quinoa flakes.

Swap the pecans for sunflower seeds and use tahini (sesame paste) instead of cashew butter.

dairy-free
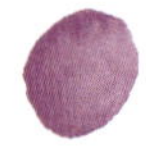

gluten-free

nut-free
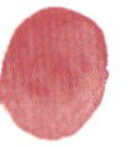

sesame-free
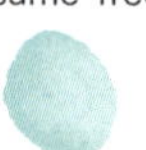

egg-free

soy-free

vegetarian
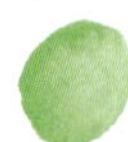

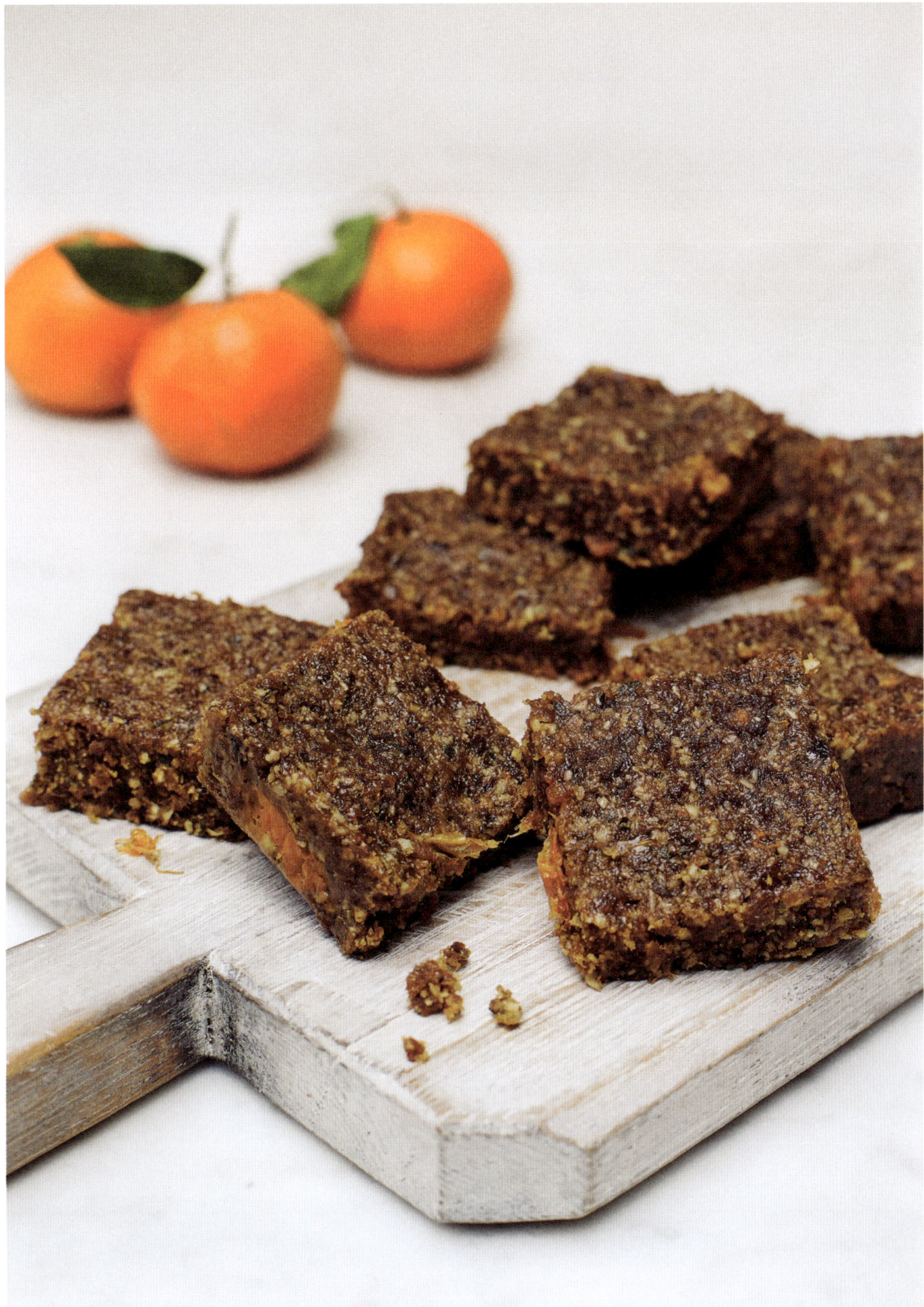

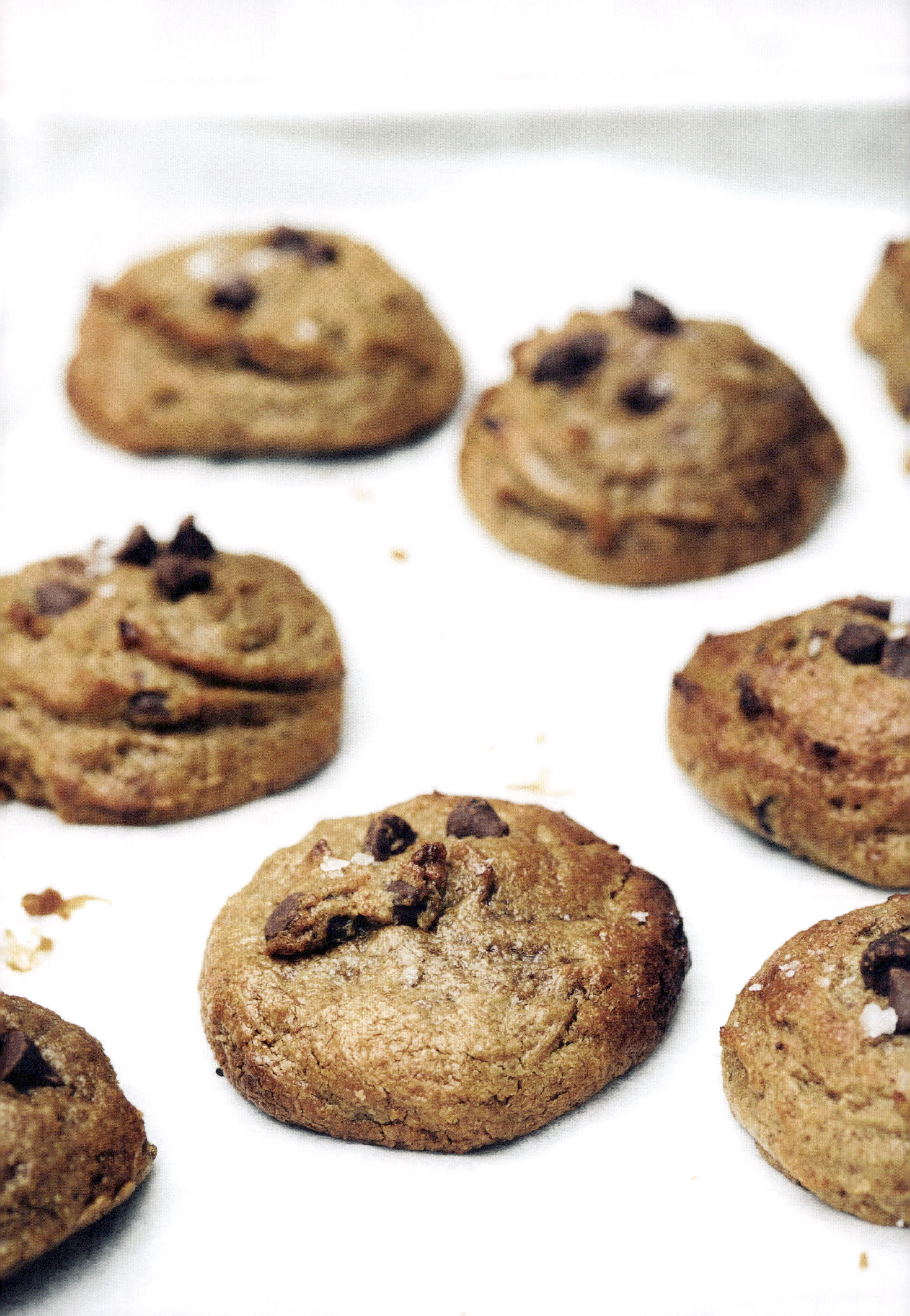

CASHEW BUTTER CHOCOLATE CHIP COOKIES

Makes 8

250g (generous 1 cup) cashew butter
1 egg, preferably free-range
90g (about ½ cup) coconut sugar or light muscovado sugar
½ tsp vanilla extract
¼ tsp sea salt flakes (kosher salt), plus extra (optional) for sprinkling
2 Tbsp dark or milk chocolate chips

Crunchy and nourishing, these chocolate chip cookies are real feel-good snacks with a creamy magnesium-packed cashew nut base.

If you don't have a jar of cashew butter to hand, you can easily make your own by roasting 2 cups of shelled cashew nuts gently in a preheated oven at 180°C/160°C/350°F/Gas mark 4 for 8–10 minutes. Let them cool a little and then grind in a food processor, blending for 10 minutes until smooth and paste-like. Stop and scrape down the sides with a spatula every couple of minutes. Halfway through add 2 teaspoons of coconut oil to make it even creamier.

Preheat the oven to 180°C/160°C/350°F/Gas mark 4 and line a baking tray with baking paper.

Combine the cashew butter, egg, coconut sugar, vanilla extract and salt in a mixing bowl until smooth. Then stir through the chocolate chips.

Divide the dough into 12 pieces, rolling each piece into a ball. Place, spaced apart, on the lined tray and squish down with a fork to flatten. Sprinkle an extra pinch of salt on top if you wish. Bake in the oven for 8–10 minutes or until they are firm at the edges and light brown. Cool on the baking tray and then transfer to a wire rack before serving.

Store for up to 3 days in an airtight container or in the freezer for up to 3 months.

Use dairy-free chocolate.

Swap the cashew butter for light tahini (sesame paste) or sunflower seed butter, which you can make in the same way as the cashew butter (see above).

Use 1 tablespoon of ground flaxseed combined with 2 tablespoons of warm water, in place of the egg.

dairy-free
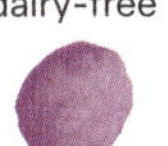
gluten-free
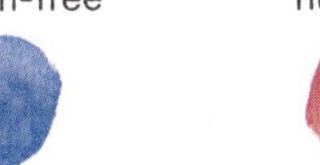
nut-free

sesame-free

egg-free

soy-free

vegetarian

BLACK BEAN TAHINI BROWNIES

Makes 9

Base
150g (5½oz) dark (plain) chocolate (70% cocoa), broken into pieces
150g (⅔ cup) butter
3 eggs, preferably free-range
125g (scant ⅔ cup) coconut sugar or light muscovado sugar
1 tsp vanilla extract
400g (14oz) can black beans, drained
sea salt flakes (kosher salt)

Tahini swirl
4 Tbsp tahini (sesame paste)
2 Tbsp date syrup or maple syrup
1 egg, preferably free-range

Brownies are always a winner and these squidgy squares are made with black beans, making them packed with protein and iron. They are a real treat for neurodivergent kids who need to bolster their nutrient intake. Top with a beautiful creamy swirl to make these brownies that bit more special.

Preheat the oven to 180°C/160°C/350°F/Gas mark 4. Grease and line a 20cm (8in) square brownie tin with baking paper.

Put the chocolate and butter into a saucepan over a very gentle heat. Leave to melt, stirring from time to time to combine well. Remove from the heat and allow to cool a little.

Crack the eggs into the jug of a high-speed blender. Add the coconut sugar and vanilla extract to the eggs and blend until the mixture is light and bubbly.

Stir in the drained black beans, the slightly cooled chocolate-butter mixture and a pinch of sea salt flakes. Blend again for a minute or two to make a nice, smooth batter. This is the base for your brownies.

To make the tahini swirl, stir the tahini, syrup and egg together in a small bowl to make a thick creamy sauce.

Pour the chocolate batter into the lined brownie tin, ensuring it fills the corners.

Spoon the tahini swirl on top of the batter and use a fork to swirl it into the chocolate base so it makes a beautiful, marbled pattern throughout – don't overmix. Sprinkle a few more salt flakes over the top, then bake for around 25 minutes, until the edges are firm but there is still a wobble in the centre. Allow to cool in the tin, then cut into 9 squares.

Store in an airtight tin for up to 3 days or the freezer for up to 3 months.

Swap the butter for a dairy-free spread or coconut oil. Use dairy-free chocolate.

Swap the tahini for cashew butter or sunflower seed butter.

For the base swap the eggs for 3 tablespoons of ground flaxseed combined with 6 tablespoons of water OR whisk 4½ tablespoons of chickpea water (known as aquafaba) for a few minutes using an electric whisk until the mixture forms soft peaks, then add to the blender. For the tahini swirl, use 1 tablespoon of ground flaxseed combined with 1 tablespoon of warm water in place of the egg.

dairy-free
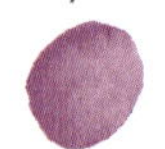
gluten-free

nut-free

sesame-free

egg-free
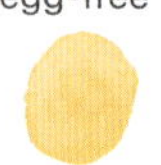
soy-free
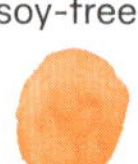
vegetarian
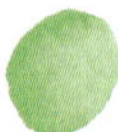

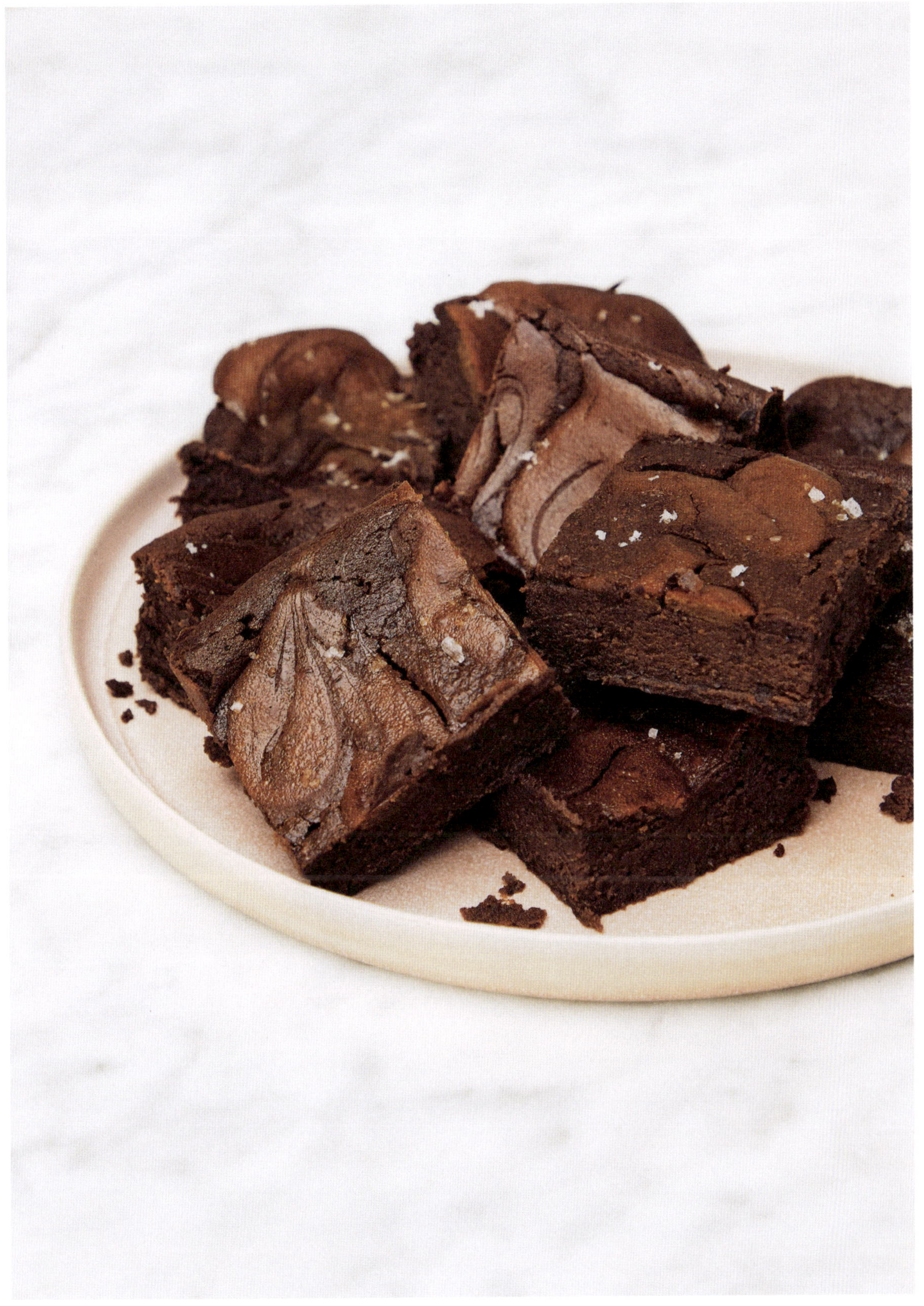

PEANUT CARAMEL BITES

Makes 12

Base
50g (½ cup) walnut pieces
50g (scant ½ cup) blanched almonds
½ tsp salt
6 pitted dates
1½ Tbsp water

Caramel
8 pitted dates
100g (scant ½ cup) almond butter
1 tsp vanilla extract
1 Tbsp maple syrup
¼ tsp salt
2 Tbsp water

Topping
50g (scant ½ cup) roasted peanuts
150g (5½oz) dark (plain) chocolate (70% cocoa), broken into pieces
1 Tbsp coconut oil

The combination of chocolate, peanuts and caramel is always a winner, and you will become very popular whenever you rustle up a batch of these no-bake bites for your family. They're incredibly nutritious and delicious – eat straight from the freezer.

Make the base by grinding up the walnuts, almonds and salt in a food processor. Add the dates and pulse until fully chopped. Add the water, a little at a time, while pulsing until a thick dough forms and starts to make a ball. (You might only need 1 tablespoon of water; only add the extra ½ tablespoon if your dates are quite dry.)

Line a 20cm (8in) square cake tin or deep-sided baking tray with baking paper and press the dough down into it until it makes a flat and even base.

Blend all the caramel ingredients together in the food processor for 3 minutes until smooth, again adding water gradually – you'll need to scrape down the sides of the food processor bowl every minute – until the mixture is nice and thick. Spread the caramel over the base with a palette knife and top with the peanuts. Freeze for at least 4 hours.

When the base is ready, put the dark chocolate and coconut oil in a small saucepan over a very low heat, stirring until melted and well combined.

Remove the base from freezer and cut it into squares. Dip each one in the melted chocolate to coat, then pop them back on the lined tray and return to the freezer for 15–20 minutes until set.

Store in the refrigerator for 3 days or the freezer for up to 3 months.

TIP
This recipe works really well with other nuts, so try pecans or cashews. You can also use organic milk chocolate or vegan chocolate if you prefer.

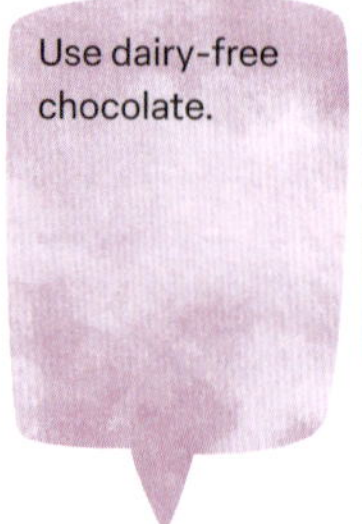

Swap the walnuts for pumpkin seeds and the almonds for sunflower seeds. Use tahini (sesame paste) instead of almond butter and replace the peanuts with goji berries, dried mulberries or chopped dried apricots.

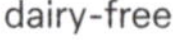

dairy-free
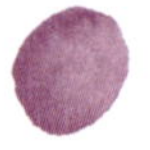

gluten-free

nut-free

sesame-free

egg-free

soy-free

vegetarian
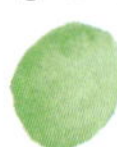

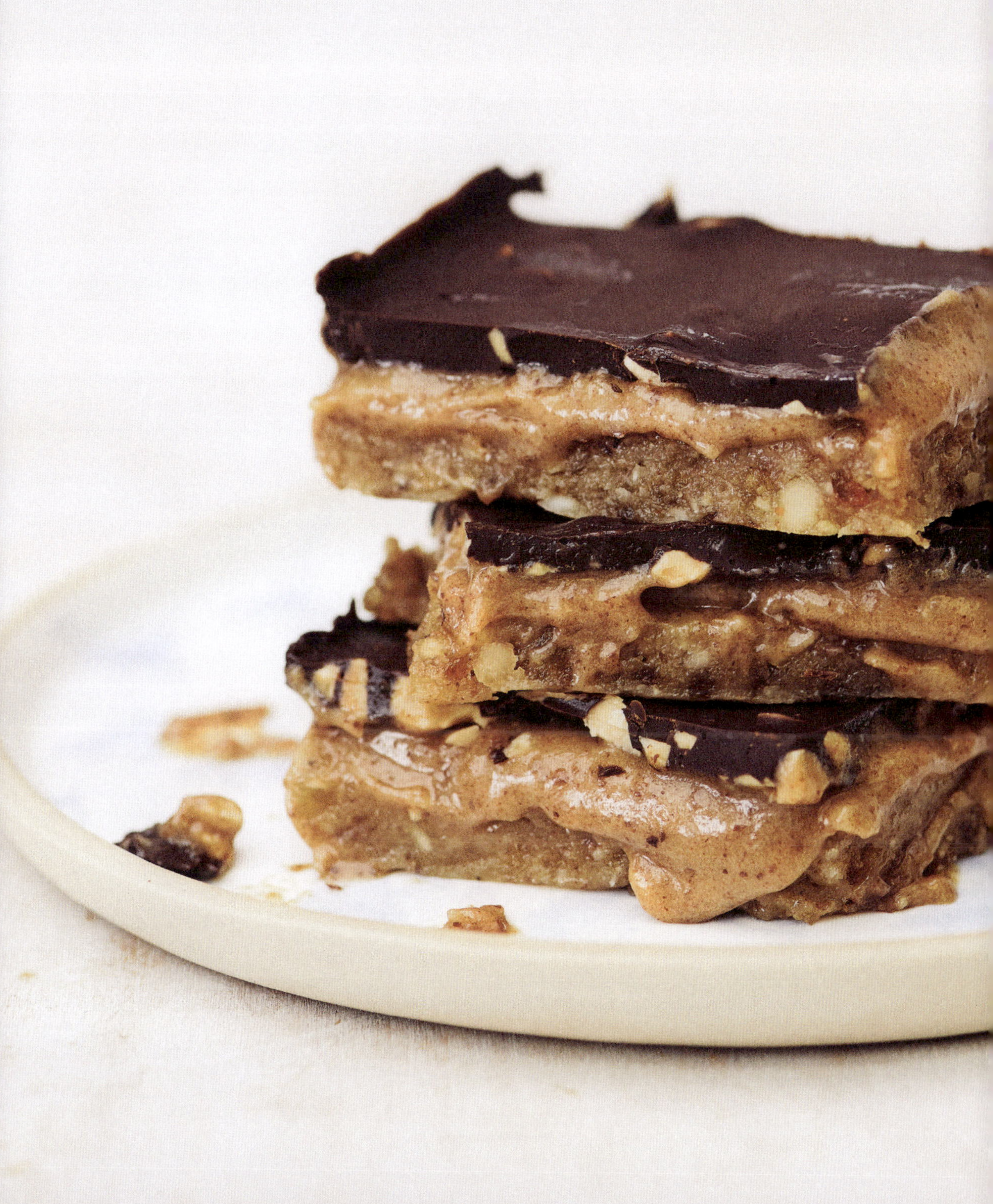

RASPBERRY CHOCOLATE MUG CAKE

Makes 1

1 Tbsp light olive oil, plus extra for greasing
30g (⅓ cup) ground (powdered) almonds
1 Tbsp cacao or unsweetened cocoa powder
¼ tsp baking powder
pinch of sea salt flakes (kosher salt)
2 Tbsp coconut sugar or light muscovado sugar (add a little more for those with a sweet tooth)
1 egg, preferably free-range, well beaten
5 raspberries
1 date stoned and finely diced or 8 raisins
1 tsp dark or milk chocolate chips

Raspberry and chocolate together are one of my favourite flavours and the combination is even better when made into a fluffy mug cake.

Many people do not have access to an oven but that doesn't exclude them from enjoying a quick, warming and nutritious brain-food snack to tide them over. A mug cake is made in under 3 minutes in a microwave, and this one is packed with nutritious goodies that keep blood glucose levels even and the brain sharp.

Grease a microwaveable mug or glass jar using a little olive oil on a piece of paper towel.

Add the ground almonds, cocoa powder, baking powder, salt and coconut sugar. Stir well, then add the beaten egg and the tablespoon of olive oil. Stir to combine the ingredients so they are evenly mixed.

Gently stir in the raspberries, dates or raisins and chocolate chips.

Place the mug in an 800W microwave and cook for 30 seconds. Remove the mug, stir the mixture again well and shake it a little to help even up the top.

Pop it back in the microwave for 60 seconds. If the top of the cake is too loose, then microwave for a further 20–30 seconds. Do not overcook, as this will make the mixture too dry.

Wait for it to cool down a bit, as the centre of the cake will be very hot, then eat with a spoon, straight from the mug! Alternatively, store, covered, for up to 3 days in the mug it was cooked in.

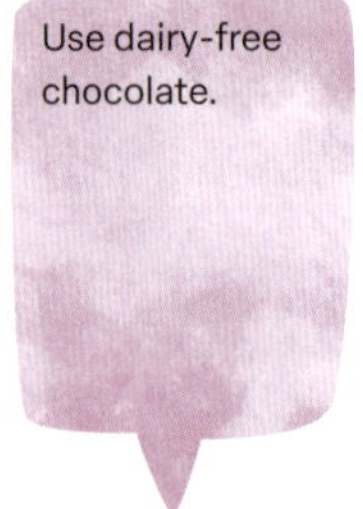

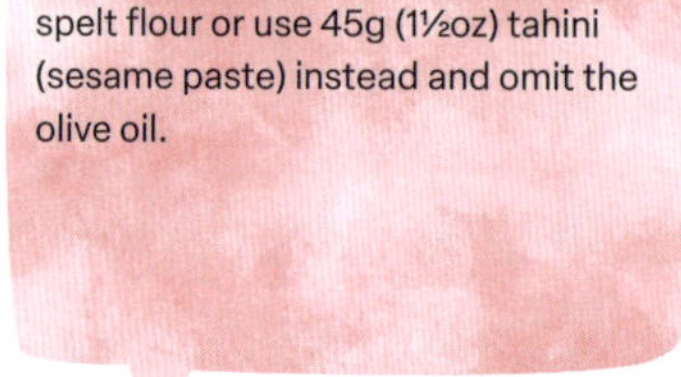

Swap the egg for 1 tablespoon of ground chia seeds or flaxseed soaked in 1 tablespoon warm water for 10 minutes before adding to the mixture.

dairy-free

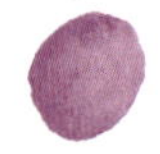

gluten-free

nut-free

sesame-free

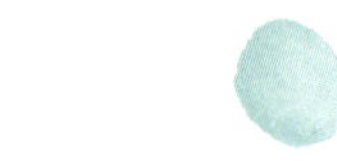

egg-free

soy-free

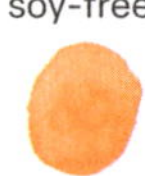

vegetarian

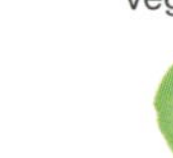

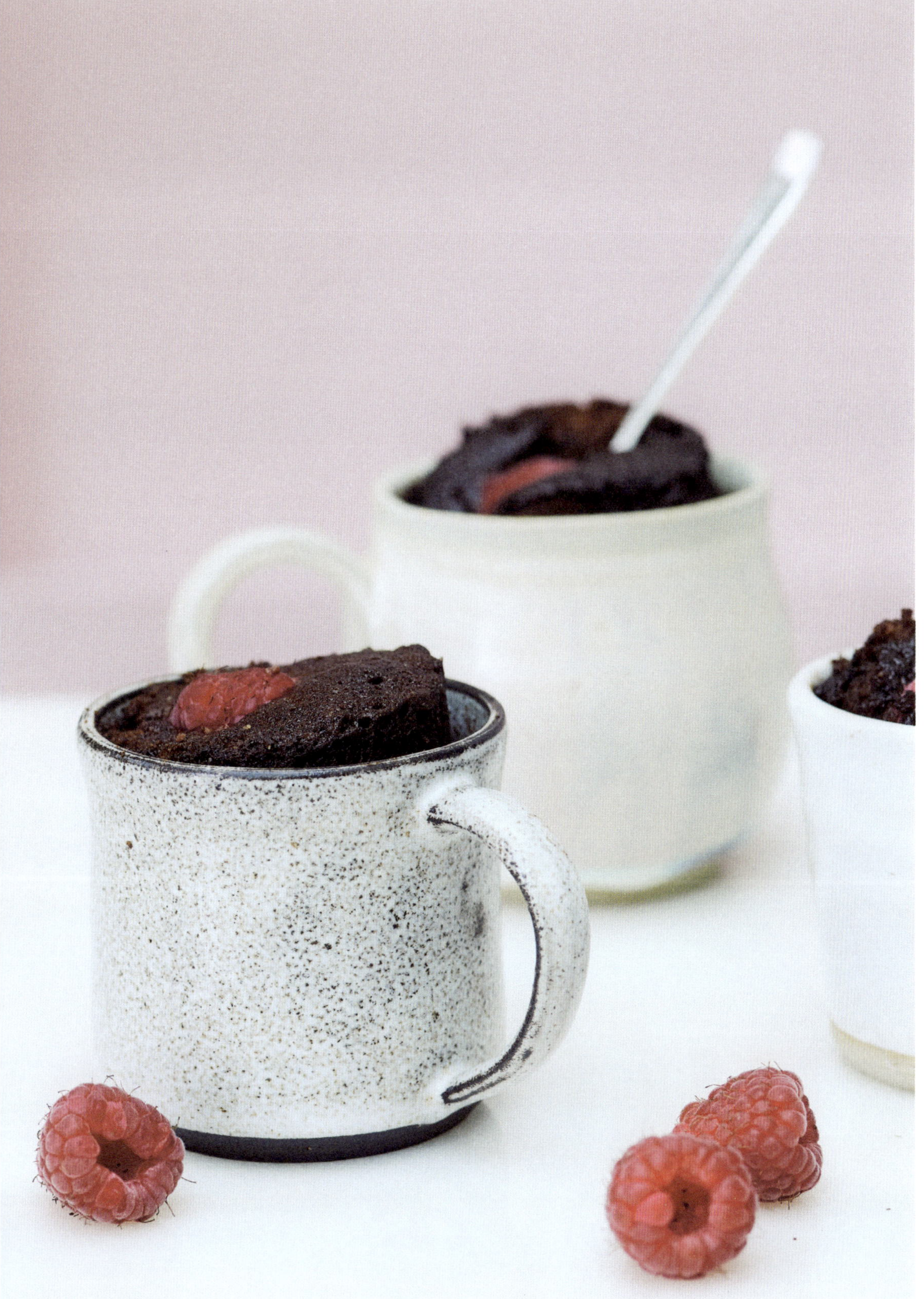

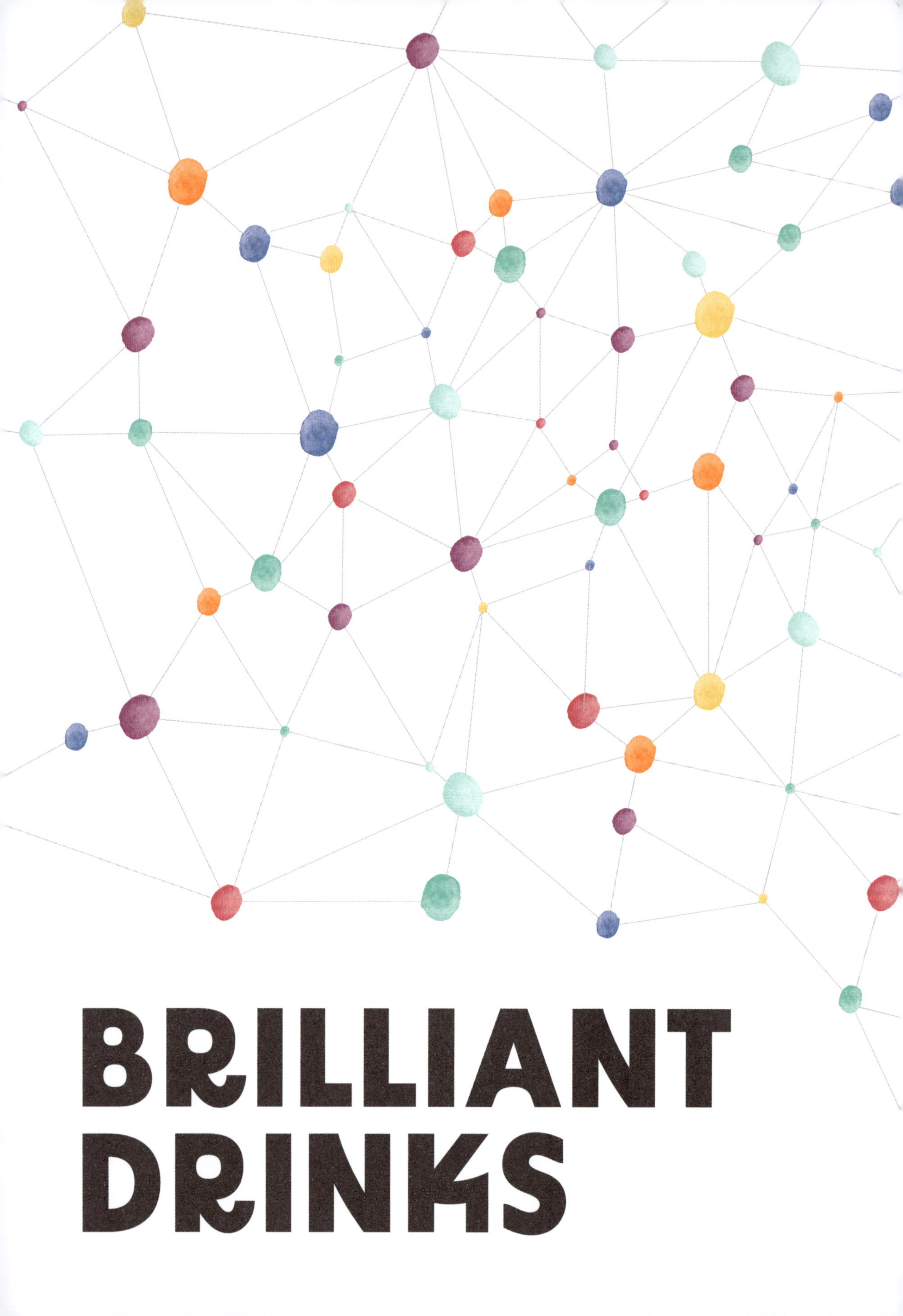
BRILLIANT
DRINKS

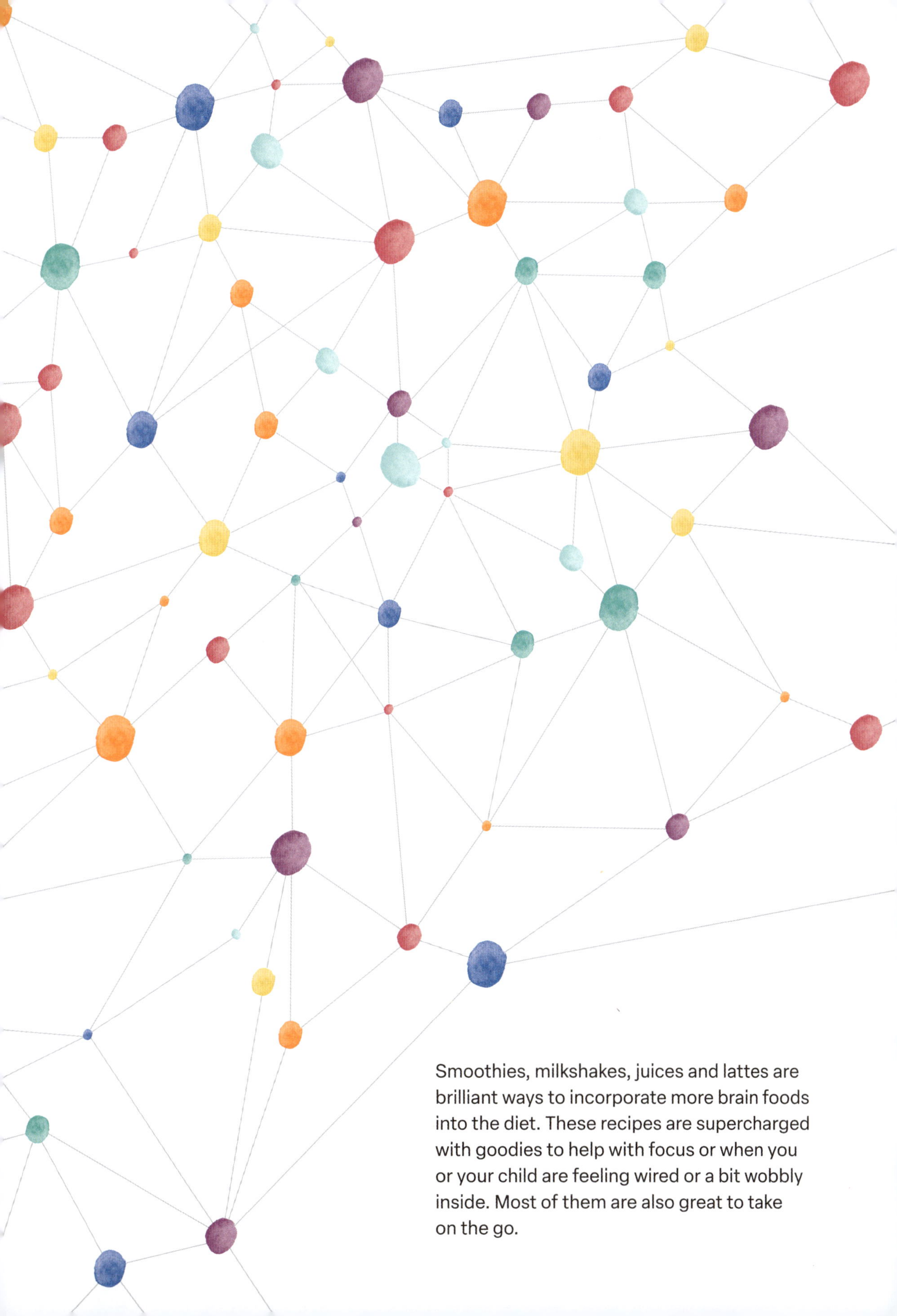

Smoothies, milkshakes, juices and lattes are brilliant ways to incorporate more brain foods into the diet. These recipes are supercharged with goodies to help with focus or when you or your child are feeling wired or a bit wobbly inside. Most of them are also great to take on the go.

CACAO & PEANUT BUTTER MILKSHAKE

Packed with filling ingredients that fuel focus, this shake makes a wholesome breakfast if you are in a rush, or try it as a great afternoon snack. You can boost it up with a tablespoon of vanilla or cacao protein powder or ½ teaspoon of lion's mane powder – supplements that will help to supercharge this smoothie further and keep the brain sharp. These powders are readily available from health shops.

Makes 1 drink

1 cup (240ml) milk of choice
2 dates, pitted
1 Tbsp cacao or unsweetened cocoa powder
1 banana (fresh or frozen), cut into chunks
2 Tbsp peanut butter
¼ tsp vanilla extract
1 Tbsp vanilla or chocolate protein powder (optional)
½ tsp lion's mane powder (optional)
3 ice cubes (optional)

Pour the milk into a high-speed blender, add the remaining ingredients except the ice, and whizz for about 1 minute until smooth.

If using ice, add it to the blender at the end and whizz again, or simply pour the smoothie over the cubes in a glass.

Serve immediately or store in the refrigerator for up to 12 hours. You can make any leftovers into ice lollies.

Use tahini (sesame paste) or sunflower seed butter instead of peanut butter.

dairy-free
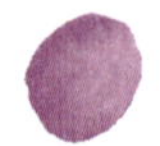
gluten-free

nut-free

sesame-free

egg-free

soy-free

vegetarian

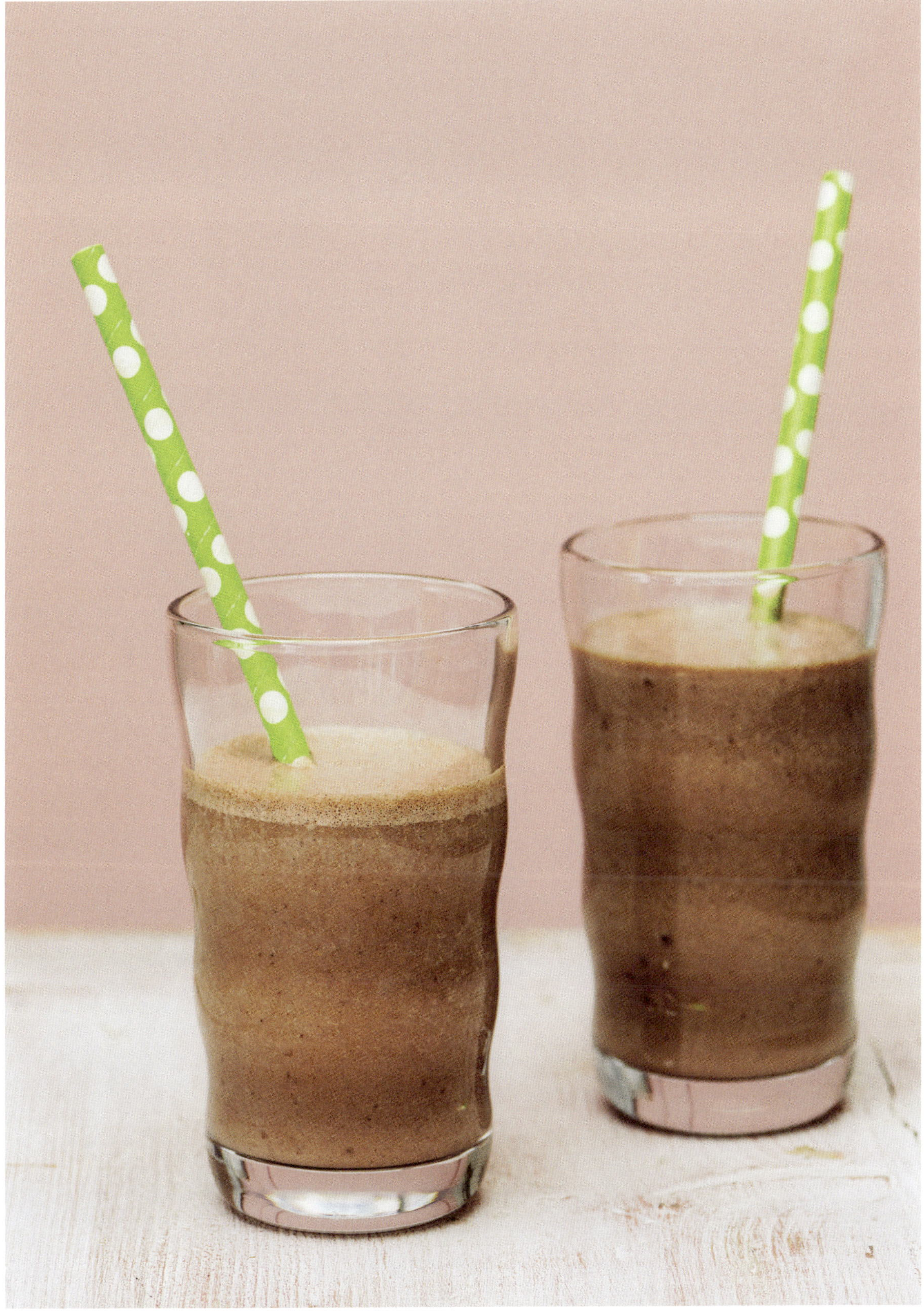

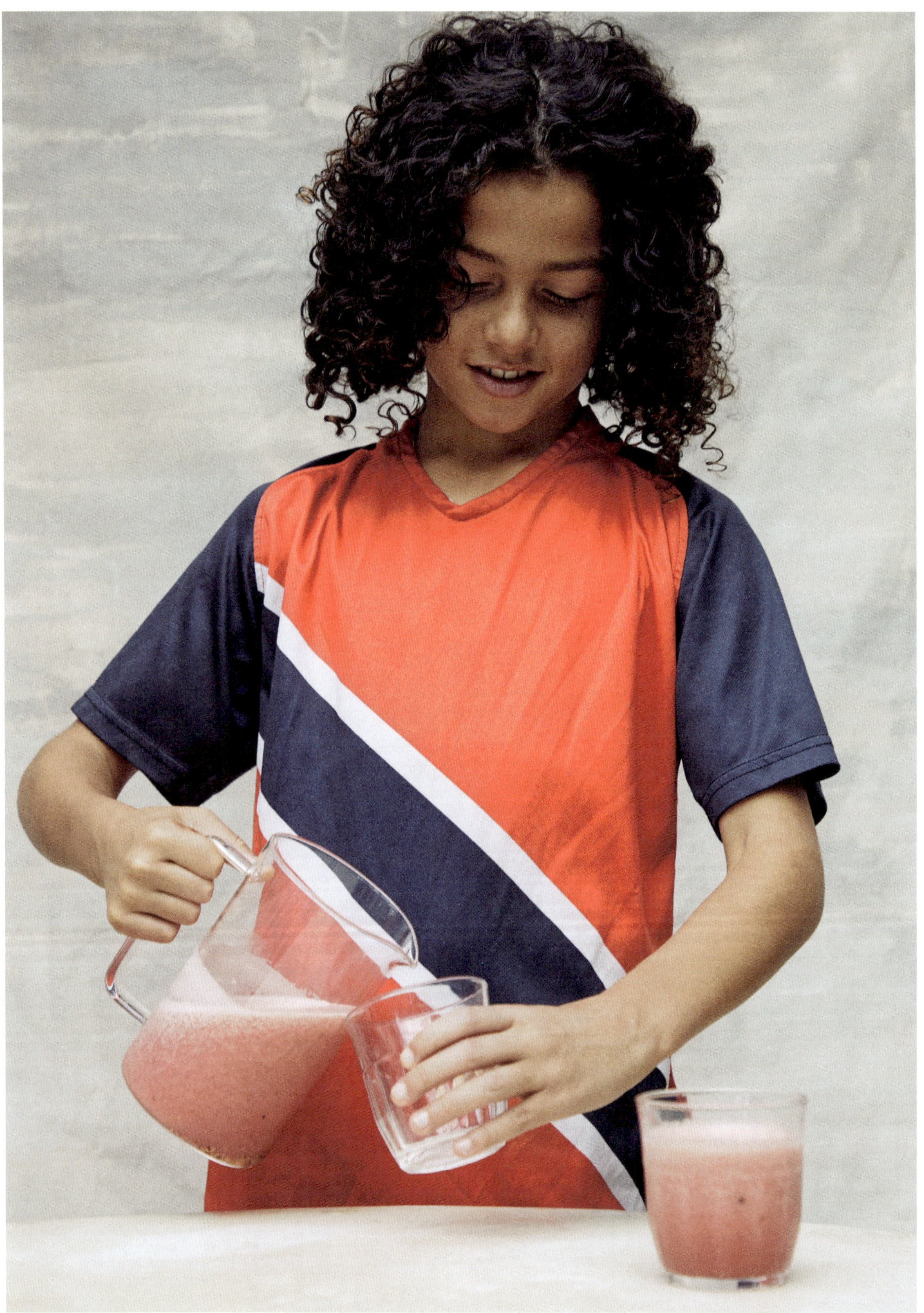

WATERMELON & RASPBERRY REFRESHER

Makes 1 drink

3 thick slices or ¼ watermelon, skin removed
100ml (scant ½ cup) coconut water
8 raspberries
4 ice cubes

Watermelon and raspberries make a delicious deep-red drink. Blended with coconut water this makes a lovely and refreshing electrolyte drink – perfect when you are feeling dehydrated or you need a boost to your energy.

Blend all the ingredients except the ice in a high-speed blender for 1 minute, then add the ice and blend again. Pour into a glass and serve immediately.

This can be stored in the refrigerator for up to 12 hours or any leftovers made into ice lollies.

dairy-free

gluten-free

nut-free

sesame-free
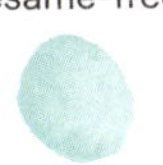
egg-free
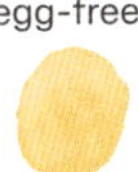
soy-free

vegetarian
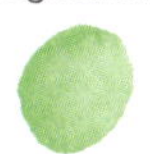

BRAINY BLUEBERRY SMOOTHIE

Makes 1 drink

100ml (scant ½ cup) milk of choice
1 Tbsp full-fat plain Greek yoghurt or kefir
50g (scant ½ cup) blueberries (fresh or frozen)
1 small banana or a handful of mango cubes, fresh or frozen
1 tsp chia seeds
1 tsp hulled hemp seeds

Use plant-based milk and swap the yoghurt/kefir for coconut yoghurt/kefir or silken tofu (beancurd).

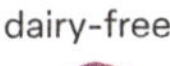

Eating blueberries at breakfast has been shown to help cognitive performance during both the morning and the afternoon. So, these nutrient-dense berries are good for your brain as well as really tasty! This smoothie is a winner that balances protein and healthy fats – and you can whizz it up in only a minute.

Pour the milk into a high-speed blender, add all the other ingredients and whizz for 1 minute. You may need to stop halfway through and scrape down the sides, especially if using frozen fruit.

Serve immediately or store in the refrigerator for up to 12 hours. You can make any leftovers into ice lollies.

TIP
When making smoothies always pour the liquid into the blender first, then add the rest of the ingredients.

pictured on page 219

dairy-free
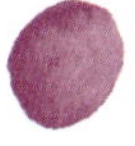
gluten-free
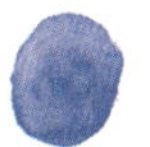
nut-free
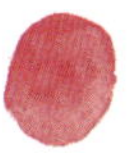
sesame-free

egg-free

soy-free

vegetarian
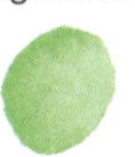

SAFFRON & CARDAMOM LATTE

Makes 1 drink

240ml (1 cup) milk of choice
1 tsp runny honey or maple syrup
1 saffron strand
1 cardamom pod (seeds only, crushed)
¼ tsp vanilla extract

A milky drink before bed is very calming, and this latte contains saffron, which is said to help focus, mood-balancing and managing stress. Cardamom is very settling on the tummy. Think of this latte as the ultimate hug in a mug when you are overwhelmed by life!

Pour the milk into a small saucepan and heat gently. Stir in the other ingredients and use a mini whisk to make it nice and frothy. Pour into a mug and drink warm. You can strain out the saffron strand and the cardamom seeds if you are particular about texture, but ideally you would consume them to maximize their therapeutic effects.

Store any leftovers in the refrigerator for up to 48 hours and reheat once. Alternatively, once cooled, you could freeze the latte into creamy ice lollies for anyone who does not like hot drinks.

dairy-free
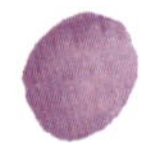
gluten-free

nut-free
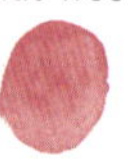
sesame-free

egg-free
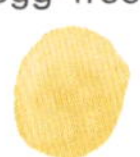
soy-free

vegetarian

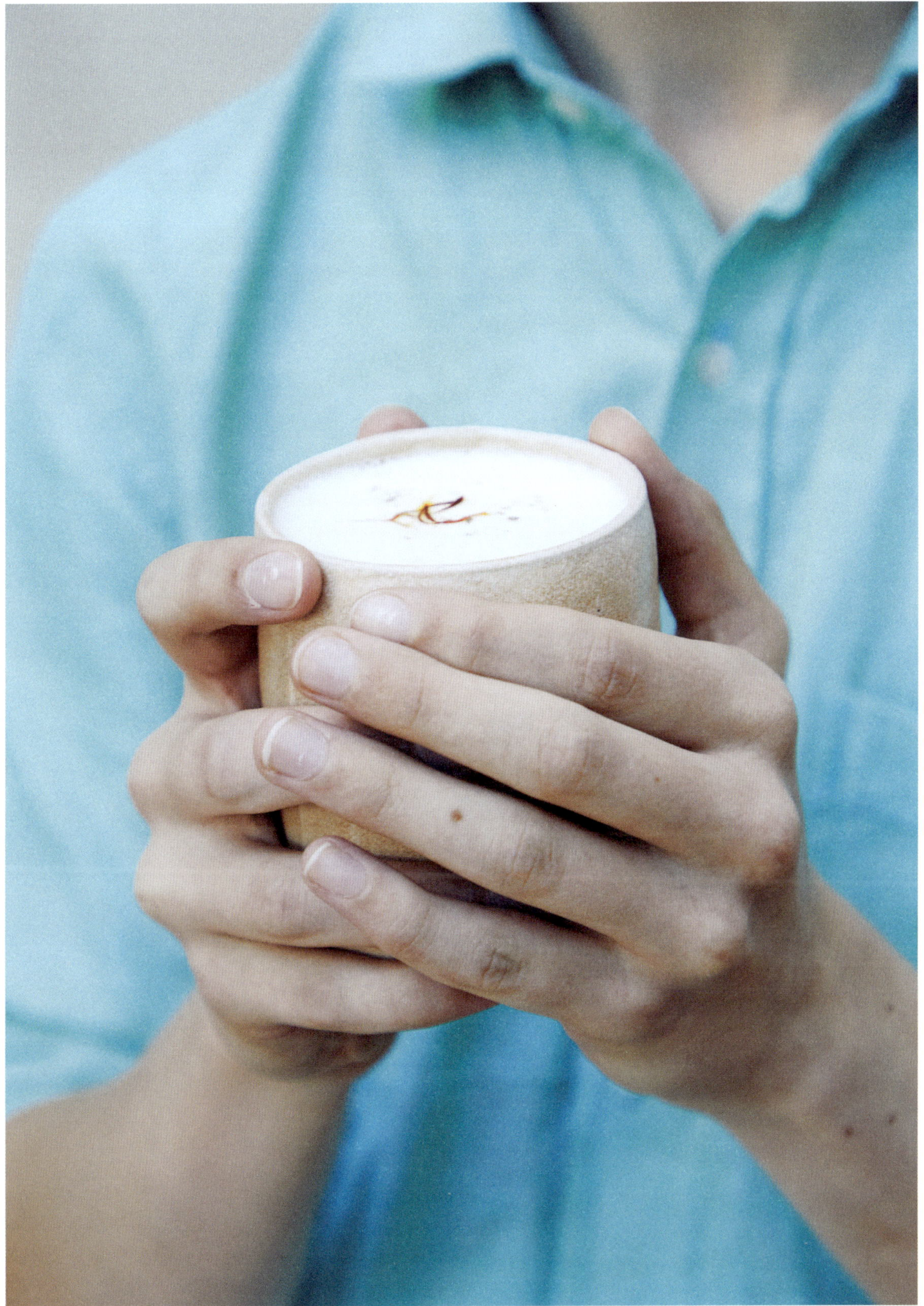

CHAMOMILE & CHERRY SLEEPY SMOOTHIE

Makes 1 drink

1 chamomile tea bag
240ml (1 cup) boiling water
2 Tbsp coconut milk or cream
2 Tbsp rolled oats
1 tsp almond butter
50g (¼ cup) pitted cherries (fresh or frozen)
1 fresh or frozen nectarine, stoned

A combination of delicious ingredients that help the body and brain to wind down in the evening, making it easier to get to sleep. Cherries are a natural source of melatonin, the sleepy hormone, and chamomile, oats and almonds contain the amino acid GABA, which helps us feel mellow and relaxed after a stressful day. Nectarine naturally sweetens this smoothie; peaches, apricots, a few raspberries, or chunks of mango, pineapple or banana would also work.

You can make a big batch of strong chamomile tea and store it in the refrigerator or freeze it in ice cube trays to speed up the process in the evening. You would need 4–5 ice cubes per serving.

Steep the chamomile tea bag in the boiling water for at least 15 minutes before removing the bag. Leave the tea to cool – add a couple of ice cubes if you want to cool it faster. The cooled brewed tea stores in the refrigerator for up to 3 days.

Blend all the ingredients in a high-speed blender for at least 1 minute until smooth and creamy.

The smoothie can be kept in the refrigerator for up to 12 hours, and you can freeze any leftovers into ice lollies for up to 6 months.

Choose gluten-free oats, quinoa flakes or millet flakes.

Swap the almond butter for tahini (sesame paste) or 1 teaspoon of sunflower seeds.

dairy-free
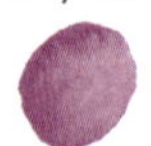

gluten-free

nut-free
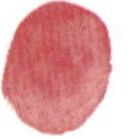

sesame-free
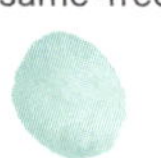

egg-free
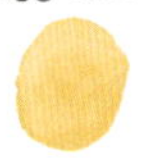

soy-free
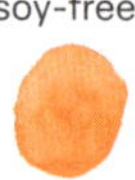

vegetarian
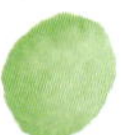

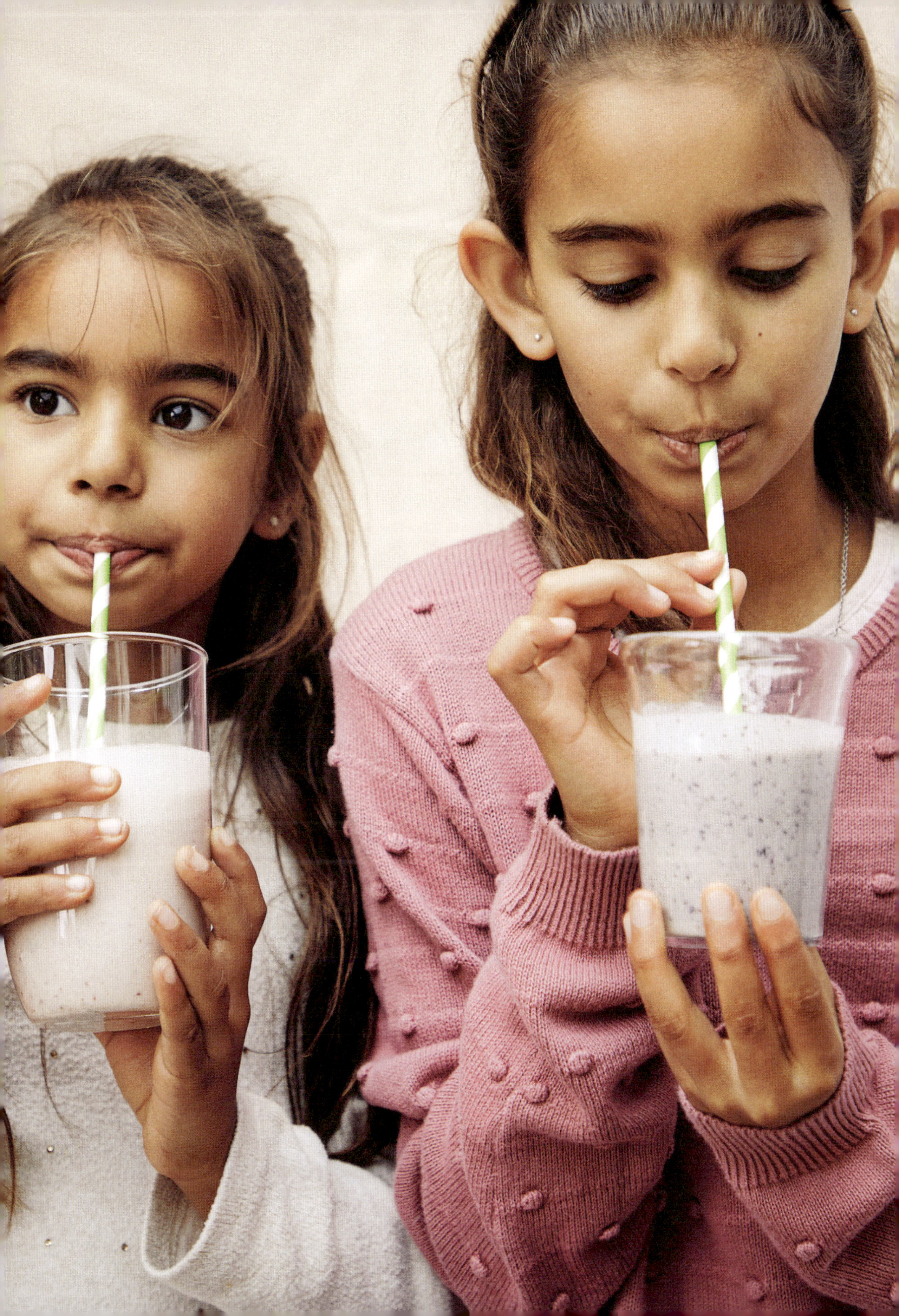

FOOTNOTES

1 Publication of 'The Prevalence of Autism (including Asperger's Syndrome) in School Age Children in Northern Ireland. Annual report 2023 https://www.health-ni.gov.uk/news/publication-prevalence-Autism-including-aspergers-syndrome-school-age-children-northern-ireland-1

2 New shocking data highlights the Autism employment gap https://www.Autism.org.uk/what-we-do/news/new-data-on-the-Autism-employment-gap

3 Outcomes for disabled people in the UK: 2020 https://www.ons.gov.uk/peoplepopulationandcommunity/healthandsocialcare/disability/articles/outcomesfordisabledpeopleintheuk/2020

4 The Role of Epigenetic Change in Autism Spectrum Disorders https://www.ncbi.nlm.nih.gov/pmc/articles/PMC4443738/

5 Epigenetic Findings in Autism: New Perspectives for Therapy https://www.ncbi.nlm.nih.gov/pmc/articles/PMC3799534/

6 From Genes to Environment: Using integrative genomics to build a 'systems level' understanding of Autism spectrum disorders https://www.ncbi.nlm.nih.gov/pmc/articles/PMC3402607/

7 Risk and Protective Environmental Factors Associated with Autism Spectrum Disorder: Evidence-Based Principles and Recommendations https://www.ncbi.nlm.nih.gov/pmc/articles/PMC6406684/

8 The contribution of environmental exposure to the etiology of Autism spectrum disorder https://www.ncbi.nlm.nih.gov/pmc/articles/PMC6420889/

9 Higher rates of Autism and attention deficit/hyperactivity disorder in American children: Are food quality issues impacting epigenetic inheritance? https://www.wjgnet.com/2219-2808/full/v12/i2/25.htm

10 Learning one's genetic risk changes physiology independent of actual genetic risk https://www.ncbi.nlm.nih.gov/pmc/articles/PMC6874306/

11 Water, drinks and hydration – NHS https://www.nhs.uk/live-well/eat-well/food-guidelines-and-food-labels/water-drinks-nutrition/

12 The Oxford-Durham study: a randomized, controlled trial of dietary supplementation with fatty acids in children with developmental coordination disorder https://pubmed.ncbi.nlm.nih.gov/15867048/

13 Omega-3 supplementation improves cognition and modifies brain activation in young adults https://pubmed.ncbi.nlm.nih.gov/24470182/

14 Docosahexaenoic acid for reading, cognition and behavior in children aged 7-9 years: a randomized, controlled trial (the DOLAB Study) https://pubmed.ncbi.nlm.nih.gov/22970149/

15 Reduced Symptoms of Inattention after Dietary Omega-3 Fatty Acid Supplementation in Boys with and without Attention Deficit/Hyperactivity Disorder https://www.ncbi.nlm.nih.gov/pmc/articles/PMC4538345/

16 The Importance of Marine Omega-3s for Brain Development and the Prevention and Treatment of Behavior, Mood, and Other Brain Disorders https://www.ncbi.nlm.nih.gov/pmc/articles/PMC7468918/

17 The Relationship of Docosahexaenoic Acid (DHA) with Learning and Behavior in Healthy Children: A Review https://www.ncbi.nlm.nih.gov/pmc/articles/PMC3738999/

18 Docosahexaenoic acid (DHA) in fetal development and in infant nutrition https://pubmed.ncbi.nlm.nih.gov/11775350/

19 Docosahexaenoic Acid and Cognition throughout the Lifespan https://www.ncbi.nlm.nih.gov/pmc/articles/PMC4772061/

20 Comparative omega-3 fatty acid enrichment of egg yolks from first-cycle laying hens fed flaxseed oil or ground flaxseed https://pubmed.ncbi.nlm.nih.gov/28108729/

21 New study finds clear differences between organic and non-organic milk and meat https://www.sciencedaily.com/releases/2016/02/160215210707.htm

22 Are all n-3 polyunsaturated fatty acids created equal? https://lipidworld.biomedcentral.com/articles/10.1186/1476-511X-8-33

23 Achieving optimal essential fatty acid status in vegetarians: current knowledge and practical implications https://pubmed.ncbi.nlm.nih.gov/12936959/

24 Microalgae as sources of omega-3 polyunsaturated fatty acids: Biotechnological aspects https://www.sciencedirect.com/science/article/abs/pii/S2211926421002290

25 Physical fatty acid deficiency signs in children with ADHD symptoms https://pubmed.ncbi.nlm.nih.gov/17825546/

26 Omega-3 Fatty Acid and Skin Diseases https://www.ncbi.nlm.nih.gov/pmc/articles/PMC7892455/

27 Phrynoderma: a manifestation of vitamin A deficiency?... The rest of the story https://pubmed.ncbi.nlm.nih.gov/15660900

28 Celiac Disease and Dermatologic Manifestations: Many Skin Clue to Unfold Gluten-Sensitive Enteropathy https://www.ncbi.nlm.nih.gov/pmc/articles/PMC3369470/

29 Vitamin A deficiency phrynoderma: Due to malabsorption and inadequate diet https://www.jaad.org/article/S0190-9622(99)70375-0/fulltext

30 Dietary intake and plasma levels of choline and betaine in children with Autism spectrum disorders https://pubmed.ncbi.nlm.nih.gov/24396597/

31 Choline and Working Memory Training Improve Cognitive Deficits Caused by Prenatal Exposure to Ethanol https://pubmed.ncbi.nlm.nih.gov/28961168/

32 Preventing childhood and lifelong disability: Maternal dietary supplementation for perinatal brain injury https://pubmed.ncbi.nlm.nih.gov/30227261/

33 Choline, Neurological Development and Brain Function: A Systematic Review Focusing on the First 1000 Days https://pubmed.ncbi.nlm.nih.gov/32531929/

34 The Role of Choline in Neurodevelopmental Disorders—A Narrative Review Focusing on ASC, ADHD and Dyslexia https://www.ncbi.nlm.nih.gov/pmc/articles/PMC10343507/

35 Neurochemistry Predicts Convergence of Written and Spoken Language: A Proton Magnetic Resonance Spectroscopy Study of Cross-Modal Language Integration https://pubmed.ncbi.nlm.nih.gov/30233445/

36 Association between Maternal Choline, Fetal Brain Development, and Child Neurocognition: Systematic Review and Meta-Analysis of Human Studies https://www.ncbi.nlm.nih.gov/pmc/articles/PMC9776654/

37 Increase of cytosolic phospholipase A2 as hydrolytic enzyme of phospholipids and Autism cognitive, social and sensory dysfunction severity https://lipidworld.biomedcentral.com/articles/10.1186/s12944-016-0391-4

38 Association between psychiatric disorders and iron deficiency anemia among children and adolescents: a nationwide population-based study https://www.ncbi.nlm.nih.gov/pmc/articles/PMC3680022/

39 Iron and Mechanisms of Emotional Behavior https://www.ncbi.nlm.nih.gov/pmc/articles/PMC4253901/

40 Frequency of anemia in chronic psychiatry patients https://www.ncbi.nlm.nih.gov/pmc/articles/PMC4622486/

41 Iron deficiency as strong predictor of attention deficit hyperactivity disorder in children https://pubmed.ncbi.nlm.nih.gov/25364604/

42 Peripheral iron levels in children with attention-deficit hyperactivity disorder: a systematic review and meta-analysis https://pubmed.ncbi.nlm.nih.gov/29335588/

43 Zinc in the central nervous system: From molecules to behavior https://www.ncbi.nlm.nih.gov/pmc/articles/PMC3757551/

44 Zinc deficiency and child development https://www.sciencedirect.com/science/article/pii/S0002916523006263

45 Developmental Dyslexia and zinc deficiency

https://www.thelancet.com/journals/lancet/article/PIIS0140-6736(04)16671-3/fulltext
46 Zinc status in attention-deficit/hyperactivity disorder: a systematic review and meta-analysis of observational studies https://www.ncbi.nlm.nih.gov/pmc/articles/PMC8285486/
47 Zinc Status and Autism Spectrum Disorder in Children and Adolescents: A Systematic Review https://www.mdpi.com/2072-6643/15/16/3663
48 Effectiveness of Methylphenidate Supplemented by Zinc, Calcium, and Magnesium for Treatment of ADHD Patients in the City of Zahedan https://brieflands.com/articles/semj-20468.html
49 Infantile zinc deficiency: Association with Autism spectrum disorders https://www.ncbi.nlm.nih.gov/pmc/articles/PMC3216610/
50 Assessment of Infantile Mineral Imbalances in Autism Spectrum Disorders (ASDs) https://www.ncbi.nlm.nih.gov/pmc/articles/PMC3863885/
51 Dynamical features in fetal and postnatal zinc-copper metabolic cycles predict the emergence of Autism spectrum disorder https://pubmed.ncbi.nlm.nih.gov/29854952/
52 Fetal and postnatal metal dysregulation in Autism https://www.nature.com/articles/ncomms15493.pdf
53 Role of zinc in the development and treatment of mood disorders https://pubmed.ncbi.nlm.nih.gov/10801965/
54 Zinc deficiency and eating disorders https://pubmed.ncbi.nlm.nih.gov/2600063/
55 Neurobiology of zinc-influenced eating behavior https://pubmed.ncbi.nlm.nih.gov/10801965/
56 Zinc supplementation in the treatment of anorexia nervosa https://pubmed.ncbi.nlm.nih.gov/11930982/
57 Leukonychia https://www.sciencedirect.com/topics/medicine-and-dentistry/leukonychia
58 Prevalence and Recurrence of Pica Behaviors in Early Childhood: Findings from the ALSPAC Birth Cohort https://www.ncbi.nlm.nih.gov/pmc/articles/PMC10275014/
59 A meta-analysis of pica and micronutrient status https://www.ncbi.nlm.nih.gov/pmc/articles/PMC4270917/
60 Relation between anemia and blood levels of lead, copper, zinc and iron among children https://www.ncbi.nlm.nih.gov/pmc/articles/PMC2887903/
61 Lead Poisoning https://www.ncbi.nlm.nih.gov/pmc/articles/PMC5528905/
62 Magnesium, hyperactivity and Autism in children https://www.ncbi.nlm.nih.gov/books/NBK507249/
63 The Therapeutic Effects of Magnesium in Insulin Secretion and Insulin Resistance https://www.ncbi.nlm.nih.gov/pmc/articles/PMC9379913/
64 Magnesium supplementation in children with attention deficit hyperactivity disorder https://www.sciencedirect.com/science/article/pii/S1110863015000555
65 Effect of Vitamin D and Magnesium Supplementation on Behavior Problems in Children with Attention-Deficit Hyperactivity Disorder https://www.ncbi.nlm.nih.gov/pmc/articles/PMC7011463/
66 The Efficacy of Magnesium Supplementation in Children With Attention Deficit Hyperactivity Disorder under Treatment With Methylphenidate: A Randomized Controlled Trial https://www.cjmb.org/uploads/pdf/pdf_CJMB_480.pdf
67 Myth or Reality—Transdermal Magnesium? https://www.ncbi.nlm.nih.gov/pmc/articles/PMC5579607/
68 Effect of Vitamin D and Magnesium Supplementation on Behavior Problems in Children with Attention-Deficit Hyperactivity Disorder https://www.ncbi.nlm.nih.gov/pmc/articles/PMC7011463/
69 The Role of Vitamin D in Brain Health: A Mini Literature Review https://www.ncbi.nlm.nih.gov/pmc/articles/PMC6132681/
70 Is there a role for vitamin D in the treatment of chronic pain? https://www.ncbi.nlm.nih.gov/pmc/articles/PMC5466150/
71 Molecular Basis Underlying the Therapeutic Potential of Vitamin D for the Treatment of Depression and Anxiety https://www.ncbi.nlm.nih.gov/pmc/articles/PMC9266859/
72 Gut instincts: vitamin D/vitamin D receptor and microbiome in neurodevelopment disorders https://www.ncbi.nlm.nih.gov/pmc/articles/PMC7574554/
73 Vitamin D status in children with attention-deficit-hyperactivity disorder https://pubmed.ncbi.nlm.nih.gov/24417979/
74 Effect of vitamin D supplementation as adjunctive therapy to methylphenidate on ADHD symptoms: A randomized, double blind, placebo-controlled trial https://pubmed.ncbi.nlm.nih.gov/27924679/
75 Serum levels of 25-hydroxyvitamin D in children with Autism spectrum disorders https://pubmed.ncbi.nlm.nih.gov/25616297/
76 The Association between Vitamin D Status and Autism Spectrum Disorder (ASD): A Systematic Review and Meta-Analysis https://www.ncbi.nlm.nih.gov/pmc/articles/PMC7824115/
77 Vitamin D and Autism, what's new? https://pubmed.ncbi.nlm.nih.gov/28217829/
78 The mTOR Signaling Pathway Activity and Vitamin D Availability Control the Expression of Most Autism Predisposition Genes https://pubmed.ncbi.nlm.nih.gov/31847491/
79 Nutritional Rickets Due to Severe Food Selectivity in Autism Spectrum Disorder https://pubmed.ncbi.nlm.nih.gov/32890122/
80 Vitamin D Levels in Sows from Five Danish Outdoor Herds https://www.ncbi.nlm.nih.gov/pmc/articles/PMC8833377/
81 Environmental and genetic factors influence the vitamin D content of cows' milk https://www.cambridge.org/core/journals/proceedings-of-the-nutrition-society/article/environmental-and-genetic-factors-influence-the-vitamin-d-content-of-cows-milk/8754AB72F72B6E5AA8C4502C3B77ADAD
82 Benefits of Sunlight: A Bright Spot for Human Health https://www.ncbi.nlm.nih.gov/pmc/articles/PMC2290997/
83 Neurological, Psychiatric, and Biochemical Aspects of Thiamine Deficiency in Children and Adults https://www.ncbi.nlm.nih.gov/pmc/articles/PMC6459027/
84 Profiling plasma levels of thiamine and histamine in Jordanian children with Autism spectrum disorder (ASD): potential biomarkers for evaluation of ASD therapies and diet https://pubmed.ncbi.nlm.nih.gov/35900205/
85 A Review of the Biochemistry, Metabolism and Clinical Benefits of Thiamin(e) and Its Derivatives https://www.ncbi.nlm.nih.gov/pmc/articles/PMC1375232/
86 Dietary Vitamin B1 Intake Influences Gut Microbial Community and the Consequent Production of Short-Chain Fatty Acids https://www.ncbi.nlm.nih.gov/pmc/articles/PMC9147846/
87 Hiding in Plain Sight: Modern Thiamine Deficiency https://www.ncbi.nlm.nih.gov/pmc/articles/PMC8533683/
88 Critical vitamin deficiencies in Autism spectrum disorder: Reversible and irreversible outcomes https://pubmed.ncbi.nlm.nih.gov/35689090/
89 Riboflavin – Science Direct https://www.sciencedirect.com/topics/biochemistry-genetics-and-molecular-biology/riboflavin
90 Riboflavin – Linus Pauling https://lpi.oregonstate.edu/mic/vitamins/riboflavin
91 Niacin – Linus Pauling https://lpi.oregonstate.edu/mic/vitamins/niacin
92 The chemistry of the vitamin B3 metabolome https://www.ncbi.nlm.nih.gov/pmc/articles/PMC6411094/
93 Why is vitamin B6 effective in alleviating the symptoms of Autism? https://pubmed.ncbi.nlm.nih.gov/29685187/
94 Vitamin B6 Deficiency Induces Autism-Like Behaviors in Rats by Regulating mTOR-Mediated Autophagy in the Hippocampus https://pubmed.ncbi.nlm.nih.gov/37200987/
95 Combined vitamin B6□magnesium treatment in Autism spectrum disorder https://www.ncbi.nlm.nih.gov/pmc/articles/PMC7003675/
96 Improvement of neurobehavioral disorders in children supplemented with magnesium-vitamin B6. II. Pervasive developmental disorder-Autism https://pubmed.ncbi.nlm.nih.gov/16846101/
97 Effects of Vitamin B6 (Pyridoxine) and a B Complex Preparation on Dreaming and Sleep https://journals.sagepub.com/doi/10.1177/0031512518770326
98 Vitamin B6 – NIH https://ods.od.nih.gov/factsheets/VitaminB6-HealthProfessional/
99 Folic Acid and Autism: A Systematic Review of the Current State of Knowledge
100 Homocysteine and MTHFR Mutations https://www.ahajournals.org/doi/10.1161/circulationaha.114.013311
101 Role of Vitamin B12 in Autistic Spectrum and Attention Deficit Hyperactivity Disorders: A Scoping Review https://www.opensciencepublications.com/fulltextarticles/IJN-2395-2326-8-240.html
102 Comparison of serum B12, folate and homocysteine concentrations in children with Autism spectrum disorder or attention deficit hyperactivity disorder and healthy controls https://www.ncbi.nlm.nih.gov/pmc/articles/PMC6689552/
103 The Effectiveness of Cobalamin (B12) Treatment for Autism Spectrum Disorder: A Systematic Review and Meta-Analysis https://www.ncbi.nlm.nih.gov/pmc/articles/PMC8400809/
104 Obsessive Compulsive Disorder as Early

Manifestation of B12 Deficiency https://www.ncbi.nlm.nih.gov/pmc/articles/PMC3271502/
105 The Effectiveness of Cobalamin (B12) Treatment for Autism Spectrum Disorder: A Systematic Review and Meta-Analysis https://www.ncbi.nlm.nih.gov/pmc/articles/PMC8400809/
106 Effects of Saffron Extract Supplementation on Mood, Well-Being, and Response to a Psychosocial Stressor in Healthy Adults: A Randomized, Double-Blind, Parallel Group, Clinical Trial https://www.ncbi.nlm.nih.gov/pmc/articles/PMC7882499/
107 Saffron (Crocus sativus L.) and major depressive disorder: a meta-analysis of randomized clinical trials https://www.ncbi.nlm.nih.gov/pmc/articles/PMC4643654/
108 Crocus Sativus for Insomnia: A Systematic Review and Meta-Analysis https://pubmed.ncbi.nlm.nih.gov/36141931/
109 Efficacy and safety of saffron as adjunctive therapy in adults with attention-deficit/hyperactivity disorder: A randomized, double-blind, placebo-controlled clinical trial https://www.sciencedirect.com/science/article/abs/pii/S2212958822000027
110 Effectivity of Saffron Extract (Saffr'Activ) on Treatment for Children and Adolescents with Attention Deficit/Hyperactivity Disorder (ADHD): A Clinical Effectivity Study https://www.ncbi.nlm.nih.gov/pmc/articles/PMC9573091/
111 Effects of Saffron Extract on Sleep Quality: A Randomized Double-Blind Controlled Clinical Trial https://www.ncbi.nlm.nih.gov/pmc/articles/PMC8145009/
112 Effects of saffron on sleep quality in healthy adults with self-reported poor sleep: a randomized, double-blind, placebo-controlled trial https://jcsm.aasm.org/doi/10.5664/jcsm.8376
113 Saffron for mood improvement in children and adolescents: a narrative review doi: 10.7363/110222
114 Comparison of the Effects of Crocus Sativus and Mefenamic Acid on Primary Dysmenorrhea https://jpc.tums.ac.ir/index.php/jpc/article/view/170
115 A Whiff of Saffron Changes Hormone Levels in Women https://www.naturalmedicinejournal.com/journal/whiff-saffron-changes-hormone-levels-women
116 The effect of Crocus sativus (saffron) on the severity of premenstrual syndrome https://www.sciencedirect.com/science/article/abs/pii/S187638201530010X
117 Saffron for the Management of Premenstrual Dysphoric Disorder: A Randomized Controlled Trial https://www.ncbi.nlm.nih.gov/pmc/articles/PMC7792881/
118 Theanine https://www.sciencedirect.com/topics/pharmacology-toxicology-and-pharmaceutical-science/theanine
119 The effects of L-theanine (Suntheanine®) on objective sleep quality in boys with attention deficit hyperactivity disorder (ADHD): a randomized, double-blind, placebo-controlled clinical trial https://pubmed.ncbi.nlm.nih.gov/22214254/
120 The science of tea's mood-altering magic doi: 10.1038/d41586-019-00398-1 https://www.researchgate.net/publication/330916774_The_science_of_tea's_mood-altering_magic
121 Green tea effects on cognition, mood and human brain function: A systematic review https://pubmed.ncbi.nlm.nih.gov/28899506/
122 The Cognitive-Enhancing Outcomes of Caffeine and L-theanine: A Systematic Review https://pubmed.ncbi.nlm.nih.gov/35111479/
123 Hericium erinaceus, an amazing medicinal mushroom https://www.researchgate.net/profile/Sylvie-Rapior/publication/281146648_Hericium_erinaceus_an_amazing_medicinal_mushroom/links/57d0180508ae5f03b4890299/Hericium-erinaceus-an-amazing-medicinal-mushroom.pdf
124 The Anti-Inflammatory Effects of Lion's Mane Culinary-Medicinal Mushroom, Hericium erinaceus (Higher Basidiomycetes) in a Coculture System of 3T3-L1 Adipocytes and RAW264 Macrophages https://pubmed.ncbi.nlm.nih.gov/26559695/
125 Hericerin derivatives activates a pan-neurotrophic pathway in central hippocampal neurons converging to ERK1/2 signaling enhancing spatial memory https://onlinelibrary.wiley.com/doi/10.1111/jnc.15767
126 Hericium erinaceus in Neurodegenerative Diseases: From Bench to Bedside and Beyond, How Far from the Shoreline? https://www.ncbi.nlm.nih.gov/pmc/articles/PMC10218917/
127 Neurohealth Properties of Hericium erinaceus Mycelia Enriched with Erinacines https://www.ncbi.nlm.nih.gov/pmc/articles/PMC5987239/
128 Bacopa monnieri https://www.ncbi.nlm.nih.gov/books/NBK589635/
129 Efficacy of Standardized Extract of Bacopa monnieri (Bacognize®) on Cognitive Functions of Medical Students: A Six-Week, Randomized Placebo-Controlled Trial https://www.ncbi.nlm.nih.gov/pmc/articles/PMC5075615/
130 An acute, double-blind, placebo-controlled cross-over study of 320 mg and 640 mg doses of Bacopa monnieri (CDRI 08) on multitasking stress reactivity and mood https://pubmed.ncbi.nlm.nih.gov/23788517/
131 Systematic Overview of Bacopa monnieri (L.) Wettst. Dominant Poly-Herbal Formulas in Children and Adolescents https://www.ncbi.nlm.nih.gov/pmc/articles/PMC5750610/
132 The sedative activity of flavonoids from Passiflora quadrangularis is mediated through the GABAergic pathway https://pubmed.ncbi.nlm.nih.gov/29454287/
133 Passiflora incarnata in Neuropsychiatric Disorders—A Systematic Review https://www.ncbi.nlm.nih.gov/pmc/articles/PMC7766837/
134 Passiflora incarnata in the treatment of attention-deficit hyperactivity disorder in children and adolescents https://www.openaccessjournals.com/articles/passiflora-incarnata-in-the-treatment-of-attentiondeficit-hyperactivity-disorder-in-children-and-adolescents.pdf
135 Role Identification of Passiflora Incarnata Linnaeus: A Mini Review https://www.ncbi.nlm.nih.gov/pmc/articles/PMC5770524/
136 Passionflower Extract Induces High-amplitude Rhythms without Phase Shifts in the Expression of Several Circadian Clock Genes in Vitro and in Vivo
137 Pilot trial of Melissa officinalis L. leaf extract in the treatment of volunteers suffering from mild-to-moderate anxiety disorders and sleep disturbances https://www.ncbi.nlm.nih.gov/pmc/articles/PMC3230760/
138 Herbal Remedies and Their Possible Effect on the GABAergic System and Sleep https://www.ncbi.nlm.nih.gov/pmc/articles/PMC7914492/
139 Hyperactivity, concentration difficulties and impulsiveness improve during seven weeks' treatment with valerian root and lemon balm extracts in primary school children https://pubmed.ncbi.nlm.nih.gov/24837472/
140 Valerian Root and Lemon Balm Extracts A Phytomedicine Compound Improves Symptoms of Hyperactivity, Attention Deficits, and Impulsivity in Children https://journals.lww.com/hnpjournal/citation/2015/11000/valerian_root_and_lemon_balm_extracts__a.9.aspx
141 A combination of valerian and lemon balm is effective in the treatment of restlessness and dyssomnia in children. https://europepmc.org/article/med/16487692
142 Dietary Neurotransmitters: A Narrative Review on Current Knowledge https://www.ncbi.nlm.nih.gov/pmc/articles/PMC5986471/
143 Glutamate: The Master Neurotransmitter and its Implications in Chronic Stress and Mood Disorders https://www.ncbi.nlm.nih.gov/pmc/articles/PMC8586693/
144 Autism Spectrum Disorder: Focus on Glutamatergic Neurotransmission https://www.ncbi.nlm.nih.gov/pmc/articles/PMC8998955/
145 GABA and glutamate in children with Tourette syndrome: A 1H MR spectroscopy study at 7 T https://www.ncbi.nlm.nih.gov/pmc/articles/PMC5815927/
146 Glutamatergic modulatory therapy for Tourette syndrome https://pubmed.ncbi.nlm.nih.gov/20022434/
147 Cortical glutamate and GABA are related to compulsive behaviour in individuals with obsessive compulsive disorder and healthy controls https://www.nature.com/articles/s41467-023-38695-z
148 Prefrontal cortex glutamate and extraversion https://academic.oup.com/scan/article/7/7/811/1675529
149 □-Aminobutyric Acid (GABA) Content of Selected Uncooked Foods https://www.researchgate.net/publication/264106529_g_-Aminobutyric_Acid_GABA_Content_of_Selected_Uncooked_Foods
150 The Gut Microbiome and the Brain https://www.ncbi.nlm.nih.gov/pmc/articles/PMC4259177/
151 Probiotic Properties, Prebiotic Fermentability, and GABA-Producing Capacity of Microorganisms Isolated from Mexican Milk Kefir Grains: A Clustering Evaluation for Functional Dairy Food Applications https://www.ncbi.nlm.nih.gov/pmc/articles/PMC8534820/
152 Natural products as safeguards against monosodium glutamate-induced toxicity https://www.ncbi.nlm.nih.gov/pmc/articles/PMC7239414/
153 Influence of Tryptophan and Serotonin on Mood and Cognition with a Possible Role of the

Gut-Brain Axis https://www.ncbi.nlm.nih.gov/pmc/articles/PMC4728667/

154 The serotonin system in Autism spectrum disorder: from biomarker to animal models https://www.ncbi.nlm.nih.gov/pmc/articles/PMC4824539/

155 Clinical Test of Pyrroles: Usefulness and Association with Other Biochemical Markers https://clinmedjournals.org/articles/cmrcr/cmrcr-2-027.pdf

156 Clinical significance and importance of elevated urinary kryptopyrroles (UKP): Self-reported observations and experience of Australian clinicians using UKP testing https://www.sciencedirect.com/science/article/abs/pii/S2212958821000252

157 Reduced violent behavior following biochemical therapy https://pubmed.ncbi.nlm.nih.gov/15451647/

158 Role of cholesterol and sphingolipids in brain development and neurological diseases https://pubmed.ncbi.nlm.nih.gov/30683111/

159 Central nervous system: cholesterol turnover, brain development and neurodegeneration https://pubmed.ncbi.nlm.nih.gov/19166320/

160 Autism: the role of cholesterol in treatment https://pubmed.ncbi.nlm.nih.gov/18386207/

161 Lowered serum cholesterol, famine and aggression: a Darwinian hypothesis https://journals.sagepub.com/doi/10.1177/053901897036002001

162 Low HDL cholesterol associates with major depression in a sample with a 7-year history of depressive symptoms https://pubmed.ncbi.nlm.nih.gov/18583011/

163 Behavior phenotype in the RSH/Smith-Lemli-Opitz syndrome https://pubmed.ncbi.nlm.nih.gov/11223857/

164 Cognitive and behavioral aspects of Smith-Lemli-Opitz syndrome https://pubmed.ncbi.nlm.nih.gov/23042585/

165 Treatment of Smith-Lemli-Opitz Syndrome and Other Sterol Disorders https://www.ncbi.nlm.nih.gov/pmc/articles/PMC3890258/

166 A new classification of foods based on the extent and purpose of their processing https://pubmed.ncbi.nlm.nih.gov/21180977/

167 Ultra-processed foods: what they are and how to identify them https://pubmed.ncbi.nlm.nih.gov/30744710/

168 Increased ultra-processed food consumption is associated with worsening of cardiometabolic risk factors in adults with metabolic syndrome: Longitudinal analysis from a randomized trial https://pubmed.ncbi.nlm.nih.gov/37343432/

169 Association of ultra-processed food consumption with incident depression and anxiety: a population-based cohort study https://pubmed.ncbi.nlm.nih.gov/37534433/

170 Processed foods and diet quality in pregnancy may affect child neurodevelopment disorders: a narrative review https://pubmed.ncbi.nlm.nih.gov/37039128/

171 Dietary patterns, brain morphology and cognitive performance in children: Results from a prospective population-based study https://pubmed.ncbi.nlm.nih.gov/37155025/

172 Binge-Eating Precursors in Children and Adolescents: Neurodevelopment, and the Potential Contribution of Ultra-Processed Foods https://pubmed.ncbi.nlm.nih.gov/37447320/

173 Ultra-processed foods (UPF) in the diets of infants and young children in the UK First Steps Nutrition Trust https://www.firststepsnutrition.org/upfs-marketed-for-infants-and-young-children

174 Trends in Consumption of Ultraprocessed Foods Among US Youths Aged 2-19 Years, 1999-2018 https://jamanetwork.com/journals/jama/fullarticle/2782866

175 Ultra-Processed Foods and Nutritional Dietary Profile: A Meta-Analysis of Nationally Representative Samples https://pubmed.ncbi.nlm.nih.gov/34684391/

176 Ultra-Processed Food Consumption and Incidence of Obesity and Cardiometabolic Risk Factors in Adults: A Systematic Review of Prospective Studies https://pubmed.ncbi.nlm.nih.gov/37299546/

177 Effect of the food processing degree on cardiometabolic health outcomes: A prospective approach in childhood https://pubmed.ncbi.nlm.nih.gov/36081298/

178 Ultra-Processed Food Addiction: An Epidemic? https://karger.com/pps/article/91/6/363/826582/Ultra-Processed-Food-Addiction-An-Epidemic

179 Ultraprocessed Food: Addictive, Toxic, and Ready for Regulation https://www.ncbi.nlm.nih.gov/pmc/articles/PMC7694501/

180 The impact of junk foods on the adolescent brain https://pubmed.ncbi.nlm.nih.gov/29251841/

181 Processed food diet in early childhood may lower subsequent IQ https://www.sciencedaily.com/releases/2011/02/110207225943.htm

182 Is there an association between dietary intake and academic achievement: a systematic review https://pubmed.ncbi.nlm.nih.gov/27599886/

183 Processed foods and effect on developing fetus' brain: Autism link? https://www.sciencedaily.com/releases/2019/06/190620121415.htm

184 The association between maternal ultra-processed food consumption during pregnancy and child neuropsychological development: A population-based birth cohort study https://pubmed.ncbi.nlm.nih.gov/36087519/

185 Association between ultra-processed food consumption and nutrient intake among low-risk pregnant women https://www.scielo.br/j/rbsmi/a/Gf6N3jm6XdtvzyhLkmqRyYR/

186 Diet during pregnancy: Ultra-processed foods and the inflammatory potential of diet https://www.sciencedirect.com/science/article/abs/pii/S0899900722000168

187 Higher rates of Autism and attention deficit/hyperactivity disorder in American children: Are food quality issues impacting epigenetic inheritance? https://www.wjgnet.com/2219-2808/full/v12/i2/25.htm

188 Data & Statistics on Autism Spectrum Disorder https://www.cdc.gov/ncbddd/Autism/data.html

189 Ultraprocessed Food Intake Is Associated With Poor Cardiovascular Fitness in US Children and Adolescents https://www.ncbi.nlm.nih.gov/pmc/articles/PMC9193634/

190 'Junk food' diet and childhood behavioural problems: Results from the ALSPAC cohort https://www.ncbi.nlm.nih.gov/pmc/articles/PMC2664919/

191 Processed meat products and snacks consumption in ADHD: A case–control study https://www.ncbi.nlm.nih.gov/pmc/articles/PMC9464840/

192 Dietary Patterns and Attention Deficit Hyperactivity Disorder Among Iranian Children: A Case-Control Study https://www.tandfonline.com/doi/abs/10.1080/07315724.2018.1473819

193 Sugar consumption, sugar sweetened beverages and Attention Deficit Hyperactivity Disorder: A systematic review and meta-analysis https://www.sciencedirect.com/science/article/abs/pii/S0965229919320540

194 Malnutrition at age 3 years and externalizing behavior problems at ages 8, 11, and 17 years https://pubmed.ncbi.nlm.nih.gov/15514400/

195 Associations between Prenatal and Early Childhood Fish and Processed Food Intake, Conduct Problems, and Co-Occurring Difficulties https://link.springer.com/article/10.1007/s10802-016-0224-y

196 Behavioral Effects of Childhood Malnutrition https://ajp.psychiatryonline.org/doi/full/10.1176/appi.ajp.162.9.1760-b

197 The Association between Ultra-Processed Foods, Quality of Life and Insomnia among Adolescent Girls in Northeastern Iran https://www.ncbi.nlm.nih.gov/pmc/articles/PMC9141842/

198 Association between the Degree of Processing of Consumed Foods and Sleep Quality in Adolescents https://www.ncbi.nlm.nih.gov/pmc/articles/PMC7071336/

199 Intake of ultra-processed foods and sleep-related outcomes: A systematic review and meta-analysis https://pubmed.ncbi.nlm.nih.gov/36470114/

200 Ultra-Processed Food Consumption and Mental Health: A Systematic Review and Meta-Analysis of Observational Studies https://www.ncbi.nlm.nih.gov/pmc/articles/PMC9268228/

201 Ultra-Processed Food Is Positively Associated With Depressive Symptoms Among United States Adults https://www.ncbi.nlm.nih.gov/pmc/articles/PMC7770142/

202 Prospective association between ultra-processed food consumption and incident depressive symptoms in the French NutriNet-Santé cohort https://pubmed.ncbi.nlm.nih.gov/30982472/

203 High ultra-processed food consumption is associated with elevated psychological distress as an indicator of depression in adults from the Melbourne Collaborative Cohort Study https://www.sciencedirect.com/science/article/pii/S0165032723006092?via%3Dihub

204 Mediterranean-DASH Intervention for Neurodegenerative Delay (MIND) study: Rationale, design and baseline characteristics of a randomized control trial of the MIND diet on cognitive decline https://pubmed.ncbi.nlm.nih.gov/33434704/

205 High ultra-processed food consumption is associated with elevated psychological distress as an indicator of depression in adults from the Melbourne Collaborative Cohort Study https://

www.sciencedirect.com/science/article/pii/S0165032723006092?via%3Dihub
206 Mind-altering microorganisms: the impact of the gut microbiota on brain and behaviour https://www.nature.com/articles/nrn3346
207 The gut microbiome and the brain https://pubmed.ncbi.nlm.nih.gov/25402818/
208 Emerging Developments in Microbiome and Microglia Research: Implications for Neurodevelopmental Disorders https://www.ncbi.nlm.nih.gov/pmc/articles/PMC6129765/
209 Current Evidence on the Role of the Gut Microbiome in ADHD Pathophysiology and Therapeutic Implications https://www.ncbi.nlm.nih.gov/pmc/articles/PMC7830868/
210 Microbiota and Microglia Interactions in ASD https://pubmed.ncbi.nlm.nih.gov/34113350/
211 Gut Microbiome–Brain Alliance: A Landscape View into Mental and Gastrointestinal Health and Disorders https://www.ncbi.nlm.nih.gov/pmc/articles/PMC10197139/
212 Altered gut microbiota profile in patients with generalized anxiety disorder https://pubmed.ncbi.nlm.nih.gov/30029052/
213 The Role of the Gut Microbiota in Dietary Interventions for Depression and Anxiety https://www.ncbi.nlm.nih.gov/pmc/articles/PMC7360462/
214 More than a Gut Feeling: the Microbiota Regulates Neurodevelopment and Behavior https://www.ncbi.nlm.nih.gov/pmc/articles/PMC4262908/
215 The gut microbiome and the brain https://www.liebertpub.com/doi/10.1089/jmf.2014.7000
216 The Gut–Brain Axis: Influence of Microbiota on Mood and Mental Health https://www.ncbi.nlm.nih.gov/pmc/articles/PMC6469458/
217 Microbiome–microglia connections via the gut–brain axis https://www.ncbi.nlm.nih.gov/pmc/articles/PMC6314531/
218 The Vagus Nerve at the Interface of the Microbiota-Gut–Brain Axis https://www.frontiersin.org/articles/10.3389/fnins.2018.00049/full
219 Vagus Nerve as Modulator of the Brain–Gut Axis in Psychiatric and Inflammatory Disorders https://www.frontiersin.org/articles/10.3389/fpsyt.2018.00044/full and https://www.frontiersin.org/files/Articles/298797/fpsyt-09-00044-HTML/image_m/fpsyt-09-00044-g001.jpg
220 Vagus Nerve and Underlying Impact on the Gut Microbiota-Brain Axis in Behavior and Neurodegenerative Diseases https://www.ncbi.nlm.nih.gov/pmc/articles/PMC9656367/
221 The Vagus Nerve at the Interface of the Microbiota-Gut–Brain Axis https://www.ncbi.nlm.nih.gov/pmc/articles/PMC5808284/
222 Gut Microbe to Brain Signaling: What Happens in Vagus… https://www.cell.com/neuron/fulltext/S0896-6273(19)30117-5
223 The Role of Gut Microbiota in Anxiety, Depression, and Other Mental Disorders as Well as the Protective Effects of Dietary Components https://www.mdpi.com/2072-6643/15/14/3258
224 Clostridium Bacteria and Autism Spectrum Conditions: A Systematic Review and Hypothetical Contribution of Environmental Glyphosate Levels https://www.ncbi.nlm.nih.gov/pmc/articles/PMC6024569/
225 Real-time PCR quantitation of clostridia in feces of autistic children https://pubmed.ncbi.nlm.nih.gov/15528506/
226 Detection of Clostridium perfringens toxin genes in the gut microbiota of autistic children https://pubmed.ncbi.nlm.nih.gov/28215985/
227 Gut Bacteria and Neurotransmitters https://www.ncbi.nlm.nih.gov/pmc/articles/PMC9504309/
228 Psychobiotics and the Manipulation of Bacteria–Gut–Brain Signals https://www.sciencedirect.com/science/article/pii/S0166223616301138#bib1075
229 Collective unconscious: How gut microbes shape human behavior https://www.sciencedirect.com/science/article/pii/S0022395615000655
230 Regulation of Neurotransmitters by the Gut Microbiota and Effects on Cognition in Neurological Disorders https://www.ncbi.nlm.nih.gov/pmc/articles/PMC8234057/
231 First Encounters: Effects of the Microbiota on Neonatal Brain Development https://www.frontiersin.org/articles/10.3389/fncel.2021.682505/full
232 Gut microbiota composition is associated with newborn functional brain connectivity and behavioral temperament https://www.sciencedirect.com/science/article/abs/pii/S0889159120323771
233 Association between Gut Microbiota and Infant's Temperament in the First Year of Life in a Chinese Birth Cohort https://www.ncbi.nlm.nih.gov/pmc/articles/PMC7285300/
234 Babies, bugs and brains: How the early microbiome associates with infant brain and behavior development https://www.ncbi.nlm.nih.gov/pmc/articles/PMC10411758/
235 Gut microbiome composition is associated with temperament during early childhood https://www.sciencedirect.com/science/article/abs/pii/S0889159114005157
236 Gut microbiota composition is associated with temperament traits in infants https://www.sciencedirect.com/science/article/pii/S0889159119300777
237 Bifidobacterium Species Colonization in Infancy: A Global Cross-Sectional Comparison by Population History of Breastfeeding https://www.ncbi.nlm.nih.gov/pmc/articles/PMC9003546/
238 Bifidobacterial Dominance of the Gut in Early Life and Acquisition of Antimicrobial Resistance https://pubmed.ncbi.nlm.nih.gov/30258040/
239 Bifidobacteria-mediated immune system imprinting early in life https://www.cell.com/cell/fulltext/S0092-8674(21)00660-7
240 Colonization by B. infantis EVC001 modulates enteric inflammation in exclusively breastfed infants https://pubmed.ncbi.nlm.nih.gov/31443102/
241 The intestinal flora of infants and young children https://onlinelibrary.wiley.com/doi/abs/10.1002/path.1700180154
242 Elevated Fecal pH Indicates a Profound Change in the Breastfed Infant Gut Microbiome Due to Reduction of Bifidobacterium over the Past Century https://journals.asm.org/doi/10.1128/msphere.00041-18
243 Gut microbiome composition and diversity are related to human personality traits https://www.sciencedirect.com/science/article/pii/S2452231719300181
244 Maternal and Early-Life Exposure to Antibiotics and the Risk of Autism and Attention-Deficit Hyperactivity Disorder in Childhood: a Swedish Population-Based Cohort Study https://pubmed.ncbi.nlm.nih.gov/37087706/
245 Meta-analysis of the effects of proton pump inhibitors on the human gut microbiota https://pubmed.ncbi.nlm.nih.gov/37337143/
246 Symbiosis and Dysbiosis of the Human Mycobiome https://www.frontiersin.org/articles/10.3389/fmicb.2021.636131/full
247 Antibiotic-induced gut metabolome and microbiome alterations increase the susceptibility to Candida albicans colonization in the gastrointestinal tract https://academic.oup.com/femsec/article/96/1/fiz187/5643884
248 Immune defence against Candida fungal infections https://www.nature.com/articles/nri3897
249 Immune Sensing of Candida albicans https://www.mdpi.com/2309-608X/7/2/119
250 Microbiota-Gut–Brain Axis: Yeast Species Isolated from Stool Samples of Children with Suspected or Diagnosed Autism Spectrum Disorders and In Vitro Susceptibility Against Nystatin and Fluconazole https://pubmed.ncbi.nlm.nih.gov/26442855/
251 Anti-Candida albicans IgG Antibodies in Children With Autism Spectrum Disorders https://www.frontiersin.org/articles/10.3389/fpsyt.2018.00627/full
252 Intestinal Dysbiosis and Yeast Isolation in Stool of Subjects with Autism Spectrum Disorders https://link.springer.com/article/10.1007/s11046-016-0068-6
253 Gut mycobiome dysbiosis and its impact on intestinal permeability in attention-deficit/hyperactivity disorder https://acamh.onlinelibrary.wiley.com/doi/full/10.1111/jcpp.13779
254 Could yeast infections impair recovery from mental illness? A case study using micronutrients and olive leaf extract for the treatment of ADHD and depression https://pubmed.ncbi.nlm.nih.gov/23784606/
255 Factors in an Auto-Brewery Syndrome group compared to an American Gut Project group: a case-control study https://pubmed.ncbi.nlm.nih.gov/34567530/
256 Auto-Brewery Syndrome: A Clinical Dilemma https://www.ncbi.nlm.nih.gov/pmc/articles/PMC7667719/
257 Drunk Without Drinking: A Case of Auto-Brewery Syndrome https://www.ncbi.nlm.nih.gov/pmc/articles/PMC6831150/
258 Auto□brewery syndrome caused by oral fungi and periodontal disease bacteria https://www.ncbi.nlm.nih.gov/pmc/articles/PMC8091436/
259 The Auto-Brewery Syndrome: A Perfect Metabolic 'Storm' with Clinical and Forensic Implications https://www.ncbi.nlm.nih.gov/pmc/articles/PMC8537665/
260 Role of microglia in fungal infections of the central nervous system https://www.tandfonline.com/doi/full/10.1080/21505594.2016.1261789
261 Traversal of Candida albicans across Human

Blood-Brain Barrier In Vitro https://journals.asm.org/doi/10.1128/iai.69.7.4536-4544.2001
262 Microglia and amyloid precursor protein coordinate control of transient Candida cerebritis with memory deficits https://www.ncbi.nlm.nih.gov/pmc/articles/PMC6320369/
263 New perspectives on the nutritional factors influencing growth rate of Candida albicans in diabetics. An in vitro study https://www.ncbi.nlm.nih.gov/pmc/articles/PMC5572443/
264 Application of Probiotic Yeasts on Candida Species Associated Infection https://www.ncbi.nlm.nih.gov/pmc/articles/PMC7711718/
265 Zinc in Human Health and Infectious Diseases https://www.ncbi.nlm.nih.gov/pmc/articles/PMC9775844/
266 Zinc supplementation reduces Candida infections in pediatric intensive care unit: a randomized placebo-controlled clinical trial https://www.ncbi.nlm.nih.gov/pmc/articles/PMC6436042/
267 The Roles of Biotin in Candida Albicans Physiology https://digitalcommons.unl.edu/cgi/viewcontent.cgi
268 The response of selenium-deficient mice to Candida albicans infection https://pubmed.ncbi.nlm.nih.gov/3701459/
269 Comparative Study of the Antimicrobial Activity of Selenium Nanoparticles With Different Surface Chemistry and Structure https://www.frontiersin.org/articles/10.3389/fbioe.2020.624621/full
270 Antibacterial and Antifungal Activities of Spices https://www.ncbi.nlm.nih.gov/pmc/articles/PMC5486105/
271 Plants' Natural Products as Alternative Promising Anti-Candida Drugs https://www.ncbi.nlm.nih.gov/pmc/articles/PMC5628516/
272 The Dietary Food Components Capric Acid and Caprylic Acid Inhibit Virulence Factors in Candida albicans Through Multitargeting https://www.liebertpub.com/doi/full/10.1089/jmf.2017.3971
273 Production from dairy cows of semi-industrial quantities of milk-protein concentrate (MPC) containing efficacious anti-Candida albicans IgA antibodies https://pubmed.ncbi.nlm.nih.gov/17466122/
274 Inhibition of Growth of Candida albicans by Iron-Unsaturated Lactoferrin: Relation to Host-Defense Mechanisms in Chronic Mucocutaneous Candidiasis https://academic.oup.com/jid/article-abstract/124/6/539/894615?login=true
275 The Antifungal Activity of Lactoferrin and Its Derived Peptides: Mechanisms of Action and Synergy with Drugs against Fungal Pathogens https://www.ncbi.nlm.nih.gov/pmc/articles/PMC5241296/
276 Chronic Inflammation https://www.ncbi.nlm.nih.gov/books/NBK493173/
277 So depression is an inflammatory disease, but where does the inflammation come from? https://www.ncbi.nlm.nih.gov/pmc/articles/PMC3846682/
278 The Role of Inflammation in Diabetes: Current Concepts and Future Perspectives https://www.ncbi.nlm.nih.gov/pmc/articles/PMC6523054/
279 Dietary Inflammatory Index and Non-Communicable Disease Risk: A Narrative Review https://www.ncbi.nlm.nih.gov/pmc/articles/PMC6722630/
280 Chronic inflammation in the etiology of disease across the life span https://www.nature.com/articles/s41591-019-0675-0
281 Introduction: Oxidation and Inflammation, A Molecular Link Between Non-communicable Diseases https://link.springer.com/chapter/10.1007/978-3-319-07320-0_1
282 Chronic inflammation and asthma https://www.ncbi.nlm.nih.gov/pmc/articles/PMC2923754/
283 Pathophysiology of atopic dermatitis: Clinical implications https://www.ncbi.nlm.nih.gov/pmc/articles/PMC6399565/
284 Association of inflammation with depression and anxiety: evidence for symptom-specificity and potential causality from UK Biobank and NESDA cohorts https://www.nature.com/articles/s41380-021-01188-w
285 The association between anxiety, traumatic stress, and obsessive–compulsive disorders and chronic inflammation: A systematic review and meta-analysis https://onlinelibrary.wiley.com/doi/10.1002/da.22790
286 Inflammation: depression fans the flames and feasts on the heat https://pubmed.ncbi.nlm.nih.gov/26357876/
287 Peripheral cytokine and chemokine alterations in depression: a meta-analysis of 82 studies https://pubmed.ncbi.nlm.nih.gov/28122130/
288 Neuroimmune mechanisms of depression https://pubmed.ncbi.nlm.nih.gov/26404713/
289 The role of inflammation in depression: from evolutionary imperative to modern treatment target https://pubmed.ncbi.nlm.nih.gov/26711676/
290 Association of serum interleukin 6 and C-reactive protein in childhood with depression and psychosis in young adult life: a population-based longitudinal study https://pubmed.ncbi.nlm.nih.gov/25133871/
291 Brain 'fog,' inflammation and obesity: key aspects of neuropsychiatric disorders improved by luteolin https://www.ncbi.nlm.nih.gov/pmc/articles/PMC4490655/
292 Long Covid brain fog: a neuroinflammation phenomenon? https://www.ncbi.nlm.nih.gov/pmc/articles/PMC9914477/
293 Depression in sleep disturbance: A review on a bidirectional relationship, mechanisms and treatment https://www.ncbi.nlm.nih.gov/pmc/articles/PMC6433686/
294 The Role of Inflammation in Depression and Fatigue https://www.ncbi.nlm.nih.gov/pmc/articles/PMC6658985
295 Peripheral and central inflammation in Autism spectrum disorders https://www.sciencedirect.com/science/article/abs/pii/S1044743112001856
296 A Review on the Role of Inflammation in Attention-Deficit/Hyperactivity Disorder https://karger.com/nim/article/25/5-6/328/229828/A-Review-on-the-Role-of-Inflammation-in-Attention
297 Inflammation and Neuro-Immune Dysregulations in Autism Spectrum Disorders https://www.ncbi.nlm.nih.gov/pmc/articles/PMC6027314/
298 Autism, Joint Hypermobility-Related Disorders and Pain https://www.ncbi.nlm.nih.gov/pmc/articles/PMC6292952/
299 Chronic Pain And Health-Related Quality Of Life In Women With Autism And/Or ADHD: A Prospective Longitudinal Study https://pubmed.ncbi.nlm.nih.gov/31695481/
300 Indifference or hypersensitivity? Solving the riddle of the pain profile in individuals with Autism https://pubmed.ncbi.nlm.nih.gov/36730631
301 'When I'm in Pain, Everything Is Overwhelming': Implications of Pain in Adults With Autism on Their Daily Living and Participation https://www.frontiersin.org/articles/10.3389/fpsyg.2022.911756/full
302 Joint Hypermobility Links Neurodivergence to Dysautonomia and Pain https://www.researchgate.net/publication/358782960_Joint_Hypermobility_Links_Neurodivergence_to_Dysautonomia_and_Pain
303 Association between Autism spectrum disorder and inflammatory bowel disease: A systematic review and meta-analysis https://pubmed.ncbi.nlm.nih.gov/34939353/
304 Autism and Migraine: An Unexplored Association? https://www.ncbi.nlm.nih.gov/pmc/articles/PMC7565535/
305 Headaches in patients with Autism spectrum disorder https://www.researchgate.net/publication/274891930_EHMTI-0290_Headaches_in_patients_with_Autism_spectrum_disorder
306 The Dietary Inflammatory Index: A New Tool for Assessing Diet Quality Based on Inflammatory Potential https://www.researchgate.net/publication/264554956_The_Dietary_Inflammatory_Index_A_New_Tool_for_Assessing_Diet_Quality_Based_on_Inflammatory_Potential
307 Low-Grade Inflammation and Ultra-Processed Foods Consumption: A Review https://www.ncbi.nlm.nih.gov/pmc/articles/PMC10058108/
308 Gut-microbiota-targeted diets modulate human immune status https://www.cell.com/cell/fulltext/S0092-8674(21)00754-6
309 Review of Anti-Inflammatory Herbal Medicines https://www.ncbi.nlm.nih.gov/pmc/articles/PMC4877453/
310 The role of yoga in inflammatory markers https://www.ncbi.nlm.nih.gov/pmc/articles/PMC8842003/
311 Mindfulness meditation and the immune system: a systematic review of randomized controlled trials https://www.ncbi.nlm.nih.gov/pmc/articles/PMC4940234/
312 Immunopsychiatry Research Group http://www.immunopsychiatry.com/
313 Prevalence and correlates of low-grade systemic inflammation in adult psychiatric inpatients: An electronic health record-based study https://www.ncbi.nlm.nih.gov/pmc/articles/PMC5910056/
314 Autoimmune Diseases and Psychotic Disorders https://www.frontiersin.org/articles/10.3389/fpsyt.2019.00131/full
315 Mast cells' involvement in inflammation pathways linked to depression: evidence in mastocytosis https://pubmed.ncbi.nlm.nih.gov/26809839/
316 Mast cell activation disease: An underappreciated cause of neurologic and psychiatric symptoms and diseases https://

www.sciencedirect.com/science/article/abs/pii/S0889159115002366
317 The Histaminergic System in Neuropsychiatric Disorders https://www.ncbi.nlm.nih.gov/pmc/articles/PMC8467868/
318 Viral infection, inflammation and schizophrenia https://www.ncbi.nlm.nih.gov/pmc/articles/PMC3408569/
319 Are some cases of psychosis caused by microbial agents? A review of the evidence https://pubmed.ncbi.nlm.nih.gov/18268502/
320 Autoimmunity in Autism https://www.ncbi.nlm.nih.gov/pmc/articles/PMC6952169
321 Atopic diseases and inflammation of the brain in the pathogenesis of Autism spectrum disorders https://www.ncbi.nlm.nih.gov/pmc/articles/PMC4931610/
322 Viruses and Autism: A Bi-mutual cause and effect https://www.ncbi.nlm.nih.gov/pmc/articles/PMC10311578/
323 Autism Spectrum Disorder and Their Anthropometric Measurements https://pubmed.ncbi.nlm.nih.gov/32130666/
324 Microglia: Housekeeper of the Central Nervous System https://pubmed.ncbi.nlm.nih.gov/28534246/
325 Microglial activation and its implications in the brain diseases https://pubmed.ncbi.nlm.nih.gov/17504139/
326 Microglia: Synaptic modulator in Autism spectrum disorder https://www.frontiersin.org/articles/10.3389/fpsyt.2022.958661/full
327 In vivo imaging of dopamine D1 receptor and activated microglia in attention-deficit/hyperactivity disorder: a positron emission tomography study https://pubmed.ncbi.nlm.nih.gov/32439845/
328 PANDAS—Questions and Answers https://www.nimh.nih.gov/health/publications/pandas
329 Pediatric Acute-onset Neuropsychiatric Syndrome and Mycoplasma Pneumoniae Infection: A Case Report Analysis with a Metabolomics Approach https://www.ncbi.nlm.nih.gov/pmc/articles/PMC8193809/
330 Epstein-Barr virus and autoimmune diseases https://www.nih.gov/news-events/nih-research-matters/epstein-barr-virus-autoimmune-diseases
331 Epstein-Barr Virus and Systemic Autoimmune Diseases https://www.frontiersin.org/articles/10.3389/fimmu.2020.587380/full
332 Epstein-Barr Virus and the Origin of Myalgic Encephalomyelitis or Chronic Fatigue Syndrome https://www.frontiersin.org/articles/10.3389/fimmu.2021.656797/full
333 Evaluation of antibodies to cytomegalovirus and Epstein-Barr virus in patients with Autism spectrum disorder https://content.iospress.com/articles/human-antibodies/hab335
334 Personality, Anxiety, and Stress in Patients with Small Intestine Bacterial Overgrowth Syndrome. The Polish Preliminary Study https://www.ncbi.nlm.nih.gov/pmc/articles/PMC9819554
335 Association of family history of autoimmune diseases and Autism spectrum disorders https://pubmed.ncbi.nlm.nih.gov/19581261/
336 Parental Autoimmune Diseases Associated With Autism Spectrum Disorders in Offspring https://www.ncbi.nlm.nih.gov/pmc/articles/PMC3115699/
337 Familial clustering of autoimmune disorders and evaluation of medical risk factors in Autism https://pubmed.ncbi.nlm.nih.gov/10385847/
338 Clinical presentation of pediatric autoimmune neuropsychiatric disorders associated with streptococcal infections in research and community settings https://pubmed.ncbi.nlm.nih.gov/25695941/
339 Clinical Evaluation of Youth with Pediatric Acute-Onset Neuropsychiatric Syndrome (PANS): Recommendations from the 2013 PANS Consensus Conference https://www.liebertpub.com/doi/10.1089/cap.2014.0084
340 Infection-triggered anorexia nervosa in children: clinical description of four cases https://pubmed.ncbi.nlm.nih.gov/10933123/
341 Disordered Eating and Food Restrictions in Children with PANDAS/PANS https://www.ncbi.nlm.nih.gov/pmc/articles/PMC4340640/
342 Prevalence of pediatric acute-onset neuropsychiatric syndrome (PANS) in children and adolescents with eating disorders https://www.ncbi.nlm.nih.gov/pmc/articles/PMC9749211/
343 A Two-to-Five Year Follow-Up of a Pediatric Acute-Onset Neuropsychiatric Syndrome Cohort https://link.springer.com/article/10.1007/s10578-021-01135-4
344 PANS/PANDAS UKhttps://www.panspandasuk.org/
345 Mold Allergens in Respiratory Allergy: From Structure to Therapy https://www.ncbi.nlm.nih.gov/pmc/articles/PMC4397360/
346 Clinical Distinctness of Allergic Rhinitis in Patients with Allergy to Molds https://www.ncbi.nlm.nih.gov/pmc/articles/PMC4906200/
347 Exposure and Health Effects of Fungi on Humans https://www.ncbi.nlm.nih.gov/pmc/articles/PMC4861659/
348 Association of mast-cell-related conditions with hypermobile syndromes: a review of the literature https://www.ncbi.nlm.nih.gov/pmc/articles/PMC9022617/
349 The challenges of chronic pain and fatigue https://www.rcpjournals.org/content/clinmedicine/21/1/19
350 Histamine Intolerance: The Current State of the Art https://www.ncbi.nlm.nih.gov/pmc/articles/PMC7463562/
351 Mast cells activated by SARS-CoV-2 release histamine which increases IL-1 levels causing cytokine storm and inflammatory reaction in COVID-19 https://pubmed.ncbi.nlm.nih.gov/32945158/
352 COVID-19: Famotidine, Histamine, Mast Cells, and Mechanism https://www.ncbi.nlm.nih.gov/pmc/articles/PMC7336703/
353 Role of Appetite Hormone Dysregulation in Symptomology and Executive Function in Adolescents With Attention Deficit Hyperactivity Disorder https://academic.oup.com/ijnp/article/26/2/91/6714002
354 Cerebral glucose metabolism in adults with hyperactivity of childhood onset https://pubmed.ncbi.nlm.nih.gov/2233902/
355 Dyslexic Children Have Abnormal Brain Lactate Response to Reading-Related Language Tasks https://www.ncbi.nlm.nih.gov/pmc/articles/PMC7657735/
356 Hypothetical molecular interconnection between type 2 diabetes and Dyslexia https://bmcneurosci.biomedcentral.com/articles/10.1186/s12868-021-00666-9
357 Sweetened Blood Cools Hot Tempers: Physiological Self-Control and Aggression https://www.ncbi.nlm.nih.gov/pmc/articles/PMC4073202/
358 Autism spectrum disorders: let's talk about glucose? https://www.ncbi.nlm.nih.gov/pmc/articles/PMC6355780/
359 Effect of a High Protein Diet at Breakfast on Postprandial Glucose Level at Dinner Time in Healthy Adults https://www.ncbi.nlm.nih.gov/pmc/articles/PMC9824806/
360 Food Order Has a Significant Impact on Postprandial Glucose and Insulin Levels https://www.ncbi.nlm.nih.gov/pmc/articles/PMC4876745/
361 Vinegar (acetic acid) intake on glucose metabolism: A narrative review https://pubmed.ncbi.nlm.nih.gov/31221273/
362 Vinegar consumption can attenuate postprandial glucose and insulin responses; a systematic review and meta-analysis of clinical trials https://pubmed.ncbi.nlm.nih.gov/28292654/
363 Impact of Diet Composition on Blood Glucose Regulation https://pubmed.ncbi.nlm.nih.gov/24219323/
364 The essential role of exercise in the management of type 2 diabetes https://pubmed.ncbi.nlm.nih.gov/28708479/
365 Effects of zinc, magnesium, and chromium supplementation on cardiometabolic risk in adults with metabolic syndrome: A double-blind, placebo-controlled randomised trial https://www.sciencedirect.com/science/article/abs/pii/S0946672X18300695
366 Influence of biotin intervention on glycemic control and lipid profile in patients with type 2 diabetes mellitus: A systematic review and meta-analysis https://www.ncbi.nlm.nih.gov/pmc/articles/PMC9659605/
367 Gastrointestinal symptoms and Autism spectrum disorder: links and risks – a possible new overlap syndrome https://www.ncbi.nlm.nih.gov/pmc/articles/PMC5683266/
368 Manifestations of food protein induced gastrointestinal allergies presenting to a single tertiary paediatric gastroenterology unit https://www.ncbi.nlm.nih.gov/pmc/articles/PMC3828665/
369 The rapidly changing world of food allergy in children https://www.ncbi.nlm.nih.gov/pmc/articles/PMC4371379/
370 Prevalence of pediatric acute-onset neuropsychiatric syndrome (PANS) in children and adolescents with eating disorders https://www.ncbi.nlm.nih.gov/pmc/articles/PMC9749211/
371 Immune response to dietary proteins, gliadin and cerebellar peptides in autistic children https://pubmed.ncbi.nlm.nih.gov/15526989/
372 Gluten-Free Casein-Free Diet for Autism Spectrum Disorders: Can It Be Effective in Solving Behavioural and Gastrointestinal Problems? https://www.ncbi.nlm.nih.gov/pmc/

articles/PMC7651765/
373 A systematic review and meta-analysis of the benefits of a gluten-free diet and/or casein-free diet for children with Autism spectrum disorder https://pubmed.ncbi.nlm.nih.gov/34617108/
374 The hidden burden of eating disorders: an extension of estimates from the Global Burden of Disease Study 2019 https://www.thelancet.com/journals/lanpsy/article/PIIS2215-0366(21)00040-7
375 Binge Eating More Common Than Other Eating Disorders, Survey Finds https://www.sciencedaily.com/releases/2007/02/070203103249.htm
376 High fructose corn syrup induces metabolic dysregulation and altered dopamine signaling in the absence of obesity https://www.ncbi.nlm.nih.gov/pmc/articles/PMC5747444/
377 Glucose variability: A physiological correlate of eating disorder behaviors among individuals with binge-spectrum eating disorders https://pubmed.ncbi.nlm.nih.gov/36305323/
378 Emotional dysregulation and Autism spectrum disorders https://pubmed.ncbi.nlm.nih.gov/28256682/
379 Emotional Dysregulation in Preschoolers with Autism Spectrum Disorder—A Sample of Romanian Children https://www.ncbi.nlm.nih.gov/pmc/articles/PMC8535493/
380 Pupil and Salivary Indicators of Autonomic Dysfunction in Autism Spectrum Disorder https://www.ncbi.nlm.nih.gov/pmc/articles/PMC3832142/
381 The Effects of Acute Stress on Core Executive Functions: A Meta-Analysis and Comparison with Cortisol https://www.ncbi.nlm.nih.gov/pmc/articles/PMC5003767/
382 Assessment of plasma cortisol level in prepubertal boy with attention deficit hyperactivity disorder and comorbid oppositional defiant disorder https://gcris.pau.edu.tr/handle/11499/4726
383 Cortisol levels at baseline and under stress in adolescent males with attention-deficit hyperactivity disorder, with or without comorbid conduct disorder https://www.ncbi.nlm.nih.gov/pmc/articles/PMC4986851/
384 The function of hypothalamus-pituitary-adrenal axis in children with ADHD https://pubmed.ncbi.nlm.nih.gov/20971091/
385 Early temperamental and biological predictors of dimensions of social withdrawal in childhood https://pubmed.ncbi.nlm.nih.gov/36426788/
386 Facial expressivity and vagal tone in 5- and 10-month-old infants https://www.sciencedirect.com/science/article/abs/pii/0163638389900015
387 Moderate baseline vagal tone predicts greater prosociality in children https://pubmed.ncbi.nlm.nih.gov/27819463/
388 Darwin revisited: The vagus nerve is a causal element in controlling recognition of other's emotions https://www.sciencedirect.com/science/article/abs/pii/S0010945217300977
389 Recognizing emotions in bodies: Vagus nerve stimulation enhances recognition of anger while impairing sadness https://www.ncbi.nlm.nih.gov/pmc/articles/PMC8563521/
390 Trusting your heart: Long-term memory for bad and good people is influenced by resting vagal tone https://www.sciencedirect.com/science/article/abs/pii/S1053810019300583?via%3Dihub
391 Children's sleep and adjustment: the moderating role of vagal regulation https://pubmed.ncbi.nlm.nih.gov/18036085/
392 Contributing factors predicting nightmares in children: Trauma, anxiety, dissociation, and emotion regulation https://pubmed.ncbi.nlm.nih.gov/29963889/
393 Ingestion of Lactobacillus strain regulates emotional behavior and central GABA receptor expression in a mouse via the vagus nerve https://www.pnas.org/doi/full/10.1073/pnas.1102999108
394 The anxiolytic effect of Bifidobacterium longum NCC3001 involves vagal pathways for gut–brain communication https://pubmed.ncbi.nlm.nih.gov/21988661/
395 Omega-3 Polyunsaturated Fatty Acids and Heart Rate Variability https://www.ncbi.nlm.nih.gov/pmc/articles/PMC3217222/
396 The gut microbiome and inflammation in obsessive-compulsive disorder patients compared to age- and sex-matched controls: a pilot study https://pubmed.ncbi.nlm.nih.gov/32307692/
397 The Role of Gut Microbiota in Anxiety, Depression, and Other Mental Disorders as Well as the Protective Effects of Dietary Components https://www.ncbi.nlm.nih.gov/pmc/articles/PMC10384867/
398 Double-blind, placebo-controlled, crossover trial of inositol treatment for panic disorder https://www.ncbi.nlm.nih.gov/books/NBK184852/
399 A meta-analysis of inositol for depression and anxiety disorders https://onlinelibrary.wiley.com/doi/10.1002/hup.2369
400 Inositol treatment of obsessive-compulsive disorder https://pubmed.ncbi.nlm.nih.gov/8780431/
401 How does the tea L-theanine buffer stress and anxiety https://www.sciencedirect.com/science/article/pii/S2213453021001324
402 L-theanine combination therapy with fluvoxamine in moderate-to-severe obsessive-compulsive disorder: A placebo-controlled, double-blind, randomized trial https://pubmed.ncbi.nlm.nih.gov/37169515/
403 The Effects of Magnesium Supplementation on Subjective Anxiety and Stress—A Systematic Review https://www.ncbi.nlm.nih.gov/pmc/articles/PMC5452159/
404 The Role and the Effect of Magnesium in Mental Disorders: A Systematic Review https://www.ncbi.nlm.nih.gov/pmc/articles/PMC7352515/
405 Alterations of serum zinc, copper, manganese, iron, calcium, and magnesium concentrations and the complexity of interelement relations in patients with obsessive-compulsive disorder https://pubmed.ncbi.nlm.nih.gov/22383079/
406 An open study evaluating the efficacy and security of magnesium and vitamin B(6) as a treatment of Tourette syndrome in children https://pubmed.ncbi.nlm.nih.gov/19087826/
407 Magnesium Status and Stress: The Vicious Circle Concept Revisited https://www.ncbi.nlm.nih.gov/pmc/articles/PMC7761127
408 Treatment of refractory obsessive-compulsive disorder with nutraceuticals (TRON): a 20-week, open label pilot study https://pubmed.ncbi.nlm.nih.gov/34165060/
409 Vitamin B6: A new approach to lowering anxiety, and depression? https://www.ncbi.nlm.nih.gov/pmc/articles/PMC9577631/
410 Use of Nutritional Supplements Based on L-Theanine and Vitamin B6 in Children with Tourette Syndrome, with Anxiety Disorders: A Pilot Study https://www.mdpi.com/2072-6643/14/4/852
411 Effect of concomitant administration of three different antidepressants with vitamin B6 on depression and obsessive compulsive disorder in mice models https://pubmed.ncbi.nlm.nih.gov/28255313
412 Vitamin D supplementation improves anxiety but not depression symptoms in patients with vitamin D deficiency https://onlinelibrary.wiley.com/doi/10.1002/brb3.1760
413 Investigation of vitamin D levels in obsessive-compulsive disorder https://www.ncbi.nlm.nih.gov/pmc/articles/PMC9435610/
414 Vitamin D status in chronic tic-disorder and comorbid obsessive-compulsive disorder and attention-deficit/hyperactivity disorder: A pan-European study https://www.medrxiv.org/content/10.1101/19012062v1.full
415 Associations between Dietary Intake of Vitamin D, Sun Exposure, and Generalized Anxiety among College Women
416 Changes of Serum Homocysteine and Vitamin B12, but Not Folate Are Correlated With Obsessive-Compulsive Disorder: A Systematic Review and Meta-Analysis of Case-421 Control Studies https://www.frontiersin.org/articles/10.3389/fpsyt.2022.754165/full
417 Obsessive Compulsive Disorder as Early Manifestation of B12 Deficiency https://www.ncbi.nlm.nih.gov/pmc/articles/PMC3271502/
418 Involuntary movements due to vitamin B12 deficiency https://pubmed.ncbi.nlm.nih.gov/24852503/

419 Impact of insufficient sleep on dysregulated blood glucose control under standardised meal conditions https://pubmed.ncbi.nlm.nih.gov/34845532/
420 Long-term HRV analysis shows stress reduction by magnesium intake https://www.ncbi.nlm.nih.gov/pubmed/27933574
421 Effect of tart cherry juice (Prunus cerasus) on melatonin levels and enhanced sleep quality https://www.ncbi.nlm.nih.gov/pubmed/22038497
422 vJoint Hypermobility Links Neurodivergence to Dysautonomia and Pain https://www.ncbi.nlm.nih.gov/pmc/articles/PMC8847158/
423 Relationship between variant connective tissue (hypermobility) and Autism sensory processing: externally oriented thinking as a mediator https://jnnp.bmj.com/content/92/8/A7.2
424 Autistic Traits Correlate with Chronic Musculoskeletal Pain: A Self-Selected Population Based Survey https://www.lidsen.com/journals/neurobiology/neurobiology-07-01-155
425 The Links Between Fibromyalgia, Hypermobility and Neurodivergence https://

www.touchimmunology.com/fibromyalgia/journal-articles/the-links-between-fibromyalgia-hypermobility-and-neurodivergence/
426 Pain Symptomatology and Management in Pediatric Ehlers–Danlos Syndrome: A Review https://www.ncbi.nlm.nih.gov/pmc/articles/PMC7552757/
427 Gastrointestinal Involvement in the Ehlers–Danlos Syndromes https://www.ehlers-danlos.com/wp-content/uploads/2022/03/Fikree_et_al-2017-American_Journal_of_Medical_Genetics_Part_C-_Seminars_in_Medical_Genetics.pdf
428 Higher prevalence of joint hypermobility in constipation predominant irritable bowel syndrome https://pubmed.ncbi.nlm.nih.gov/29687534/
429 Ehlers-Danlos Syndrome, Hypermobility Type: An Underdiagnosed Hereditary Connective Tissue Disorder with Mucocutaneous, Articular, and Systemic Manifestations https://www.ncbi.nlm.nih.gov/pmc/articles/PMC3512326/
430 An Overview of Mitochondrial Protein Defects in Neuromuscular Diseases https://www.ncbi.nlm.nih.gov/pmc/articles/PMC8615828/
431 Mitochondrial dysfunction in Autism spectrum disorders: a systematic review and meta-analysis https://www.ncbi.nlm.nih.gov/pmc/articles/PMC3285768/
432 Carnitine Inborn Errors of Metabolism https://www.ncbi.nlm.nih.gov/pmc/articles/PMC6766900/
433 Effect of Core Stability Exercises on Hand Functions in Children With Hemiplegic Cerebral Palsy https://www.ncbi.nlm.nih.gov/pmc/articles/PMC7960954/
434 A novel therapeutic strategy for Ehlers-Danlos syndrome based on nutritional supplements https://pubmed.ncbi.nlm.nih.gov/15607555/
435 Nutritional Implications of Patients with Dysautonomia and Hypermobility Syndromes https://link.springer.com/article/10.1007/s13668-021-00373-1#ref-CR83
436 Vitamin C promotes wound healing through novel pleiotropic mechanisms https://onlinelibrary.wiley.com/doi/10.1111/iwj.12484
437 Use of complementary and alternative medicine by patients with hypermobile Ehlers–Danlos Syndrome: A qualitative study https://www.frontiersin.org/articles/10.3389/fmed.2022.1056438/full
438 New Targets in Pain, Non-Neuronal Cells, and the Role of Palmitoylethanolamide https://www.researchgate.net/publication/274190929_New_Targets_in_Pain_Non-Neuronal_Cells_and_the_Role_of_Palmitoylethanolamide
439 Clinical applications of palmitoylethanolamide in pain management: protocol for a scoping review https://systematicreviewsjournal.biomedcentral.com/articles/10.1186/s13643-018-0934-z
440 Therapeutic effect of quercetin in collagen-induced arthritis https://pubmed.ncbi.nlm.nih.gov/28342364/
441 Quercetin inhibits collagen-stimulated platelet activation through inhibition of multiple components of the glycoprotein VI signaling pathway https://pubmed.ncbi.nlm.nih.gov/12871380/
442 Phytomedicine in Joint Disorders https://pubmed.ncbi.nlm.nih.gov/28275210/
443 The effect of Omega-3 polyunsaturated fatty acid supplementation on exercise-induced muscle damage https://pubmed.ncbi.nlm.nih.gov/33441158/
444 Omega-3 fatty acids in health and disease and in growth and development https://pubmed.ncbi.nlm.nih.gov/1908631/
445 Hearing Loss, Tinnitus, and Dizziness in COVID-19: A Systematic Review and Meta-Analysis
446 Magnesium and Hearing https://www.researchgate.net/publication/10595530_Magnesium_and_Hearing
447 Pyridoxine and Magnesium Administration–Induced Hyperactivity in Two Children With Autism Spectrum Disorder: Case Reports From a Clinical Trial https://www.sciencedirect.com/science/article/abs/pii/S0149291820304604
448 Electrophysiological effects of fenfluramine or combined vitamin b6 and magnesium on children with autistic behaviour https://onlinelibrary.wiley.com/doi/abs/10.1111/j.1469-8749.1989.tb04067.x
449 Efficacy of vitamin B6 and magnesium in the treatment of Autism: A methodology review and summary of outcomes https://link.springer.com/article/10.1007/bf02178295
450 Hericium erinaceus enhances neurotrophic factors and prevents cochlear cell apoptosis in senescence accelerated mice https://www.sciencedirect.com/science/article/pii/S1756464620300566
451 Effects of erinacine A-enriched Hericium erinaceus on elderly hearing-impaired patients: A double-blind, randomized, placebo-controlled clinical trial https://www.sciencedirect.com/science/article/pii/S1756464622002900
452 Hericium erinaceus enhances neurotrophic factors and prevents cochlear cell apoptosis in senescence accelerated mice https://www.sciencedirect.com/science/article/pii/S1756464620300566
453 The magnocellular theory of developmental Dyslexia https://pubmed.ncbi.nlm.nih.gov/11305228
454 Working memory: Its role in Dyslexia and other specific learning difficulties https://onlinelibrary.wiley.com/doi/abs/10.1002/dys.278
455 Working memory in children with developmental disorders https://pubmed.ncbi.nlm.nih.gov/19380495/
456 Zinc deficiency in children with Dyslexia: Concentrations of zinc and other minerals in sweat and hair https://www.researchgate.net/publication/20029212_Zinc_deficiency_in_children_with_Dyslexia_Concentrations_of_zinc_and_other_minerals_in_sweat_and_hair
457 Zinc Deficiency and Dyslexia https://pediatricneurologybriefs.com/articles/10.15844/pedneurbriefs-2-3-12
458 The associations of zinc and GRIN2B genetic polymorphisms with the risk of Dyslexia https://pubmed.ncbi.nlm.nih.gov/32937172/
459 The combined effect between BDNF genetic polymorphisms and exposure to metals on the risk of Chinese Dyslexia https://www.sciencedirect.com/science/article/abs/pii/S0269749122008545?via%3Dihub
460 Urine metals concentrations and Dyslexia among children in China https://www.sciencedirect.com/science/article/pii/S016041201934810X
461 Exposure to multiple metals and the risk of Dyslexia – A case control study in Shantou, China https://www.sciencedirect.com/science/article/abs/pii/S0269749122007321
462 Status and High Anemia Prevalence https://www.ncbi.nlm.nih.gov/pmc/articles/PMC5040806/
463 Membrane fatty acids, reading and spelling in dyslexic and non-dyslexic adults https://www.sciencedirect.com/science/article/abs/pii/S0924977X06001325?via%3Dihub
464 The Relationship of Docosahexaenoic Acid (DHA) with Learning and Behavior in Healthy Children: A Review https://www.ncbi.nlm.nih.gov/pmc/articles/PMC3738999/
465 Biochemical Differences in People with Irlen Syndrome https://www.irlen.be/paper-brugge_Greg_Robinson2004.pdf
466 Plasma cholesterol levels and Irlen syndrome: preliminary study of 10- to 17-yr.-old students https://pubmed.ncbi.nlm.nih.gov/14738334/
467 Antioxidants and vision health: facts and fiction https://pubmed.ncbi.nlm.nih.gov/24311110/
468 Lutein across the Lifespan: From Childhood Cognitive Performance to the Aging Eye and Brain https://www.ncbi.nlm.nih.gov/pmc/articles/PMC6629295/
469 Eye Nutrition in Context: Mechanisms, Implementation, and Future Directions https://www.ncbi.nlm.nih.gov/pmc/articles/PMC3738983/
470 The Photobiology of Lutein and Zeaxanthin in the Eye https://www.ncbi.nlm.nih.gov/pmc/articles/PMC4698938/
471 Lutein: more than just a filter for blue light https://pubmed.ncbi.nlm.nih.gov/22465791/
472 A diagnostic marker for speech delay associated with otitis media with effusion: the intelligibility-speech gap https://pubmed.ncbi.nlm.nih.gov/14608797/
473 Prevalence and severity of voice and swallowing difficulties in mitochondrial disease https://pubmed.ncbi.nlm.nih.gov/22268906/
474 Speech-Stimulating Substances in Autism Spectrum Disorders https://www.ncbi.nlm.nih.gov/pmc/articles/PMC6616660/
475 Polyunsaturated fatty acids supplementation can improve specific language impairment in preschool children: a pilot study https://ejnpn.springeropen.com/articles/10.1186/s41983-020-0158-8
476 Effect of Omega-3 and -6 Supplementation on Language in Preterm Toddlers Exhibiting Autism Spectrum Disorder Symptoms https://pubmed.ncbi.nlm.nih.gov/28748334/
477 Effectiveness of Methylcobalamin and Folinic Acid Treatment on Adaptive Behavior in Children with Autistic Disorder Is Related to Glutathione Redox Status https://www.hindawi.com/journals/aurt/2013/609705/
478 The Effectiveness of Cobalamin (B12) Treatment for Autism Spectrum Disorder: A Systematic Review and Meta-Analysis https://www.ncbi.nlm.nih.gov/pmc/articles/PMC8400809/

479 Vitamin D and Autism, what's new? https://link.springer.com/article/10.1007/s11154-017-9409-0
480 Autism, will vitamin D treat core symptoms? https://pubmed.ncbi.nlm.nih.gov/23725905/
481 Beneficial Effects of Palmitoylethanolamide on Expressive Language, Cognition, and Behaviors in Autism: A Report of Two Cases https://pubmed.ncbi.nlm.nih.gov/26491593/
482 A case series of a luteolin formulation (NeuroProtek®) in children with Autism spectrum disorders https://pubmed.ncbi.nlm.nih.gov/22697063/
483 Streptococcal Infection as a Major Historical Cause of Stuttering: Data, Mechanisms, and Current Importance https://pubmed.ncbi.nlm.nih.gov/33304252/
484 Streptococcal Infection as a Major Historical Cause of Stuttering: Data, Mechanisms, and Current Importance https://www.ncbi.nlm.nih.gov/pmc/articles/PMC7693426/
485 Stuttering and Word-Finding Difficulties in a Patient With COVID-19 Presenting to the Emergency Department https://pubmed.ncbi.nlm.nih.gov/33409021/
486 Stuttering-Like Dysfluencies as a Consequence of Long COVID-19 https://pubmed.ncbi.nlm.nih.gov/36749838
487 Neurological and neuropsychiatric complications of COVID-19 in 153 patients: a UK-wide surveillance study https://www.thelancet.com/journals/lanpsy/article/PIIS2215-0366(20)30287-X/fulltext
488 The concentrations of bioelements in the hair samples of Jordanian children who stutter https://pubmed.ncbi.nlm.nih.gov/30055725/
489 Biochemical studies in stuttering in children https://pubmed.ncbi.nlm.nih.gov/2067858/
490 A Consideration of Thiamin Supplement in Prevention of Stuttering in Preschool Children https://pubs.asha.org/doi/10.1044/jshd.1604.327
491 A Study of the effects of thiamine on children with speech non-fluency https://ufdc.ufl.edu/UF00098033/00001
492 The effects of vitamin D supplementation on ADHD (Attention Deficit Hyperactivity Disorder) in 6–13 year-old students: A randomized, double-blind, placebo-controlled study https://www.sciencedirect.com/science/article/abs/pii/S1876382018301975
493 The Effect of Vitamin D3 Supplementation on Serum BDNF, Dopamine, and Serotonin in Children with Attention-Deficit/Hyperactivity Disorder https://pubmed.ncbi.nlm.nih.gov/31269890/
494 Zinc sulfate as an adjunct to methylphenidate for the treatment of attention deficit hyperactivity disorder in children: a double blind and randomized trial https://pubmed.ncbi.nlm.nih.gov/15070418/
495 Effectiveness of Methylphenidate Supplemented by Zinc, Calcium, and Magnesium for Treatment of ADHD Patients in the City of Zahedan https://brieflands.com/articles/semj-20468.html
496 Sunlight in the morning Dopaminergic modulation of retinal processing from starlight to sunlight https://www.sciencedirect.com/science/article/pii/S1347861319310448
497 ADHD Prevalence: Altitude or Sunlight? Better Understanding the Interrelations of Dopamine and the Circadian System https://brainclinics.com/wp-content/uploads/2019/04/Arns-2015-ADHD-Prevalence-Altitude-or-Sunlight-B.pdf
498 Effects of physical exercise on children with attention deficit hyperactivity disorder https://pubmed.ncbi.nlm.nih.gov/34856393/
499 Bidirectional Association between Physical Activity and Dopamine Across Adulthood—A Systematic Review https://www.ncbi.nlm.nih.gov/pmc/articles/PMC8301978/
500 Intensely pleasurable responses to music correlate with activity in brain regions implicated in reward and emotion https://pubmed.ncbi.nlm.nih.gov/11573015/
501 Dopamine modulates the reward experiences elicited by music https://www.pnas.org/doi/full/10.1073/pnas.1811878116
502 Neurophysiological, cognitive-behavioral and neurochemical effects in practitioners of transcendental meditation – A literature review https://pubmed.ncbi.nlm.nih.gov/31166449/
503 https://www.develop.bc.ca/the-reverse-flynn-effect/
504 Are dietary patterns in childhood associated with IQ at 8 years of age? A population-based cohort study https://pubmed.ncbi.nlm.nih.gov/21300993/
505 Dietary patterns at 6, 15 and 24 months of age are associated with IQ at 8 years of age https://pubmed.ncbi.nlm.nih.gov/22810299/
506 Who benefits most from a prenatal HEPA filter air cleaner intervention on childhood cognitive development? The UGAAR randomized controlled trial https://pubmed.ncbi.nlm.nih.gov/37121346/
507 Portable HEPA Filter Air Cleaner Use during Pregnancy and Children's Cognitive Performance at Four Years of Age: The UGAAR Randomized Controlled Trial https://pubmed.ncbi.nlm.nih.gov/35730943/
508 Half of US population exposed to adverse lead levels in early childhood https://www.pnas.org/doi/abs/10.1073/pnas.2118631119
509 The effect of lead exposure on IQ test scores in children under 12 years: a systematic review and meta-analysis of case-control studies https://systematicreviewsjournal.biomedcentral.com/articles/10.1186/s13643-022-01963-y
510 The relationship between childhood blood lead levels below 5 µg/dL and childhood intelligence quotient (IQ): Protocol for a systematic review and meta-analysis https://www.sciencedirect.com/science/article/pii/S0160412022004020?via%3Dihub
511 CDC updates blood lead reference value to 3.5 µg/dL https://www.cdc.gov/nceh/lead/news/cdc-updates-blood-lead-reference-value.html
512 Blood Lead Levels in Children https://www.cdc.gov/nceh/lead/docs/lead-levels-in-children-fact-sheet-508.pdf
513 Recommendations on Management of Childhood Lead Exposure https://www.pehsu.net/_Library/facts/PEHSU_Fact_Sheet_Lead_Management_Health_Professionals_9_2021.pdf
514 Healthy Diet & Lead Poisoning Prevention https://www.tn.gov/health/health-program-areas/mch-lead/for-parents/lead-prevention.html
515 The role of modified citrus pectin as an effective chelator of lead in children hospitalized with toxic lead levels https://pubmed.ncbi.nlm.nih.gov/18616067/
516 Discharge of lead contamination by natural compounds pectin and chitin: biochemical analysis of DNA, RNA, DNase, RNase and GOT in albino rat as an early bio-marker of lead-toxicity https://www.sciencedirect.com/science/article/abs/pii/S2221169111601603
517 Cellular and molecular toxicity of lead in bone https://www.ncbi.nlm.nih.gov/pmc/articles/PMC1519349.
518 A pharmacokinetic model of lead absorption and calcium competitive dynamics https://www.nature.com/articles/s41598-019-50654-7
519 Overcome procrastination: Enhancing emotion regulation skills reduce procrastination https://www.sciencedirect.com/science/article/pii/S1041608016302187
520 Apathy: Why Care? https://neuro.psychiatryonline.org/doi/10.1176/jnp.17.1.7
521 Brain mechanisms underlying apathy https://jnnp.bmj.com/content/90/3/302
522 Neural Correlates for Apathy: Frontal-Prefrontal and Parietal Cortical- Subcortical Circuits https://www.ncbi.nlm.nih.gov/pmc/articles/PMC5145860/
523 Apathy and the Functional Anatomy of the Prefrontal Cortex–Basal Ganglia Circuits https://academic.oup.com/cercor/article/16/7/916/425683
524 Apathy and the basal ganglia https://pubmed.ncbi.nlm.nih.gov/17131230/
525 Causal Link between n-3 Polyunsaturated Fatty Acid Deficiency and Motivation Deficits https://www.sciencedirect.com/science/article/pii/S1550413120300711
526 N-3 (omega-3) fatty acids: effects on brain dopamine systems and potential role in the etiology and treatment of neuropsychiatric disorders https://www.ncbi.nlm.nih.gov/pmc/articles/PMC6563911/
527 Influence of dietary choline and tryptophan on motivational state https://www.emerald.com/insight/content/doi/10.1108/00346650110385864/full/html
528 Alpha-Glycerylphosphorylcholine Increases Motivation in Healthy Volunteers: A Single-Blind, Randomized, Placebo-Controlled Human Study https://www.ncbi.nlm.nih.gov/pmc/articles/PMC8235064/
529 Zinc, the brain and behavior https://pubmed.ncbi.nlm.nih.gov/7082716/
530 Mood disorder with mixed, psychotic features due to vitamin b12 deficiency in an adolescent: case report https://capmh.biomedcentral.com/articles/10.1186/1753-2000-6-25

APPENDIX

DAILY NUTRIENT INTAKE

The figures below are general guidelines, and you must consider all sources of these nutrients, both through diet and food supplements when assessing the needs of your child. Recommended daily amounts and upper tolerable levels differ slightly from country to country so please keep this in mind.

The Recommended Daily Allowance (RDA) is often called the Nutrient Reference Value (NRV), which is the average general nutritional needs for a child to avoid serious nutrient deficiencies. Children will not need this much every single day, so long as they average it out over time. But I see this as the absolute minimum average because kids can thrive so much better when they are nourished more than just the bare minimum.

The UTL is the Upper Tolerable Limit, which is the highest daily intake recommended taken over long periods of time to avoid mild to moderate side effects or toxicity. It's OK to have more than this for short periods of time. Some nutrients do not have a UTL, as no serious side effects or toxicity have been found even when taken at very high amounts, and these are marked with Not Established (N/E).

Ideally, nutrient levels are tested regularly and guided by a health professional such as a medical doctor, nutritional therapist or naturopath. Occasionally, when a marked deficiency or metabolic problem has been identified, your health professional may recommend higher therapeutic doses for short periods of time.

Generally, taking therapeutic levels (higher than RDA but within UTL) daily for 3 months is safe.

Source: National Institutes of Health

	TODDLER 1–3 YEARS		SCHOOL 4–8 YEARS		TWEENS 9–13 YEARS		TEENS 14–18 YEARS	
	RDA	UTL	RDA	UTL	RDA	UTL	RDA	UTL
Iron	7mg	40mg	10mg	40mg	8mg	40mg	11mg M, 15mg F	45mg
Vitamin D	15 mcg (600 IU)	63 mcg (2,500 IU)	15 mcg (600 IU)	75 mcg (3,000 IU)	15 mcg (600 IU)	100 mcg (4,000 IU)	15 mcg (600 IU)	100 mcg (4,000 IU)
Zinc	3mg	7mg	5mg	12mg	8mg	23mg	11mg M, 9mg F	34mg
Magnesium	80mg	N/E	130mg	N/E	250mg	N/E	410mg M, 360mg F	N/E
Vitamin B6	0.5mg	30mg	0.6mg	40mg	1.0mg	60mg	1.3mg	80mg
Folate (B9)	150mcg	300mcg	200mcg	400mcg	300mcg	600mcg	400mcg	800mcg
Vitamin B12	0.9mcg	N/E	1.2mcg	N/E	1.8mcg	N/E	2.4mcg	N/E
Omega-3	700mg	N/E	900mg	N/E	1,200mg M 1,000mg F	N/E	1,600mg M, 1,100mg F	N/E
Choline	200mg	1,000mg	250mg	1,000mg	375mg	2,000mg	550mg M, 400mg F	3,000mg

HOW TO GIVE SUPPLEMENTS

You may be a bit overwhelmed on how to give your child a supplement. There are many which come in drop form that can be added to juice, or as a tasty chewable. However sometimes you need to open up capsules and mix them into a food or a drink. If they are reluctant to take supplements, then here are some top tips to help you get over this roadblock:

Smoosh them: Use a thick fruit juice like orange or tropical, a fruit smoothie, fruit purée/baby food or yoghurt that your child loves. This forms the base from which to give the supplement. But apple juice does not work well for powders or fish oils. Mix the purée and supplement together in a shot glass, ramekin or egg cup and give it via a spoon or medicine syringe. Sometimes a resealable food pouch works well for storage.

Try a straw: If the supplement is particularly strong tasting, even when added to juice, then try giving it through a straw (cut the straw in half so less suck-power is needed to get the contents into the mouth and less is wasted). A plastic cup with a lid and a straw can mask many new smells or colours.

Three-day intro: If your youngster is reluctant to take a supplement off a spoon or a via a medicine syringe then start with giving that fruit purée without the supplement for 3 days in a row, before adding in the supplement. Then start adding in a pinch of the contents of a capsule or one drop of a liquid supplement. Build this up pinch by pinch or drop by drop every day or so until you reach the recommended dosage.

Tasteless ones first: Start with supplements with little to no taste. Probiotics, zinc and multiple minerals usually have a neutral taste. They can be added to fruit purée, smoothies, milk or yoghurt – again start drop by drop or pinch by pinch of powder.

Bake with them: Minerals such as calcium, zinc and magnesium supplements, as well as protein powders, are not broken down by the cooking process, so you can add these to pancake mix, muffin recipes or porridge. However, never cook or heat probiotics, vitamins, antioxidants or essential fatty acids.

Frozen lollies: You can buy mini frozen lolly (popsicle) moulds. Once you have blended up some juice or fresh fruit with the supplements, freeze them in the moulds and bring one out every day for your youngster to enjoy.

Ice-cream: Transfer ice cream into ice cube trays and mix the supplement into each compartment so that each cube is equal to one day's dose of the supplement. Freezing food supplements preserves their goodness.

A sweet spoonful: If you must, try a teaspoon of sugar-free jam, organic chocolate spread, maple syrup or honey. These can be a magic way of hiding the stronger-tasting supplements. You can give the sweet-tasting spoonful with the supplement, or as a 'chaser' afterwards to take any nasty tastes away.

Home-made gummies: Make vitamin gummy sweets (candy) by combining gelatine powder with fruit juice and the supplement. Set them in cute silicone moulds and store them in the refrigerator, or in the freezer if you are making these in large batches. This is a particularly good way of hiding liquid supplements and fish oils.

Savoury disguises: If your child has a more savoury palate, then mix the supplement into peanut butter, almond butter or cashew butter. You could also try hummus, mashed potato or puréed vegetables.

INDEX

ACKNOWLEDGEMENTS

I'd like to firstly thank my incredible husband and kids for simply being their own beautiful unique selves – I have always said we never bred sheep! Christopher, Barney, Lara and Charlie, we make a fantastic team and thanks for being my greatest cheerleaders. I love you all to the moon and back!

Also, enormous thanks to the team at Quadrille – my commissioning editor, Sophie Allen, for encouraging me to write *Brain Brilliance* in the first place, and to Stephanie Evans for steering the editing in the right direction. To Katherine Case for her incredible design of this beautiful book. Also, to the styling and photography team steered by Ali Allen with her stunning photographs, and including Holly Cowgill for her deft and clever food styling. And to Sarah Epton for proofreading at the end.

Huge thanks also go to our NatureDoc food stylist Jenny Whittingham, who was a great sounding block for some of the recipes. And to all the members of my NatureDoc neurodivergence clinical team for offering their insights into the various drafts of this book – particular thanks go to Dr Liz Giles, Katy Gordon-Smith, Sophie Henderson, Daisy York and Tash Pepper and for all your valuable input.

Thank you, Kirstin Contaroudas, for reading through the first draft and giving me such helpful input.

A particularly special thanks goes to Dr Richard Fry, who has taught me so much about paediatric psychiatry. Your ongoing support of my work has always been invaluable.

Thank you to Dr Alexandra Davidson for giving your medical oversight. Also thank you to all the children involved: Charlie, Oscar AC, Iris, Melody, Zeb, Marius, Joshua, Zachary, Isobel, Indira, Oscar R, Rosalind, Poppy and Alma.

And to all the thousands of families we have worked with over the years. It has been a total honour to help so many parents navigate the often-bumpy road with their child's nutrition, and to see so many kids blossom and become the best versions of themselves. Three cheers to you and thank you to your children for being my greatest teachers!

ABOUT THE AUTHOR

Lucinda Miller is the clinical lead of NatureDoc and has over 25 years' experience as a family Naturopath and Functional Medicine practitioner. She runs a UK-wide team of Nutritional Therapists specialising in child nutrition and neurodiversity. Lucinda regularly lectures on both. She is also a coach and mentor for kids with ADHD and Autism.

Known as the children's nutrition hero, Lucinda is the author of two books on feeding family's nutritious food: *The Good Stuff* and *I Can't Believe It's Baby Food*!

She has ADHD herself and is the mum of three teen and adult kids, two of whom have neurodivergent brains. She lives in Wiltshire, UK.
@naturedockids

PUBLISHING DIRECTOR
Sarah Lavelle

EDITORIAL DIRECTOR
Sophie Allen

DESIGNER
Katherine Case

PHOTOGRAPHER AND PROPS STYLIST
Ali Allen

FOOD STYLIST
Holly Cowgill

PRODUCTION DIRECTOR
Stephen Lang

PRODUCTION CONTROLLER
Martina Georgieva

Quadrille, Penguin Random House UK, One Embassy Gardens, 8 Viaduct Gardens, London SW11 7BW

Quadrille Publishing Limited is part of the Penguin Random House group of companies whose addresses can be found at global.penguinrandomhouse.com
Published in 2024 by Quadrille Publishing Limited

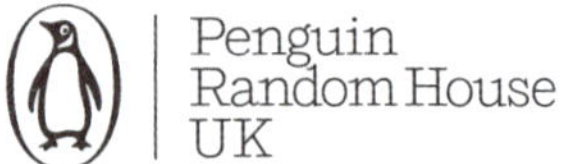

Published by Quadrille in 2024

www.penguin.co.uk

A CIP catalogue record for this book is available from the British Library

Cover Illustrations © OIDm_Shop via Creative Market and Adobe Stock

ISBN 9781837831975
10 9 8 7 6 5 4

Colour reproduction by F1
Printed in China by C&C Offset Printing Co., Ltd.

The authorised representative in the EEA is Penguin Random House Ireland, Morrison Chambers, 32 Nassau Street, Dublin D02 YH68.

Penguin Random House is committed to a sustainable future for our business, our readers and our planet. This book is made from Forest Stewardship Council® certified paper.

DISCLAIMER:
The information contained in this book is provided for general purposes only. It is not intended as, and should not be relied upon as, medical advice. The publisher and author are not responsible for any specific health needs that may require medical supervision. If you or your family have underlying health problems, or have any doubts about the advice contained in this book, you should contact a qualified medical, dietary or appropriate professional. While in some instances the author has provided suggestions for alternatives to common allergens, if you or your family have any allergies or require foods free of certain allergens, please carefully check recipe ingredients and the labels of the products you are using. Neither the author nor the publisher can be held responsible for any claim or damage arising out of the use, or misuse, of the information and suggestions made in this book.

"Lucinda has a thorough understanding of what it is we need to do to nourish the neurodivergent mind. Not only does this book give a comprehensive and understandable insight into how and why our brains may work more uniquely to others, but the recipes are practical, delicious and suitable for the whole family. Having worked with Lucinda navigating my own experiences of how challenging ADHD can be as an adult and as a mother of a neurodiverse child, her knowledge and approach to supporting people navigate this has been invaluable."

Kate Rowe-Ham, Author

"An indispensable read for better brain health, packed with important, helpful information. Highly recommended."

Liz Earle MBE